Sports Medicine

in the Pediatric Office

A Multimedia Case-Based Text With Video

2nd Edition

Jordan D. Metzl, MD, FAAP
Sports Medicine
Hospital for Special Surgery
New York, NY

WITH

David T. Bernhardt, MD, FAAP
Greg Canty, MD, FAAP
Thomas L. Devries, MD
Nicholas M. Edwards, MD, MPH, FAAP
Cassidy MacDowell Foley, DO, FAAP
Benton E. Heyworth, MD
Joseph Janosky, MS, PT, ATC
Hamish Kerr, MD, MSc, FAAP, FACSM
Derrick M. Knapik, MD
Peter Kriz, MD, FACSM, FAAP
Shaina A. Lipa, MD
Robert G. Marx, MD, MSc, FRCSC
Teri McCambridge, MD, FAAP
Kathryn Dunn McElheny, MD, FAAP
Suzy McNulty, MD, FAAP
Joshua A. Metzl, MD
Jeffrey M. Mjaanes, MD, FAAP, FACSM
Drago Novkovic, ATC
Katherine H. Rizzone, MD, MPH, FAAP
Amanda Sparrow, PT
Sarah A. Vengal, MD
James E. Voos, MD
Kristina Wilson, MD, MPH, CAQSM, FAAP
Mark Wu, BS
Tracy Zaslow, MD, FAAP, CAQSM
Stessie Dort Zimmerman, MD

WITH FOREWORD BY

Lewis R. First, MD, FAAP

American Academy of Pediatrics Publishing Staff

Mark Grimes, *Director, Department of Publishing*

Peter Lynch, *Manager, Digital Strategy and Product Development*

Theresa Wiener, *Manager, Publishing and Production Services*

Amanda Helmholz, *Editorial Specialist*

Linda Diamond, *Manager, Art Direction and Production*

Mary Lou White, *Chief Product and Services Officer/SVP, Membership, Marketing, and Publishing*

Linda Smessaert, *Brand Manager, Clinical and Professional Publications*

Published by the American Academy of Pediatrics

141 Northwest Point Blvd

Elk Grove Village, IL 60007-1019

Telephone: 847/434-4000

Facsimile: 847/434-8000

www.aap.org

The recommendations in this book and video do not indicate an exclusive course of treatment or serve as a standard of medical care. Variations, taking into account individual circumstances, may be appropriate.

Statements and opinions expressed in this book and video are those of the authors and not necessarily those of the American Academy of Pediatrics.

Listing of resources does not imply an endorsement by the American Academy of Pediatrics (AAP). The AAP is not responsible for the content of external resources. Information was current at the time of publication.

Products and Web sites are mentioned for informational purposes only and do not imply an endorsement by the American Academy of Pediatrics. Web site addresses are as current as possible but may change at any time.

Brand names are furnished for identification purposes only. No endorsement of the manufacturers or products mentioned is implied.

The publishers have made every effort to trace the copyright holders for borrowed materials. If they have inadvertently overlooked any, they will be pleased to make the necessary arrangements at the first opportunity.

This book has been developed by the American Academy of Pediatrics. The authors, editors, and contributors are expert authorities in the field of pediatrics. No commercial involvement of any kind has been solicited or accepted in the development of the content of this book and video.

Disclosures: Dr Joshua Metzl indicated that he has a consultant relationship with Arthex. Dr Marx indicated that he has an editorial duties relationship with *The Journal of Bone and Joint Surgery.* Dr Voos indicated that he has an educational consultant relationship with Arthex.

First edition published 2008; 2nd, 2018.

Printed in the United States of America

9-398/0917   1 2 3 4 5 6 7 8 9 10

MA0842

ISBN: 978-1-61002-122-7

eBook: 978-1-61002-123-4

Cover design by Linda Diamond

Book design by Linda Diamond

Library of Congress Control Number: 2016960415

This book is dedicated to

health care professionals around the world

who care each day for children and adolescents.

Contributors

Jordan D. Metzl, MD, FAAP
Sports Medicine
Hospital for Special Surgery
New York, NY

David T. Bernhardt, MD, FAAP
Professor
Department of Pediatrics, Orthopedics and Rehab
Division of Sports Medicine
University of Wisconsin School of Medicine and
    Public Health

Greg Canty, MD, FAAP
Medical Director, Center for Sports Medicine
Fellowship Director, Pediatric Sports Medicine
Assistant Professor of Orthopedics & Pediatrics,
    University of Missouri Kansas City
Children's Mercy Kansas City

Thomas L. Devries, MD
Department of Pediatrics
University of Wisconsin Hospital and Clinics

Nicholas M. Edwards, MD, MPH, FAAP
Adjunct Assistant Professor of Orthopaedics
University of Minnesota

Cassidy MacDowell Foley, DO, FAAP
Pediatric Orthopedic Associates
Next Level Sports Medicine
Children's Healthcare of Atlanta
Atlanta Ballet

Benton E. Heyworth, MD
Assistant Professor, Harvard Medical School
Attending Orthopaedic Surgeon, Division of
    Sports Medicine, Boston Children's Hospital

Joseph Janosky, MS, PT, ATC
Director, Sports Safety
Hospital For Special Surgery
New York, NY

Hamish Kerr, MD, MSc, FAAP, FACSM
Associate Professor, Internal Medicine/Pediatrics
Fellowship Director, Sports Medicine
Albany Medical College

Derrick M. Knapik, MD
Resident Physician, PGY-II
Department of Orthopaedic Surgery
University Hospitals Cleveland Sports
    Medicine Institute

Peter K. Kriz, MD, FACSM, FAAP
Assistant Professor (Clinical)
Division of Sports Medicine
Rhode Island Hospital/Hasbro Children's Hospital
Warren Alpert Medical School, Brown University

Shaina A. Lipa, MD
Harvard Combined Orthopaedic Residency
    Program/Massachusetts General Hospital

Robert G. Marx, MD, MSc, FRCSC
Professor of Orthopedic Surgery
Weill Cornell Medicine
Hospital for Special Surgery

Teri McCambridge, MD, FAAP
Assistant Professor
Department of Pediatrics and Orthopedics
University of Maryland Medical System

Kathryn Dunn McElheny, MD, FAAP
Hospital for Special Surgery

Suzy McNulty, MD, FAAP
Mia Bella Pediatrics
General Pediatrics and Sports Medicine
CHOC Children's Concussion Clinic
Pediatric Concussion Specialist

Joshua A. Metzl, MD
Steadman Hawkins Clinic - Denver

Jeffrey M. Mjaanes, MD, FAAP, FACSM
Northwestern University
Director of Sports Medicine/Head Team

Drago Novkovic, ATC

Katherine H. Rizzone, MD, MPH, FAAP
Assistant Professor, Orthopaedics, Rehabilitation
    and Pediatrics
University of Rochester Medical Center
Rochester, NY

Amanda Sparrow, PT

Sarah A. Vengal, MD
Primary Care Sports Fellow

James E. Voos, MD
Jack and Mary Herrick Endowed Director,
    Sports Medicine
Associate Professor, Case Western Reserve
    University School of Medicine
Division Chief, Sports Medicine
Department of Orthopaedic Surgery
Head Team Physician, Cleveland Browns
University Hospitals Cleveland Sports
    Medicine Institute

Kristina Wilson, MD, MPH, CAQSM, FAAP
Medical Director, Pediatric and Adolescent
    Sports Medicine
Center for Pediatric Orthopaedics, Phoenix
    Children's Hospital
Co-Director, Brain Injury and Concussion Program
Barrow Neurologic Institute at Phoenix Children's
    Hospital
Assistant Clinical Professor, Department of
    Child Health
University of Arizona College of Medicine, Phoenix

Mark Wu, BS
M.D. Candidate 2018/Harvard Medical School

Tracy Zaslow, MD, FAAP, CAQSM
Children's Orthopaedic Center (COC) at Children's
    Hospital Los Angeles
Medical Director, COC Sports Medicine and
    Concussion Program
Assistant Professor, University of Southern
    California
LA Galaxy, Team Physician

Stessie Dort Zimmerman, MD
Johns Hopkins All Children's Hospital

Contents

Foreword

How often do we hear *"See one, do one, teach one,"* the usual expression for the learner trying to master something new? Yet in this superb revision of *Sports Medicine in the Pediatric Office: A Multimedia Case-Based Text With Video,* this famous phrase gets a whole new attitude.

My job as a department chair and chief of our children's hospital puts in me contact regularly with numerous pediatric health care professionals who often tell me about the many questions they get from parents asking about their child or an adolescent involved in sports, from requests for preventive strengthening exercises to concerns about how to evaluate and treat ankle or shoulder pain. Answering these concerns requires a familiarity with anatomy along with knowledge of orthopedic physical examination maneuvers (which I've often found described with complicated text and pictures). Then there are the requests from trainees as well as from peers to gain expertise in proper splinting techniques or what exercises should be done for a particular sports medicine problem.

Until the first edition of *Sports Medicine in the Pediatric Office: A Multimedia Case-Based Text With Video* arrived, I had difficulty recommending to colleagues one reference that could answer all sports medicine inquiries in one volume. But this book not only presents the information clearly and succinctly but also provides clear demonstrative videos for proper examination of an injured extremity, so that pediatric health care professionals can avoid having to search on the Internet for these educational aids. The second edition of *Sports Medicine in the Pediatric Office: A Multimedia Case-Based Text With Video* has been updated by one of the nation's leading experts and educators in pediatric sports medicine, Jordan D. Metzl, MD, FAAP, along with several of his colleagues from across the country. The use of written text supplemented by clear illustrations, clear images, and extremely easy-to-understand video demonstrations of the points highlighted in the revised text provides any learner, from novice to expert, with what he or she needs to know about common sports medicine problems that children and teenagers experience.

The second edition continues to offer case-based examples to highlight common injuries of the upper and lower extremities, the hips, and the spine and allows the learner to apply the fundamentals stressed at the start of each chapter. This well-written revised multimedia text also incorporates information on sports physical and head injuries to the athlete, provides new chapters focusing on specific sports, and gives updates on key issues that have arisen in sports medicine since the first edition. This book ensures that the clinician knows how to examine, diagnose, and manage a sports injury and, at the same time, instructs the patient on what to do to recover and prevent further injury upon return to play.

Thanks to what Dr Metzl and his team have created, now a learner such as myself can "see one" as many times as needed and even use the videos to "teach one" to others, while becoming much more skilled at the actual "doing," thanks to the interactive way the information is provided in this book. In many ways, this book remains a great resource for informational "strength training"—something we have all been waiting for when it comes to improving our knowledge and clinical skills in the field of sports medicine. For that reason, I congratulate the authors on revising what was an already terrific educational text into an even more outstanding up-to-date volume that will put us all in much better shape when it comes to knowing what to do when the next patient comes in with a sports medicine concern. If you liked the first edition, you'll love this second edition even more!

Lewis R. First, MD, FAAP

Professor and Chair
Department of Pediatrics
University of Vermont
The Robert Larner, M.D. College of Medicine
Chief of Pediatrics
University of Vermont Children's Hospital
Burlington
Editor in Chief, *Pediatrics*

Preface

Dear Friends,

Thank you so much for looking at our updated version of *Sports Medicine in the Pediatric Office.* When we published the first version of this book more than 10 years ago, child and youth sport specialization had an upward trend, more young athletes were participating in sports than ever before, and pediatric health care professionals (including pediatricians, pediatric emergency medicine physicians, school and office-based pediatric nurses, athletic trainers, and team physicians) were faced with an ever-increasing number of sports medicine issues in the office. Thanks to readers like you, our first edition helped guide many pediatric health care professionals in navigating these new challenges and opportunities.

Today, the field of pediatric sports medicine has grown considerably, as has the science supporting the best ways to both manage and prevent injuries in the young athlete. Our goal with the updated version of *Sports Medicine in the Pediatric Office* is to bring pediatric health care professionals from around the globe up to speed on the changes that have been made over the past 10 years.

In today's health care world, pediatric and adolescent athletes are flocking to their pediatric health care professionals in high numbers, seeking guidance on the best ways to stay healthy on and off their field of choice. In this edition, we've included a series of new chapters dealing with specific sports scenarios, and we've expanded the body-specific areas and examination tools. We have also included new sections on prevention so health care professionals are better able to counsel their active patients on the subjects of preventive health.

The videos with musculoskeletal examinations were featured on a DVD in our first edition. They are now featured in an online library that we hope you will use as a supplement to the written text. Reading about knee injuries is one thing, but seeing how to examine someone's knee in a video is a different method of learning. We hope you'll take advantage of both methods in this new edition.

Finally, I'd like to thank our contributing authors, both returning authors from the first edition, who have updated their chapters, and new authors, many from the American Academy of Pediatrics Council on Sports Medicine and Fitness, who have joined this effort for the first time. Each author has graciously donated his or her time and expertise in an effort to better educate health care professionals about the optimal care and treatment of young athletes. I am so deeply appreciative of their help; thank you, everyone.

On behalf of the American Academy of Pediatrics and each of our outstanding authors, I hope you benefit from this updated version of *Sports Medicine in the Pediatric Office* as you care for active patients in your office.

Jordan D. Metzl, MD, FAAP
Sports Medicine
Hospital for Special Surgery
New York, NY

Introduction

Please view video clip:
"Welcome to the Video Component of Sports Medicine in the Pediatric Office."

Welcome to the workbook component of *Sports Medicine in the Pediatric Office.* We hope that this workbook and video will allow you to take better care of the hundreds of athletic children and teens who come into your office every year.

The field of pediatric sports medicine has evolved greatly over the past 30 years, and it is growing quickly, along with the number of children and teens who are involved in recreational and competitive sports in the United States and around the world.

For pediatricians, pediatric medical subspecialists, and pediatric surgical specialists (collectively referred to as *pediatricians* from this point on), the demands of taking care of athletic patients have changed considerably. The "stay off it until it gets better" approach used to be the accepted formula for taking care of athletic children. Patients would come in with an injury, and often the advice was, "Just stay off it until it gets better." As children and teens have become more active, the role of the pediatrician in the lives of athletic patients has changed, and that approach is no longer accepted by patients and families who are eager for safe return to play. Increasingly, patients and their families are looking for ways to reduce injury time, return to play, and prevent problems in the future.

So, let's talk about this workbook. This is not the be-all and end-all of sports medicine guides. Each topic addressed here is suitable for an entire book (and many such books already exist). The workbook and video provide a multimedia approach to basic sports medicine for the pediatric health care professional, resident, or medical student. The workbook is designed to be used interactively with the video; the intent is for you to view the video clips as you read through the corresponding text sections within the book (look for the special "video clip" icons throughout the text). By having both written and video materials, you will be able to see and practice specific examination techniques, see certain preventive strengthening exercises, and, ultimately, take better care of athletic patients.

In our updated version of this book, we have also included specific sections on prevention and sport-specific chapters. Both are designed to teach pediatric health care professionals how to better care for specific athletes in their office and to offer current recommendations that pertain to each specific sport.

Objectives

The pediatric health care professional, resident, or medical student using this book will be able to

- Better care for athletic patients.
- Display a greater feeling of comfort in dealing with sports medicine issues.
- Better serve as a resource for athletic children and teens and for the sports community.

Part ➊
Overview and Prevention

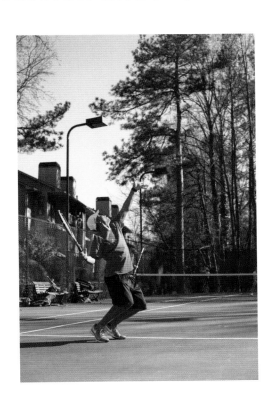

CHAPTER 1
The Basics of Sports Injury Evaluation

Jordan D. Metzl, MD, FAAP

Taking the Patient History of a Sports-Related Injury

1. Mechanism of Injury
2. Swelling
3. Level of Disability
4. Return to Play

Keys to Physical Examination of a Sports-Related Injury

1. Inspection
2. Observation
3. Palpation
4. Active Motion (Muscle Strength)
5. Passive Motion (Joint Function)
6. Special Tests and Assessments
   - **Ligamentous Stability**
   - **Neurologic Function**
   - **Specific Function**

Obtaining Specific Images, Scans, and Test Results to Evaluate a Sports-Related Injury

1. Radiographs
2. Magnetic Resonance Image
3. Computed Tomography Scan
4. Bone Scan
5. Single-Photon Emission Computed Tomography Scan
6. Dual-Energy X-ray Absorptiometry Image
7. Ultrasound Image
8. Neurocognitive Test Results
9. Complete Blood Cell Count

Referring an Athlete for Physical Therapy

Returning an Athlete to Play

1. Full Understanding of the Injury
2. Guidelines for Return to Play
3. Guidelines for Prevention

Taking the Patient History of a Sports-Related Injury

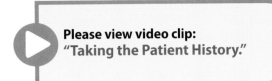

Please view video clip:
"Taking the Patient History."

As attested by our experience teaching hundreds of pediatric residents, they do not seem as comfortable taking the history of a sports-related injury as they do dealing with a medical issue, such as an asthma exacerbation. Any difference in level of comfort felt by a pediatric health care professional, resident, or medical student between taking the history of a sports injury and the history of other medical issues would be unfortunate. Of all the issues discussed in this book, patient history is likely the most important. The way in which an injury occurs is the hallmark of the type of problem that is encountered in the office. For example, an ankle injury is often characterized by the mechanism of injury (ie, how the injury happened). The way the ankle rolls speaks volumes about the type of injury that might be anticipated when examining the patient.

Following are a few of the factors that are essential in taking the history of a sports-related injury:

1. Mechanism of Injury

The mechanism of injury is how an injury happens. This is the way in which an injury occurs, which should always be one of the first considerations in evaluating any injury in an athlete. This consideration, hopefully, should include questions such as, "How did the injury happen?" Through this knowledge, the examiner can gain a much better idea of the type of problem that might have resulted. Throughout this workbook and video, we have tried to present common injuries with common mechanisms. Sometimes, patients can essentially recreate the injury in the office, using the uninjured contralateral appendage, which is often helpful as well.

2. Swelling

Swelling is a helpful indicator that leads to the proper diagnosis of many sports-related injuries. The location and timing of the onset of swelling are important clues toward diagnosis. As is discussed in Chapter 4, Knee and Lower Leg Injuries in the Young Athlete, swelling that occurs quickly, typically within 1 hour of an injury, is likely blood related. When this bleeding occurs inside a joint, it is known as an acute hemarthrosis. Fractures, because of the readily available blood supply inside of bone, also swell quickly. As such, swelling onset is a helpful clue (ie, the quicker an injury swells, the more serious it is likely to be).

3. Level of Disability

Assessing the level of disability from an injury is helpful during evaluation of both acute traumas and overuse injuries. The rules here are simple: If an injury is limiting an athlete's ability to participate in sports, "hold the athlete out" until a clear diagnosis is reached and a treatment plan is implemented. If an athlete is having trouble participating in sports because of pain, do not clear the athlete to participate until a full understanding about the severity of the injury, as well as potential ramifications from participation, is understood. For children, when in doubt, "hold them out."

> ### Basic Rule
> If an athlete is having trouble participating in sports because of pain, do not clear the athlete to participate until a full understanding about the severity of the injury, as well as potential ramifications from participation, is understood.
>
> For children, when in doubt, "hold them out."

4. Return to Play

When returning an athlete to play from an injury, the same issues discussed previously are important. A clear understanding of the injury and the knowledge that the appropriate preventive or physical therapy measures have been implemented are essential; examples are a preventive strengthening program for an athlete who has sprained his or her ankle or the implementation of a diet rich in calcium and vitamin D for an athlete who is being treated for a stress fracture. In both cases, the key to a safe and healthy return to play is remedy of the existing problem. The more knowledgeable health care professionals are about return-to-play decisions, the better able they are to make informed decisions on safe and effective return to play.

Keys to Physical Examination of a Sports-Related Injury

 Please view video clip: "Basics of Physical Examination of a Sports Injury."

Physical examination of the patient with a musculoskeletal concern should follow the same premise as the general physical examination. Before a health care professional examines the patient, a history (in this case, a targeted patient history) should precede the hands-on portion of the examination. However, in sports medicine, because the problems are injury- or concern-specific in most cases, the keys to proper examination are having a good concept of the mechanism and type of concern before the physical examination and possessing the skills to perform the targeted physical examination comfortably. As is the case with other skills, such as cardiac auscultation, the more times these examinations are repeated, the more effective the information-gathering skills become.

We stress that not every injury and physical examination needs to entail each of the categories discussed in the following text. However, these provide a helpful guideline from which the examiner can start to work. In general, physical examination is divided into the following portions:

1. Inspection

The inspection process starts the moment the examiner observes the patient. How is the patient moving? Is he or she using an injured extremity? Is associated swelling significant? These are all important considerations.

2. Observation

Observation pertains to watching the patient for function.

3. Palpation

Palpation is the actual (hands-on) portion of the examination. During palpation, the examiner, knowledgeable about the specific bony and soft-tissue landmarks, attempts to find pertinent areas of tenderness that can give clues to the specific diagnosis. For example, in the ankle, pain on focal palpation of the distal fibular physis is suggestive of a distal fibular physeal fracture, while pain to palpation of the anterior talofibular ligament (ATFL) is suggestive of an ATFL sprain. Palpation becomes a key issue in deciding management as well. For example, pain in the anatomical snuff-box on palpation, even in the presence of negative radiographic findings, mandates presumptive treatment for a scaphoid fracture, through the use of thumb spica splinting.

4. Active Motion (Muscle Strength)

Active motion applies to functional joint examination, during which the power of movement is performed by the patient, not the examiner. In this type of scenario, the joint or body part is actively moved by the patient and, as such, gives important clues about the integrity of the muscular attachments into bone. In young athletes, examinations primarily pertain to apophyseal attachments, such as the origin of the flexor muscle mass at the medial epicondyle of the elbow. When the elbow is flexed and the wrist is volar flexed, traction is placed on the medial elbow, which reproduces pain caused by traction.

5. Passive Motion (Joint Function)

Passive motion, the way in which a joint moves when the power is applied by the examiner, is an essential part of joint examination. Passive motion is especially important in joints, such as that of the hip, in which a limitation of passive motion during the rotational portion of the examination can indicate the presence of a structural problem in the joint, such as a slipped capital femoral epiphysis. In addition, limitation of passive flexion in the hip can be indicative of a structural problem in the anterior-inferior iliac spine, the apophyseal origin of the rectus femoris, which sits on the anterior-superior portion of the hip joint.

6. Special Tests and Assessments

Some special tests and assessments are tailored to specific parts of the body. Some of these special tests and assessments are reviewed in the following text:

Ligamentous Stability

For certain areas of the body, ligamentous examination provides important clues about the structural stability of a joint. For example, the athlete who experiences an inversion injury to the ankle generally injures the lateral ankle, and, if the athlete is skeletally mature, that often means a sprain of the ATFL. The anterior drawer test is used to assess laxity in the ATFL and is important to help grade the amount of joint laxity and the likelihood of further injury.

Neurologic Function

Neurologic assessment is also important for certain areas of the body, mainly as related to cervical or lumbar spine injury or, occasionally, with peripheral nerve injury, such as ulnar nerve subluxation in the cubital tunnel. Neurologic assessment generally includes muscle-strength testing, reflex testing, and sensory examination. These are often considered in the setting of an associated injury, such as an upper-extremity strength, reflex, and sensory loss in an athlete, such as a football player who has experienced an axial-load injury to the cervical spine. Mechanism and history of injury are important in helping assess these types of problems.

Specific Function

Finally, functional testing becomes important as athletes are ready to return to play. For example, before returning to play, the athlete who has experienced the ATFL sprain described previously will often be asked to stand for 30 seconds, with his or her eyes closed, on the injured foot or ankle. This is especially important because the ability or inability to perform this task is a good predictor of injury risk going forward.

Obtaining Specific Images, Scans, and Test Results to Evaluate a Sports-Related Injury

Please view video clip:
"When to Obtain Images, Scans, and Test Results to Evaluate a Sports Injury."

Knowing what image, scan, or test result to get, when to get it, and what to do with the information is tremendously important. The following text will review some of the common images, scans, and test results used in sports medicine:

1. Radiographs

Radiographs are an essential part of the evaluation of many sports-related injuries. The keys to getting proper radiographs are knowing when to get them, knowing what views to get, and developing a comfort level in evaluating musculoskeletal images. Because education regarding skeletal radiographic evaluation is minimal during many primary care residency programs, getting proper radiographs is sometimes difficult. When ordering bone radiographs, it is important to have an idea of the mechanism of injury as well as the age-appropriate findings in a particular patient. Furthermore, although not required for every injury, contralateral radiographs can aid in the comparison of injury (the injured as compared with the uninjured side). Generally, we find that repeated review of normal radiographic findings aids significantly in the ability to recognize abnormal findings.

In each section in the video, we have tried to provide the appropriate views for each body part. Although more views are needed in specific cases (and at times the opposite extremity is radiographed for comparison in evaluation of a growth plate injury), most basic information can be obtained through the radiographic screening views listed in Table 1-1. Each view is explained during the video portion of the material.

Table 1-1. Standard Radiographic Views to Screen for a Sports Injury

Body Part	Radiographic Views
Ankle	AP, lateral, mortise
Foot	AP; lateral; oblique; sesamoid (for suspected sesamoid injury)
Knee	AP, lateral, tunnel, Merchant
Tibia or fibula	AP, lateral
Shoulder	AP, axillary (for most screening examinations)
Clavicle	AP, 10° tilt
Wrist	AP; lateral; scaphoid (for suspected scaphoid fracture)
Hip	AP pelvis (for apophyseal injury), frog-leg lateral (for suspected SCFE)
Lumbar spine	AP, lateral, oblique (any for suspected spondylolysis)
Thoracic spine	AP, lateral
Cervical spine	AP, lateral, flexion, extension, odontoid (AP and lateral for basic screening, all for suspected instability)

Abbreviations: AP, anteroposterior; SCFE, slipped capital femoral epiphysis.

A radiograph is not only a helpful image for diagnosing bone injury but also the preferred image for diagnosing most apophyseal injuries, such as apophyseal avulsion fractures. These commonly occur in the hip, the knee, and the elbow, as discussed in the video examination.

2. Magnetic Resonance Image

Magnetic resonance imaging (MRI) has changed the face of medicine in the past 25 years. In many specialties, sports medicine included, MRI has allowed physicians to look inside the body, to avoid either delays or incorrect diagnoses. Because this is a magnetic-based study, it does not expose patients to radiation.

For the sports medicine physician, and for the primary care physician, obtaining and using an MRI is an important and helpful tool. However, please note and understand that an MRI is only as good as the context in which it is obtained. For example, an MRI can be a tremendously helpful tool in diagnosing conditions such as stress fractures (before they show on radiograph), edema in the capitellum if osteochondritis dissecans development is a concern in the lateral elbow of throwing athletes, and ligament or cartilage injuries in areas such as knees, shoulders, hips,

ankles, and elbows. However, an MRI can also show information that does not necessarily pertain to the clinical picture, such as the presence of a small inter-substance meniscus tear in a patient with patellofemoral knee pain. Although the meniscus tear is present, it is not contributing to the cause of knee pain.

Therefore, the key to obtaining and using an MRI is realizing when to use MRI and what to do with the information. Magnetic resonance imaging is most helpful as a secondary study, to assess injuries that do not show on radiograph. The information from MRI, however, should be considered only in the context of an associated clinical scenario. The key to assessing if an MRI finding is significant is by assessing the patient history, physical examination, and MRI findings together. Throughout the workbook and video, we have tried to illustrate when and how MRI is helpful as a diagnostic tool.

A rule that was taught in residency applies here, as with many studies: if you are not comfortable interpreting the results of a test, it is probably best not to order that test. Many clinicians around the world have become comfortable interpreting an MRI; as such, this is a helpful image to obtain for further clarification. However, if the MRI findings are not part of your normal clinical practice, results should be interpreted with caution.

Basic Rule

If you are not comfortable interpreting the results of a test, it is probably best not to order that test.

3. Computed Tomography Scan

Computed tomography (CT) scan is a helpful method for providing close-up, detailed information of bony anatomy. Like radiography, CT scan is a radiation-based study. The radiation dose is considerably higher during CT scan as compared with radiography, so these studies should always be performed with thoughtful consideration. Computed tomography scan is rarely used in the primary care setting, but, in sports medicine and all fields of orthopedic surgery, CT scan is helpful in providing further information about suspected bone injury. It is the scan of choice for evaluation of bone injuries, such as assessment of the anatomy of a spondylolysis lesion (in the spine) or the anatomical assessment and location of osteoid osteoma, a benign tumor that occurs in bone. Computed tomography scan also has the unique capability to provide 3-dimensional reconstruction views, which are especially helpful in the evaluation of trauma to bone.

4. Bone Scan

Radionuclide bone scan is a time-delayed scan that is used to screen for occult bone lesions. This scan involves injecting a radionuclide dye intravenously. A radiation-based scan is performed several hours later to screen for dye uptake. Bone scan used to be the scan of choice for diagnosing stress fracture before the age of MRI. However, if the origin of the bone-related pain is unclear, such as with suspected bone tumor, bone scan still has tremendous usefulness. In sports medicine, bone scan is a helpful screening device, but it has largely been replaced by MRI for many cases, unless the specific focus of the pain is unknown. Since the first edition of this book, bone scan use has thankfully decreased in the field of orthopedics and sports medicine and has largely been replaced by MRI.

5. Single-Photon Emission Computed Tomography Scan

Single-photon emission computed tomography (SPECT) scan is essentially a combination of bone scan and CT scan. In sports medicine, the SPECT scan has been used historically as a method to assess spondylolysis. The study is used similarly to bone scan in that it offers a time-delayed presence of dye uptake, and the CT imagery is particularly sensitive to the spinal anatomy. Increasingly, MRI has replaced this as well in many areas of the country. The image quality from MRI remains variable; as such, MRI diagnosis of spondylolysis is not universally available. In these cases, the SPECT scan is still a scan of value. Since the first edition of this book, SPECT bone scan use has thankfully decreased in the field of orthopedics and sports medicine and has largely been replaced by MRI.

6. Dual-Energy X-ray Absorptiometry Image

Dual-energy x-ray absorptiometry (DEXA) is a low-dose radiation study used to assess bone density and to screen for osteopenia and osteoporosis. These studies have been used more often for screening in the young athlete population in the past several years for several reasons, including the increasing recognition of the importance of diagnosing bone density abnormalities in teens and improved DEXA values that are now specific for adolescents. The DEXA study provides 2 scores: T and Z scores. T scores provide a comparison of bone mass between sex and race. Z scores compare bone mass by age.

The concern with DEXA has been that the developmental stage of an adolescent is not age based but rather sexual maturity rating based. As such, T and Z scores are highly variable between adolescents of the same age. Recently, however, DEXA values have been published for adolescents on the basis of sexual maturity rating, which has made this study more meaningful for teens.

Dual-energy x-ray absorptiometry studies are helpful to screen for low bone density, osteopenia (defined as a T score between −1 and −2.5 SDs from the mean), and osteoporosis (defined at less than −2.5 from the mean). In the clinical setting,

DEXA is often used to obtain a baseline value on a patient who is suspected to be at risk for low bone density, such as a teenaged athlete who has experienced a femoral stress fracture. If these values are low, a follow-up study 18 to 24 months after intervention will provide meaningful information about the trend in bone density value since the initial reading. This is often performed in an intervention setting, such as the implementation of a calcium and vitamin D supplement.

7. Ultrasound Image

Used for many years in Europe, musculoskeletal ultrasound is rapidly gaining popularity as a diagnostic study in sports medicine in the United States. Similar to the ultrasound used for fetal evaluation, diagnostic musculoskeletal ultrasound is a device that is especially helpful for evaluating soft-tissue abnormalities, such as tendon injuries. The benefit of ultrasound is that it is a dynamic study; the images it projects are moveable. This capability is especially important for tendon injuries, which, through the use of ultrasound, can be visualized easily while the affected extremity is moved. In some cases, such as iliopsoas tendinitis in dancers whose physical therapy has failed, ultrasound can be coupled with a therapeutic injection into a small area, such as the iliopsoas tendon sheath. At present, musculoskeletal ultrasound is a somewhat specialized procedure that is mostly found at some major medical centers. Since the first edition of this book, ultrasound use has increased in the fields of orthopedics and sports medicine because of ease of use, low cost, and assistance with the diagnosis and management of musculoskeletal injury.

8. Neurocognitive Test Results

Neurocognitive testing is a newer testing device used to assess athletes who have a concussion. First studied in professional football players, neurocognitive testing is becoming increasingly common in high-contact sports, which carry a higher risk of concussion. This type of testing allows for more objective decision-making when deciding whether to return an athlete to play. Neurocognitive testing works best when compared to a baseline for each individual athlete, so, if use of neurocognitive testing is indicated, such as for an athlete who has had several concussions, these tests are best administered in the preseason period. Increasingly, online computer programs are available to provide remote neurocognitive testing. Since the first edition of this book, use of neurocognitive testing has dramatically increased as a tool for evaluating concussion in pediatric and adolescent athletes.

9. Complete Blood Cell Count

A complete blood cell count is useful in many clinical situations outside of sports medicine. We have chosen to include this because, although they may look immune to infection in their sports outfits, athletes are equally prone to medical conditions such as infection and anemia, both of which can be diagnosed with a complete blood cell count. With increasing prevalence of methicillin-resistant *Staphylococcus aureus* in athletes of sports with padding, such as football and lacrosse, it is important to remind athletes that hygiene and regular cleaning of equipment are helpful preventive measures.

Referring an Athlete for Physical Therapy

In general, physical therapists are extremely helpful when caring for many musculoskeletal problems, and they can help fix the mechanical factors that are causing an injury or, sometimes, are the result of an injury.

Please note that some schools have on-site certified athletic trainers (they have earned an ATC credential) who provide a similar role inside the school. When a certified athletic trainer is available for this purpose, this scenario provides a tremendous benefit for the athletes and families at the school. Physical therapy can be used for the cases that are too time-consuming to be handled inside the school setting.

When referring a patient for physical therapy, it is helpful to ascertain if the therapist has a particular interest in treating young athletes, and also expertise in a particular type of activity. For example, a physical therapist who knows about dance is well suited to aid the young dancer, while a physical therapist who works frequently with baseball players is well suited to work with them.

Physical therapy prescriptions should include a diagnosis and a frequency of treatment. In general, it is best to see patients again after roughly 4 to 6 weeks of them starting physical therapy to ascertain progress. For athletic children and adolescents, a sports-minded physical therapist tends to provide optimal results.

Returning an Athlete to Play

1. Full Understanding of the Injury

The ultimate responsibility (and liability) for making the decision to clear an athlete for return to play rests with the physician, even though the decision is often made with input from a physical therapist or certified athletic trainer. The keys to authorizing this return to play are a full understanding of the injury and the knowledge that the appropriate preventive measures have been taken to reduce risk of repeat injury. In sports medicine, this type of clearance can be everything from the return to play of a football player after a concussion (from the sideline while the game is in progress or from the office) to a return to play of a ballet dancer to full dance after a stress fracture. The keys in all cases are knowledge of what the injury is, how it has occurred, and the level of healing of the athlete.

2. Guidelines for Return to Play

Guidelines are available for many types of injuries, and we have tried to include many of these in the context of this book. The key point here, however, is that every injury is different, as is every athlete (eg, although an injury such as traction apophysitis at the medial epicondyle in a pitcher might initially present with the same physical examination findings in 2 athletes [pain with throwing and tenderness to palpation at the medial epicondyle], both injuries may heal at quite different rates). This altered healing response has many causes, including

biological considerations (eg, the cellular healing rate), as well as extrinsic factors (eg, underlying strength and throwing mechanics). As such, there is no absolute rule for any injury. The main point is that return to play is an individual decision for each athlete and depends on issues such as presence of ongoing symptoms, ability to perform at one's pre-injury level of ability, and ability to protect oneself when on the sports field.

3. Guidelines for Prevention

Guidelines for prevention are also an important part of sports medicine. For example, an athlete with a history of several ankle sprains requires not only absence of symptoms before returning to play but a clear plan of preventive exercises to reduce the likelihood of this injury happening again. Giving guidelines for prevention (eg, the need for maintaining an ongoing ankle-strengthening program when the ankle is uninjured) is an essential part of the safe and healthy return of athletes to play.

CHAPTER 2

Trends in Prevention of Sports Injury in the Young Athlete

Cassidy MacDowell Foley, DO, FAAP, and Kathryn Dunn McElheny, MD, FAAP

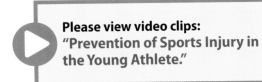

Please view video clips: "Prevention of Sports Injury in the Young Athlete."

As the field of sports medicine grows, there is a particular need to devise preventive strategies to keep young athletes safe and on their field of choice. This chapter examines some of the various areas in which prevention can make a difference for young athletes.

According to the 2008 National Council of Youth Sports' report on trends and participation in organized child and youth sports, 60 million 6- to 18-year-olds participated in organized sports compared with 45 million in 1997 (Brenner). This increase in participation allows more children and youths to benefit from the numerous well-recognized gains of child and youth sports participation, including socialization with peers, lifelong physical activity skills, teamwork and leadership skill development, improving self-esteem, having fun, and the decreased risk of major chronic diseases, including diabetes, cardiovascular (CV) disease, colon cancer, and osteoporosis. The growing popularity of child and youth sports is also increasing awareness among general pediatricians of sports medicine injuries in young athletes and the need for preventive measures.

Preventive medicine is a focal point of pediatric training and a crucial aspect of how pediatricians care for patients. Pediatricians can take an active role in starting or recommending prevention programs for their patients. Resources such as the Centers for Disease Control and Prevention Web site on Heads Up Concussion and the American Academy of Pediatrics (AAP) Council on Sports Medicine and Fitness have an abundance of resources for injury prevention and education.

This chapter will focus on trends in prevention, in the areas of sport specialization and burnout, concussions, heat illness, CV screening, spine injuries, anterior cruciate ligament (ACL) injuries, and bone health and energy deficiency as they relate to stress fracture prevention and metabolic needs of young athletes.

Sport Specialization

Case 1
Is sport specialization always a good idea?

Description
A 9-year-old female diver presents to her primary care professional's office with one month of progressively distracting wrist pain. She is diving 3 hours a day, 4 days a week, and getting only 2 hours a week of free play or dry land training.

The diver is in a sport whose participants may benefit from early specialization. However, to decrease her risk of injury, the pediatrician recommends decreasing her training hours to less than her years of age (9 years). The health care professional also recommends increasing hours of free play to achieve closer to a 2:1 ratio of organized training to free play. Last, she will be monitored closely for indicators of burnout, overuse, injury, or potential decrements in performance caused by overtraining.

Workup and Management
Caused by exposure of athletes to competition at earlier ages, a hot topic among young athletes is the trend toward sport specialization. Sport specialization is intensive, year-round training in a single sport at the exclusion of other sports. An emphasis on competitive success has become more widespread, including increased pressure to begin high-intensity training at younger ages, with select travel leagues starting as young as 7 years of age. Often the motivation for early specialization seems to stem from the athlete or parent, or both, wanting to capture a piece of the very small "pie," namely, the end goal of collegiate and professional-level athletics. Unfortunately, 70% of children and adolescents drop out of organized sports by 13 years of age; between 3% and 11% of high school athletes compete at the college level, with only 1% receiving scholarships; and only 0.03% to 0.50% of high school athletes will go on to reach professional-level sports (Figure 2-1).

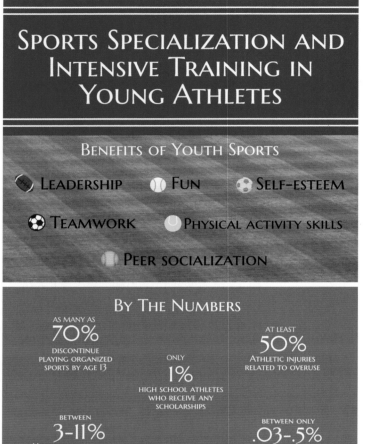

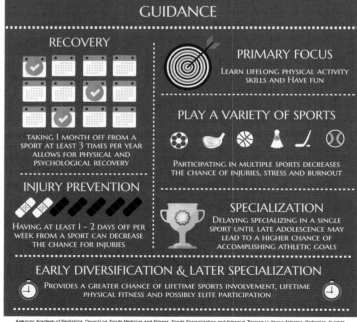

FIGURE 2-1

From Brenner JS. Sports specialization and intensive training in young athletes. *Pediatrics*. 2016;138(3):e20162148. Reproduced with permission.

One of the most concerning disadvantages of specialization is the accompanying increased rates of overuse injuries. Jayanthi et al in 2015 demonstrated that sport specialization was an independent risk factor for injury. More so than increasing growth rates, age and hours spent in sports activity were related to an increased risk of injury (Figure 2-2). Athletes who participated in more hours of organized sports per week than their age in years, and whose ratio of organized sports to free play time was greater than 2:1, had an increased risk of an overuse injury. Early specialization (before puberty) may also be correlated with reports of decreased general health and decreased psychological well-being, with increasing rates of social isolation, anxiety, depression, and burnout.

It is important to recognize that not all sport specialization is potentially harmful, as the timing of this specialization plays a crucial role. Some sports may require earlier specialization; gymnastics, figure skating, and diving may be a few. If this timing is appropriate, it has the potential of leading to higher athletic "success." However, in most endurance sports and team sports, athletes may benefit from later adolescent specialization (Table 2-1). Studies have demonstrated that Division I National Collegiate Athletic Association athletes are more likely to have played multiple sports in high school, and their first organized sport was likely different than their current one. Jayanthi et al and Côté et al have demonstrated that for most sports, late specialization with early diversification is the most likely combination to lead to elite status. As of 2016, the AAP recommends early diversification in sports and later specialization (post-puberty), as this provides a greater chance for lifetime sports involvement and physical fitness, as well as the possibility of elite participation. Participating in multiple sports early on minimizes drop-outs while maximizing sustained participation, results in fewer overuse injuries, and causes less burnout among young athletes. Emphasis should be placed on using individualized plans that capitalize on the ABCs of physical literacy (agility, balance, coordination, and speed), as opposed to being largely focused on competition-specific, specialized training. Finally, the AAP recognizes the role for earlier specialization in sports during which peak performance occurs prior to full physical maturation. This includes figure skating, gymnastics, rhythmic gymnastics, and diving. Unfortunately, long-term risks to health and well-being are not known in these populations. Although their training did not seem to affect pubertal growth and maturation, or adult height, female athletes in some of these sports that require earlier specialization were found to have a higher risk of overuse injuries and of the female athlete triad (see section in this chapter on Bone Health and Energy Deficiency).

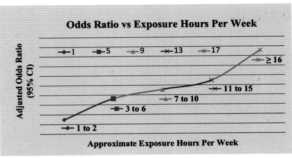

FIGURE 2-2

Relationship of injury to exposure hours in high school athletes.

From Jayanthi N, Pinkham C, Dugas L, Patrick B, Labella C. Sports specialization in young athletes: evidence-based recommendations. *Sports Health.* 2013;5(3):251–257. Reproduced with permission.

As the field of medicine and our pediatric athletes move toward the trend of specialization, once again, it is important for us to recognize the powerful role of prevention. By educating young athletes about the risks and benefits of sport specialization, primary care professionals can prevent some of the associated overuse injuries and emotional disadvantages.

Table 2-1. Recommendations for Stage of Specialization and Sport

Type of Sport	Recommended Stage of Specialization
Gymnastics, diving, figure skating	Early adolescence
Team sports, tennis, golf	Middle adolescence
Endurance sports, track, distance events	Late adolescence

From Myer GD, Jayanthi N, DiFiori JP, et al. Sports specialization, part II: alternative solutions to early sport specialization in youth athletes. *Sports Health.* 2016;8(1):65–73. Reproduced with permission.

TAKE-HOME POINTS

▶ The primary focus of sports in the pediatric athlete population should be to have fun and learn invaluable, lifelong physical activity skills.

▶ Early diversification and later specialization provides for a greater chance of sustained sports participation and attainment of athletic goals.

Burnout

Case 2
How to recognize burnout in a young athlete

Description

A 13-year-old dancer presents to his pediatrician's office, again, with ankle pain. He is dancing for more than 16 hours per week. There is no mechanism of injury described, no swelling on examination, and no focal symptoms. There are multiple areas of tenderness that "will not get better." The patient record indicates that the patient has recently been seen for shoulder pain, and he has described frequent episodes of abdominal pain and headaches in the past 6 months.

Once other causes of his distress are excluded, it is deduced that he would benefit from rest and decreased hours of training, as training for more than 16 hours a week increases the risk of injury and burnout. It is recommended that the athlete take 3 months off a year in 1-month increments from his sport. Also, 1 to 2 days off a week from his sport can decrease the chance for injuries. The patient is also recommended to discuss with his parents or a sports psychologist ways to make his experience more enjoyable.

Workup and Management

Burnout is defined as a response to chronic stress in which a young athlete ceases to participate in a previously enjoyable activity. The main difference in burnout in children compared with that in adults is the more prominent psychological component.

Symptoms of burnout may include fatigue, depression, loss of motivation or interest, sleep disturbances, weight loss, irritability, anxiety, nausea, or frequent illness. Factors related to burnout include both intrinsic and extrinsic factors, namely, individual attributes and environmental influences, respectively. Personal characteristics associated with an increased likelihood of burnout include perfectionism, an innate need to please others,

unassertiveness, self-conceptualization solely as an athlete, low self-esteem, and high perception of stress (high anxiety). Environmental factors include exorbitant training volumes, significant time demands, challenging performance expectations imposed by self or others, frequent and intense competition, inconsistent coaching practices, little personal control in sport decision-making, early sport specialization, and negative performance evaluations.

The treatment for burnout is multifaceted, but the key is early recognition. First and foremost, any possible underlying organic disease should be excluded, or addressed directly if present. Once burnout has been diagnosed, rest is a crucial first step in management. Mental health experts and sports psychologists also play an important role in this multifactorial treatment approach, as they encourage young athletes to develop realistic and positive perceptions of competence. Emphasis should be placed on skill development, as opposed to competition and winning.

Regarding burnout prevention, modifications in training workload and in strength and conditioning regimens should be implemented, and rest periods should be scheduled. It is important to limit weekly or yearly participation time and to limit sport-specific, repetitive movements (hence the importance of instituting policies such as pitch count limits) (tables 2-2 and 2-3). The AAP recommends having at least 3 total months off throughout the year, in increments of 1 month, from the athlete's sport of interest, allowing time for physical and psychological recovery. It is also recommended that young athletes have at least 1 to 2 days off per week from their primary sport to decrease burnout and diminish injury incidence. Finally, there should be careful monitoring of training workloads during the adolescent growth spurt, as this is a particularly vulnerable time for injuries. Incorporating both preseason conditioning programs and pre-practice neuromuscular training can also help prevent these potential injuries from occurring.

Table 2-2. Little League Baseball 2010 Pitching Guidelines: Maximum Pitches per Game

10 y and younger	75 pitches per d
11–12 y	85 pitcher per d
13–16 y	95 pitches per d
17–18 y	105 pitches per d

From Rice SG, Congeni JA; American Academy of Pediatrics Council on Sports Medicine and Fitness. Baseball and softball. *Pediatrics.* 2012;129(3):e842–e856. Reproduced with permission.

Table 2-3. Little League Baseball 2010 Pitching Guidelines: Rest Requirements for Pitchers

Pitchers 14 y and younger	
66 or more pitches in a day	Four (4) calendar days
51–65 pitches in a day	Three (3) calendar days
36–50 pitches in a day	Two (2) calendar days of rest must be observed
21–35 pitches in a day	One (1) calendar day of rest must be observed
1–20 pitches in a day	NO (0) calendar day of rest must be observed
Pitchers 15–18 y	
76 or more pitches in a day	Four (4) calendar days
61–75 pitches in a day	Three (3) calendar days
46–60 pitches in a day	Two (2) calendar days of rest must be observed
31–45 pitches in a day	One (1) calendar day of rest must be observed
1–30 pitches in a day	NO (0) calendar day of rest must be observed

From Rice SG, Congeni JA; American Academy of Pediatrics Council on Sports Medicine and Fitness. Baseball and softball. *Pediatrics.* 2012;129(3):e842–e856. Reproduced with permission.

TAKE-HOME POINTS

▶ Treatment for burnout is multifactorial, but the key is early recognition.

▶ Rest, development of positive perceptions of competence, and emphasizing skill development over competition and winning are crucial aspects of addressing burnout in pediatric athletes.

Concussion

Case 3
Differences in concussions among young athletes

Description

A 12-year-old male football player experienced a head injury during a Friday night football game. He was dizzy following the injury and sidelined for the rest of the game. No focal neurologic symptoms were present, and the patient's dizziness was improving; however, the family still went to the emergency department. The patient was diagnosed there as having a concussion. They are following up with their pediatrician on Monday morning, and he is symptom-free. This is the patient's third lifetime concussion, and his mother is wondering if he should consider "retiring" from football.

The pediatrician informs the family that symptoms of patients with dizziness may take longer to recover (2.6 times longer). The pediatrician counsels them that neuroimaging is recommended only if there is suspicion of serious intracranial pathology, such as a bleed, or if they notice a prolonged disturbance in level of consciousness, focal neurologic deficits, or worsening symptoms. With a young athlete, there needs to be a conversation about how many concussions is too many. Typically, these conversations revolve around symptom recovery and the burden of symptoms on the patient's day-to-day activities and skills. Symptom burden tends to increase with number of concussions, as does the duration of symptoms. A low level of activity may be beneficial for the patient, but there may be a reason to discuss return to noncontact play if the patient's symptom burden is great.

Workup and Management

Sports-related concussions are a significant public health concern in young athletes. The newest research regarding concussion risk is evaluating contributing factors such as young age, sex, obesity, anxiety, depression, visual symptoms, and high-frequency of concussions. Treatment options have been further investigated recently, including bracing options, vestibular and oculomotor therapy, and incorporating early exercise into treatment.

Diagnoses that precede a concussion, such as obesity, anxiety, and depression, seem to negatively affect recovery. Obesity seems to affect symptomatology and duration of recovery. From 2013 to 2014, adolescent and young adult athletes (13–20 years) with obesity were found to have a greater median time of return to baseline with respect to reaction time. They reported more symptoms on a post-concussion symptom scale, and they experienced symptoms longer, until they reached overall recovery. Regarding symptoms, verbal memory, visual motor speed, reaction time, and scale score of these athletes, fewer obese athletes returned to baseline in 2 weeks when compared with normal weight athletes (Lee). Patients with a prior diagnosis of anxiety and depression also tend to have a longer recovery. In a younger population (5–18 years), patients with anxiety took more than twice as long to be fully cleared compared with those without anxiety. Patients with depression took 2.2 times longer to become symptom-free compared with norms and to be fully cleared for return to play. The patient population with anxiety also experienced a prolongation of symptoms, past 4 weeks (Corwin).

Younger age is not always associated with prolongation of symptoms. It is a general trend that clinicians are more conservative with their treatment of younger athletes. In a study of children and youth aged 5 to 18 years, the group aged 13 to 14 years took longer to return to school than the youngest population (≤12 years) and the 15- to 16-year-olds were the second slowest to return. The participants with younger ages required less school accommodations and reported decline in grades less frequently. Decline in grades seemed more common with increasing age. However, in that study, the youngest patients took the longest for symptom recovery. Multiple comparison studies demonstrate a small (a few days) but important difference in recovery time for adolescent athletes compared with young adults following a sport-related concussion. Some studies also conclude a slower recovery for pediatric athletes compared with adolescent athletes. However, studies did not find prolonged (>4 weeks) recovery in the younger population compared to the older cohorts.

Symptoms at the time of a concussion that were associated with prolonged recovery included dizziness, loss of consciousness, and oculomotor symptoms. Like those with anxiety, patients with dizziness at presentation were more likely to have their symptoms for greater than 4 weeks and to require school accommodations. Loss of consciousness at the time of injury was associated with 1.8 times longer for symptoms to resolve. Patients with dizziness took the longest time to become symptom-free (2.6 times longer). Symptoms provoked after oculomotor examination were associated with symptom prolongation, delayed full recovery, decline in grades, and need for school accommodations. Please see Box 2-1 for stepwise return activity recommendations.

Box 2-1
Return to Play Progression

There are five gradual steps to help safely return an athlete to play:

Baseline: No symptoms
As the baseline step of the Return to Play Progression, the athlete needs to have completed physical and cognitive rest and not be experiencing concussion symptoms for a minimum of 24 hours. *Keep in mind, the younger the athlete, the more conservative the treatment.*

Step 1
Light aerobic activity

The Goal: Only to increase an athlete's heart rate.

The Time: 5 to 10 minutes.

The Activities: Exercise bike, walking, or light jogging. Absolutely no weight lifting, jumping, or hard running.

Step 2
Moderate activity

The Goal: Limited body and head movement.

The Time: Reduced from typical routine.

The Activities: Moderate jogging, brief running, moderate-intensity stationary biking, and moderate-intensity weight lifting.

Step 3
Heavy, non-contact activity

The Goal: More intense but non-contact.

The Time: Close to typical routine.

The Activities: Running, high-intensity stationary biking, the player's regular weight-lifting routine, and non-contact sport-specific drills. This stage may add some cognitive component to practice in addition to the aerobic and movement components introduced in Steps 1 and 2.

Step 4
Practice & full contact

The Goal: Reintegrate in full contact practice.

Step 5
Competition

The Goal: Return to competition.

From Centers for Disease Control and Prevention, National CenterFor Injury Prevention and Control, Division of Unintentional Injury Prevention. Managing return to activities: information for health care professionals; returning to play (sports and recreation). CDC Heads Up Web site. https://www.cdc.gov/headsup/providers/return_to_activities.html. Updated February 8, 2016. Accessed June 29, 2017.

Significant strides in research have been made comparing the pathophysiologic difference between the child or adolescent brain to the adult brain following a concussion. Research regarding imaging of concussions reveals that findings from clinical neuroimaging following a sports-related concussion are normal in most cases. Magnetic resonance imaging should be considered for pediatric patients with persistent symptoms for which the definition is unclear. There may be an indication to retire from contact sports if a patient is found to have a traumatic lesion on neuroimaging following a sports-related concussion. Changes on post-concussive CT scans may show contusion or a cyst in children (like in our clinical case) but will likely not restrict return to full play.

Using a mice model, adolescent mice show a distinct pattern of functional deficits after injury compared with adult mice. Injured mice had a longer loss of consciousness, impaired balance, increased impulsivity, and worsening of their spatial memory compared with adult mice. Research is aimed at discovering a biomarker that may provide diagnostic, prognostic, and monitoring information for concussions. The study of these biomarkers is rapidly evolving, as are their roles. It is hoped that they will assist in clinical decision-making by clarifying injury severity and monitoring the patient through recovery. They may play a role in prognosis of patients with repetitive injury and in return to duty, work, or play.

As concussion awareness spreads, frequency of concussion and how many concussions is "too many" has become a growing concern, particularly in players of sports such as football and hockey. History of a prior concussion is significantly associated with increased odds of repeat injury. Patients with 2 or more prior concussions are linked with longer durations of recovery, more than twice as long to become symptom-free. Those with 3 or more prior concussions took 3.6 times longer to return to school full-time compared with those without prior concussion. However, one paper reported that patients who play soccer, ice hockey or skating, and basketball are at a significantly higher risk of subsequent concussion compared with those who play football.

Sex-based differences in concussion reporting and recovery have become a current topic in concussion research. Females tend to report more symptoms than males at baseline and post-concussion. However, the recovery trajectory for females and males has been found to be identical. Increased symptom frequency, particularly higher baseline levels of migraine and neuropsychological symptoms, is noted in female concussion patients compared with males.

Protective equipment has made progress in decreasing the number of catastrophic injuries through sports, but the effects on concussion prevalence and severity are largely unproven. Recent evidence suggests that helmeted athletes do not have better relative clinical outcome and protection against concussion than un-helmeted athletes.

Last, the effect of the concussion on the young athlete must be understood during the treatment process. Young athletes most often report loss of activity to be the worst part of a concussion. Young athletes were more bothered by the loss of activity than by the symptoms (68 patients vs 17). Young age (<20 years) seems to be associated with second impact syndrome, as well as male sex and participation in American football. Therefore, return to contact play may need to be limited slightly longer for younger athletes, but return to low-intensity aerobic exercise may be of benefit. After a period of rest, low-level exercise and multimodal physiotherapy may be of benefit for children and youths who are bothered by the loss of their activities. Please see advice for professionals treating concussions (Box 2-2).

Box 2-2
Important Concussion Information for Professionals

Before the start of the season, health care professionals should learn about state, league, or sports governing body's laws or policies on concussion.

Some policies may require health care professionals to take a training program or provide written clearance as part of the return-to-play process for young athletes.

Remember, while most athletes will recover quickly and fully following a concussion, some will have symptoms for weeks or longer. Health care professionals should consider referral to a concussion specialist if:

1. The symptoms worsen at any time,

2. The symptoms have not gone away after 10-14 days, or

3. The patient has a history of multiple concussions or risk factors for prolonged recovery. This may include a history of migraines, depression, mood disorders, or anxiety, as well as developmental disorders such as learning disabilities and ADHD.

From Centers for Disease Control and Prevention, National Center for Injury Prevention and Control, Division of Unintentional Injury Prevention. Managing return to activities: information for health care professionals; when to refer to a specialist. CDC Heads Up Web site. https://www.cdc.gov/headsup/providers/return_to_activities.html. Updated February 8, 2016. Accessed June 29, 2017.

TAKE-HOME POINTS

▶ Age and symptom burden before and after a concussion are all important prognostic factors.

▶ Helpful resources are available from the Centers for Disease Control and Prevention Heads Up program and the American Academy of Pediatrics Council on Sports Medicine and Fitness.

Heat Illness

Case 4
Heat illness in young athletes

Description

A 14-year-old boy with obesity presents with collapse and mental status changes after football practice in full pads at 2:00 pm in August. His rectal temperature in the field is 40.6°C (105°F). This is the first week of high school football training for this freshman athlete. All his preceding summer workouts have been largely strength-training based in an air-conditioned gym.

This athlete had many risk factors for exertional heat stroke (EHS), some of which could have been avoided. He was practicing on a humid day in August in full pads at 2:00 pm with a lack of prior acclimatization. Obesity, aerobic deconditioning, and dehydration were likely contributing factors as well. Possible adjustments that might have prevented this EHS include holding practice early in the morning or later in the evening, both during cooler times of the day; starting some of the initial practices without tackle and pads as part of the acclimatization process; ensuring pre- and intra-practice hydration; and player education regarding clinical symptoms of heat stroke.

Workup and Management

Heat-related illness remains one of the leading causes of death of young athletes. Deaths from EHS were higher during the period of 2005 to 2009 than any other 4-year period in the past 35 years. On the basis of data from the National High School Sports-Related Injury Surveillance Study that sampled 100 schools over this 4-year period, the Centers for Disease Control and Prevention estimated 9,237 cases per year of exertional heat illness in high school athletes. The highest rate of time-loss heat illness was among football players, 4.5 per 100,000 athlete exposures, a rate 10 times higher than the average rate (0.4) for other sports.

Time-loss heat illnesses occurred most frequently during August (66.3%). Furthermore, according to the annual survey of catastrophic American football injuries presented in 2008, 31 players have died of EHS since 1995 (Mueller).

This increasing incidence and associated mortality risk make the prevention of heat-related illness a priority among coaches and physicians who care for young athletes. To understand the mechanism behind prevention tactics, it is first important to discuss the etiology and classification of heat illness.

Hyperthermia is defined as an elevation in core body temperature above diurnal range of 36.0°C to 37.5°C (96.8°F–99.5°F) caused by failure of thermoregulation. The body's heat load results from both metabolic processes and absorption of heat from the environment. As core temperature rises, the preoptic nucleus of the anterior hypothalamus stimulates efferent fibers of the autonomic nervous system to produce sweating and cutaneous vasodilatation. Core body temperature is therefore maintained within a narrow range by balancing heat load with heat dissipation. There are 4 main mechanisms of dissipation.

1. Evaporation occurs when water vaporizes from the skin and respiratory tract. This is the body's most effective cooling mechanism, but it becomes ineffective above a relative humidity of 75% (Broses).
2. Radiation is the emission of electromagnetic heat waves.
3. Convection is the transfer of heat to a gas or liquid moving over the body that is colder than the body.
4. Conduction is the direct transfer of heat to an adjacent, cooler object.

Evaporation is the primary dissipation mechanism, as the other 3 modes of heat transfer are inefficient when environmental temperature exceeds skin temperature.

In pediatrics, there are additional physiologic considerations that put children at an increased risk for heat-related illness. Children produce more metabolic heat per kilogram of body weight, have a smaller absolute blood volume (thereby limiting dissipation), have lower rates of sweating, are less likely to replace fluid losses, and have slower rates of physiologic acclimatization when compared with their adult counterparts. Other contributing factors that increase the risk of heat-related illness that are not specific to children include obesity, poor physical fitness, dehydration, lack of acclimatization, strenuous exercise in humid conditions, medications and dietary supplements, and preexisting conditions such as cystic fibrosis, ectodermal dysplasia, anorexia nervosa, and sickle cell trait.

Heat illness can be further classified into 10 categories of heat disorders, according to the *International Classification of Diseases* published by the World Health Organization. Four of these diagnoses, namely, heat cramps, heat syncope, heat exhaustion, and heat stroke, are more commonly seen in athletes and soldiers who engage in vigorous activity in humid environmental conditions. For the purposes of this chapter, we will focus on the identification, prompt management, and prevention of heat exhaustion and heat stroke (Box 2-3).

Heat exhaustion is characterized by the inability to maintain adequate cardiac output caused by strenuous exercise and environmental heat stress. Core temperature may be normal or slightly elevated, but, by definition, it will be less than or equal to 40°C (104°F). The athlete should have a normal mental status. Clinical signs include profuse sweating, mild dehydration, nausea, headache, and light-headedness or dizziness. Blood pressure is typically normal, although tachycardia and tachypnea may be present.

Heat stroke is defined as a core temperature more than 40°C to 41°C (104.0°F–105.8°F) along with central nervous system dysfunction, which will typically manifest as abnormal mental status, or seizures, in the context of tachycardia, with hypotension and moderate to severe dehydration. There are many overlapping features of heat exhaustion and heat stroke, including dizziness, nausea, vomiting, and headache. Temperature elevation is accompanied by an increased oxygen consumption and metabolic rate, thereby resulting in hyperpnea and tachycardia in cases of both heat exhaustion and heat stroke. However, once the temperature exceeds 42°C (107.6°F), oxidative phosphorylation becomes uncoupled, resulting in enzyme dysfunction, putting athletes at risk for multiorgan failure that can result from EHS. Morbidity and mortality are directly related to the duration of core temperature elevation above the critical threshold of 40.5°C to 41.0°C (104.9°F–105.8°F). Therefore, prompt recognition and treatment is critical. If there is any suspicion of EHS, in other words, any neurologic abnormality, clinicians should assume the diagnosis to be EHS and treat accordingly as quickly as possible.

Box 2-3
Heat Exhaustion Versus Heat Stroke

Heat Exhaustion
- Mild dehydration
- Core temperature 100.4° to 104°F (38° to 40°C)[a]
- Profuse sweating
- Thirst, nausea, vomiting, confusion, headache
- Feels faint or has collapsed

Heat Stroke
- Usually severe dehydration
- Core temperature may be >104°F (40°C)[a]
- Flushed with hot, dry skin
- Dizziness, vertigo, syncope, confusion, delirium
- May be unconscious
- Shock

[a] Core temperature may have fallen substantially by the time the patient reaches a medical facility.
From Jardine DS. Heat illness and heat stroke. *Pediatr Rev.* 2007;28(7):249–258. Reproduced with permission.

Rapid cooling is the most effective strategy for minimizing morbidity and mortality from EHS, and it should be initiated as soon as possible, within 30 minutes of presentation. On the basis of available evidence, cold water submersion has been shown to be most effective in dropping the core temperature rapidly. If you suspect heat stroke, the key steps to rapidly and effectively cooling an athlete in the field include

- Activate the emergency medical system.
- Remove all excess equipment and clothing, and obtain core temperature rectally, as oral, axillary, aural, and temporal methods of obtaining temperature are not validated.
- If possible, begin ice water immersion (water temperature should be 2°C–15°C [35.6°F–59.0°F], with colder being better).
- If available, monitor rectal temperature using rectal thermistor (continuous flexible thermometer) or take rectal temperature every 10 minutes.
- Cease cooling when rectal temperature reaches 38.3°C to 38.9°C (100.9°F–102.0°F).
- Avoid antipyretics, as they are ineffective and can worsen acute kidney injury.
- Give chilled salt-containing liquids to drink if athletes are neurologically capable of protecting their airway.

If immersion is not possible, other interventions may include a cold shower; application of cold, wet towels to as much of the body surface as possible; laying the patient down on a tarp that is covered in ice; or seeking shade while simultaneously maximizing evaporative cooling by spraying tepid water over the patient's body and using fans to blow air over the moist skin. If you do not have a thermometer available, cool until the patient begins to shiver or treat with cold water immersion for 15 to 20 minutes, assuming a typical cooling rate of 0.21°C (0.38°F) per minute (Casa).

Fortunately, exertional heat illness is often preventable. Coaching staff and athletes should therefore be educated about heat illness, and institution-wide preventive policies should be put into place when possible.

First and foremost, it is important to determine when exercise in certain weather conditions should be avoided. This is best determined by a wet bulb globe temperature (WBGT). A WBGT considers humidity, heat, and solar radiation, whereas the heat index considers only heat and humidity. Given that up to 70% of heat illness is attributable to humidity, reflecting the critical importance of evaporative cooling, it is important to have this index available when determining safety for outdoor exercise. Refer to Table 2-4 for heat illness risk and suggested actions. Alternatives may include early morning or evening or indoor practices.

If allowed to participate, athletes should be provided with frequent shady breaks for hydration and cooling. For every 1% of body mass lost from dehydration, there is a concomitant increase in core body temperature of 0.22°C (0.4°F), making pre-activity and intra-activity hydration crucial to preventing heat illness. Similarly, athletes with fever or a recent gastrointestinal illness that has resulted in dehydration should be excluded from activity in extreme heat and humidity until their hydration status has normalized. Athletes should drink 6 mL of fluid per kilogram of body mass every 2 to 3 hours, starting 4 to 6 hours prior to the workout or competition. A good rule of thumb for intra- and post-event fluid intake is to consume 237 mL (8 oz) of fluid for every pound lost during the event. Pre-cooling and intra-event cooling with cooling vests or ice towels around the neck can also be implemented, especially in sports such as cycling and long-distance running that involve sustained exercise in hot environments.

Careful attention should be paid to athletes with large mass to skin surface ratios (obesity) and to those with any history suggestive of prior heat illness or preexisting medical conditions that put them at a greater risk for heat illness.Furthermore, players should be screened for any medications or substances they may be taking that might put them at a higher risk for experiencing heat illness (eg, anticholinergics, antiepileptics, antihistamines and decongestants, tricyclic antidepressants, amphetamines, stimulants, lithium, diuretics, beta-adrenergic blocking agents, alcohol use). Clothing should be loose fitting, allowing for adequate ventilation and evaporative cooling, and equipment that hinders heat loss in humid conditions should be minimized. Athletes should be educated to stop exercising immediately if they begin to experience extreme exhaustion, light-headedness, or other symptoms concerning to their teammates or coaching staff.

Finally, and perhaps most important, heat acclimatization provides the best protection against heat exhaustion and heat stroke. Physiologic adaptations allow for increased heat tolerance. These include increased rate of sweating, lower temperature threshold for sweating, reduced electrolyte loss in sweat, lower heart rate, improved cutaneous blood flow, increased aldosterone production with decreased urinary sodium concentration and plasma volume expansion, and lower core and skin temperatures. Children reach their physiologic acclimatization endpoint more slowly than adults, typically requiring 10 to 14 days to achieve said adaptations. See the sample acclimatization program for American football (Box 2-4), based on "Preseason Heat-Acclimatization Guidelines for Secondary School Athletics" (Casa).

Table 2-4. Heat-Illness Risk Factors and Recommended Responses (Actions)

Risk Factors	Actions[a]

• Hot and/or humid weather
• Poor preparation
  – Not heat-acclimatized
  – Inadequate prehydration
  – Little sleep/rest
  – Poor fitness
• Excessive physical exertion
  – Insufficient rest/recovery time between repeat bouts of high-intensity exercise (eg, repeat sprints)
• Insufficient access to fluids and opportunities to rehydrate
• Multiple same-day sessions
  – Insufficient rest/recovery time between practices, games, or matches
• Overweight/obese (BMI ≥ 85th percentile for age) and other clinical conditions (eg, diabetes) or medications (eg, attention-deficit/hyperactivity disorder medications)
• Current or recent illness (especially if it involves/involved gastrointestinal distress or fever)
• Clothing, uniforms, or protective equipment that contributes to excessive heat retention
	• Provide and promote consumption of readily accessible fluids at regular intervals before, during, and after activity
	• Allow gradual introduction and adaptation to the climate, intensity, and duration of activities and uniform/protective gear
	• Physical activity should be modified
	  – Decrease duration and/or intensity
	  – Increase frequency and duration of breaks (preferably in the shade)
	  – Cancel or reschedule to cooler time
	• Provide longer rest/recovery time between same-day sessions, games, or matches
	• Avoid/limit participation if child or adolescent is currently or was recently ill
	• Closely monitor participants for signs and symptoms of developing heat illness
	• Ensure that personnel and facilities for effectively treating heat illness are readily available on site
	• In response to an affected (moderate or severe heat stress) child or adolescent, promptly activate emergency medical services and rapidly cool the victim

With any of these risk factors or other medical conditions adversely affecting exercise-heat safety present, some or all of the actions listed may be appropriate responses to reduce exertional heat-illness risk and improve well-being.

[a] As environmental conditions become more challenging (heat and humidity increase) and as additional other listed risk factors are present, the possible actions to improve safety become more urgent. Note that each listed action does not necessarily correspond or apply to any particular or every listed risk factor.

From Bergeron MF, Devore C, Rice SG; American Academy of Pediatrics Council on Sports Medicine and Fitness and Council on School Health. Climatic heat stress and exercising children and adolescents. *Pediatrics*. 2011;128(3):e741–e747. Reproduced with permission.

Box 2-4
Sample Acclimatization Program for American Football Based on Preseason Heat-Acclimatization Guidelines for Secondary School Athletics

- Days 1–5 of the heat-acclimatization period consist of the first 5 d of formal practice. During this time, athletes may not participate in >1 practice per day.

- If a practice is interrupted by inclement weather or heat restrictions, the practice should recommence once conditions are deemed safe. Total practice time should not exceed 3 h in any 1 d.

- A 1-h maximum walk-through is permitted during days 1–5 of the heat-acclimatization period. However, a 3-h recovery period should be inserted between the practice and walk-through (or vice versa).

- During days 1–2 of the heat-acclimatization period, for sports requiring helmets or shoulder pads, a helmet should be the only protective equipment permitted (goalies, as in the case of field hockey and related sports, should not wear full protective gear or perform activities that would require protective equipment). During days 3–5, only helmets and shoulder pads should be worn. Beginning on day 6, all protective equipment may be worn and full contact may begin.

- Football only: On days 3–5, contact with blocking sleds and tackling dummies may be initiated.

- Full-contact sports: 100% live contact drills should begin no earlier than day 6.

- Beginning no earlier than day 6 and continuing through day 14, double-practice days must be followed by a single-practice day. On single-practice days, 1 walk-through is permitted, separated from the practice by at least 3 h of continuous rest. When a double-practice day is followed by a rest day, another double-practice day is permitted after the rest day.

- On a double-practice day, neither practice should exceed 3 h in duration, and student-athletes should not participate in >5 total hours of practice. Warm-up, stretching, cooldown, walk-through, conditioning, and weight-room activities are included as part of the practice time. The 2 practices should be separated by at least 3 continuous hours in a cool environment.

- Because the risk of exertional heat illnesses during the preseason heat-acclimatization period is high, we strongly recommend that an athletic trainer be on site before, during, and after all practices.

TAKE-HOME POINTS

▶ Heat illness is one of the leading preventable causes of death of young athletes.

▶ If it is difficult to tell whether an athlete has heat exhaustion or heat stroke and there is *any* clinical suspicion for heat stroke, treat the patient for heat stroke.

▶ Rapid cooling with cold water immersion is the best way to prevent morbidity and mortality from heat stroke.

▶ Hydration status, wet bulb globe temperature, premorbid conditions, and acclimatization status are all important factors to consider in heat illness prevention.

Cardiovascular Screening

Case 5
Cardiovascular disease in young athletes

Description

An 18-year-old African American male collegiate freshman basketball player collapses in the middle of a game and is found to be in ventricular fibrillation. The patient is appropriately treated on the court where he collapsed. When a rhythm is not detected, cardiopulmonary resuscitation is initiated immediately. The automatic external defibrillator is brought onto the court and a shock is provided. Cardiopulmonary resuscitation is resumed awaiting a read, and the patient is found to have a pulse and a heart rhythm. He is sent immediately by ambulance to the nearest emergency department.

Upon review of his past medical history, it is noted that he has a history of a murmur and concerns of intermittent palpitations and dyspnea. Upon further questioning, it is learned that his father died of unclear reasons at a young age. He is found to have hypertrophic cardiomyopathy on cardiac ultrasound, most likely genetic in his case.

Workup and Management

The annual incidence of all sudden cardiac arrest (SCA) and sudden cardiac death (SCD) is approximately 1 in 80,000 among high school athletes and 1 in 50,000 among college athletes. Exercise is a known trigger and can unmask cardiac disease. Studies indicate that 56% to 80% of SCA and SCD of young athletes occurs during exercise, with the remainder considered non-exertional, such as at rest or during sleep. Incidence rates tend to be higher among male and African American athletes. Male college basketball players have the highest reported overall risk of SCD, at 1 in 9,000 per year, while male African American college athletes have a reported SCD risk of 1 in 16,000 per year. Studies also report that 2 sports alone, men's basketball and football, account for 50% to 61% of all identified cases of SCA and SCD. An aspect to be mindful of is that there is no mandatory reporting system

for SCA and SCD of athletes, and cases may go unreported, leaving current incidence estimates lower that the true risk.

The most commonly reported causes of SCA and SCD of athletes include hypertrophic cardiomyopathy, anomalous coronary arteries, idiopathic left ventricular hypertrophy, arrhythmogenic right ventricular cardiomyopathy, dilated cardiomyopathy, myocarditis, long QT syndrome, ventricular pre-excitation and Wolff-Parkinson-White syndrome, aortic dissection, and atherosclerotic coronary artery disease (Figure 2-3). Of note, up to 44% of athletes who experienced SCA did not have any identified structural cardiac abnormalities on autopsy. These cases, known as autopsy-negative sudden unexplained death, are likely caused by primary abnormal electrical conditions and inherited arrhythmia syndromes. Hypertrophic cardiomyopathy represents 8% to 36% of cases in US athletes.

The best strategy of screening for SCA and SCD of young athletes remains controversial. However, CV screening of athletes is thoroughly recommended and routinely performed. Cardiovascular screening is a fundamental component of the pre-participation evaluation (PPE) and is of paramount importance. Overall, the primary goal of the PPE is to evaluate the health of an athlete for optimal safety in sports participation, including determining current and future health risks. Risk factors considered include age, sex, race, sport, and level of competition. Objectives of the PPE include

- Identifying factors that predispose athletes to serious injury, illness, or sudden death
- Early detection of athletes at risk for SCA and SCD
- Identifying underlying cardiac disorders increasing the risk for SCA and SCD, with the goal of minimizing morbidity and mortality

Ideally, the PPE is conducted in the primary care setting, serving as a health care home base for the young athlete and an opportunity for education, counseling, and intervention for injury prevention, CV health, and general well-being.

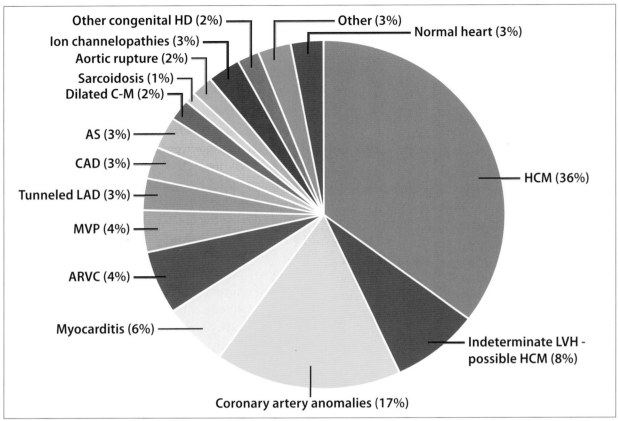

Distribution of cardiovascular causes of sudden death in 1435 young competitive athletes. From the Minneapolis Heart Institute Foundation Registry, 1980 to 2005. ARVC indicates arrhythmogenic right ventricular cardiomyopathy; AS, aortic stenosis; CAD, coronary artery disease; C-M, cardiomyopathy; HCM, hypertrophic cardiomyopathy; HD, heart disease; LAD, left anterior descending; LVH, left ventricular hypertrophy; and MVP, mitral valve prolapse.

From Maron BJ, Thompson PD, Ackerman MJ, et al. Recommendations and considerations related to preparticipation screening for cardiovascular abnormalities in competitive athletes: 2007 update; a scientific statement from the American Heart Association Council on Nutrition, Physical Activity, and Metabolism: endorsed by the American College of Cardiology Foundation. *Circulation*. 2007;115(12):1643–1655. Reproduced with permission.

The criterion standard for PPE includes a comprehensive history questionnaire and physical examination (Box 2-5). The history and review of systems establish a minimum standard to evaluate multiple organs that may affect safety in sports participation. The physical examination may pick up abnormalities that may not have provoked symptoms currently or in the past.

The addition of a resting 12-lead electrocardiogram (ECG) routinely to the PPE remains in question and has potential benefits and potential risks. Potential benefits of ECG use include identifying athletes with potential CV symptoms, such as exertional syncope, a family history of SCA and SCD, or other inherited cardiac conditions. The ECG increases early detection of some of these cardiac disorders associated with SCA and SCD before an event occurs. An estimated 60% of the disorders associated with SCA and SCD of young athletes may have detectable ECG abnormalities. An abnormal ECG finding may bring awareness of vague symptoms the athlete may have been experiencing or relevant family history that previously went unreported. In addition, approximately 80% of athletes who experience SCA and SCD have no documented

Box 2-5
The 12-Element AHA Recommendations for Preparticipation Cardiovascular Screening of Competitive Athletes

Medical History[a]

Personal History

1. Exertional chest pain/discomfort

2. Unexplained syncope/near-syncope[b]

3. Excessive exertional and unexplained dyspnea/fatigue, associated with exercise

4. Prior recognition of a heart murmur

5. Elevated systemic blood pressure

Family History

6. Premature death (sudden and unexpected, or otherwise) before age 50 years due to heart disease, in ≥1 relative

7. Disability from heart disease in a close relative <50 years of age

8. Specific knowledge of certain cardiac conditions in family members: hypertrophic or dilated cardiomyopathy, long-QT syndrome or other ion channelopathies, Marfan syndrome, or clinically important arrhythmias

Physical Examination

9. Heart murmur[c]

10. Femoral pulses to exclude aortic coarctation

11. Physical stigmata of Marfan syndrome

12. Brachial artery blood pressure (sitting position)[d]

[a] Parental verification is recommended for high school and middle school athletes.

[b] Judged not to be neurocardiogenic (vasovagal); of particular concern when related to exertion.

[c] Auscultation should be performed in both supine and standing positions (or with Valsalva maneuver), specifically to identify murmurs of dynamic left ventricular outflow tract obstruction.

[d] Preferably taken in both arms.

From Maron BJ, Thompson PD, Ackerman MJ, et al. Recommendations and considerations related to preparticipation screening for cardiovascular abnormalities in competitive athletes: 2007 update; a scientific statement from the American Heart Association Council on Nutrition, Physical Activity, and Metabolism: endorsed by the American College of Cardiology Foundation. *Circulation.* 2007;115(12):1643–1655. Reproduced with permission.

warning symptoms at the time of PPE screening and may be missed using history and physical alone. Potential risks of ECG use include variable ECG interpretation accuracy and reliability, depending on use of modern criteria and experience of the interpreting physician, leading to an increase in false-positive results. The screening leads to an increase in costlier secondary screening, anxiety related to the diagnosis, and potential for unnecessary interventions, including sports restriction and prohibiting exercise when they are not indicated. Misinterpretation of physiologic adaptations in athletes may also contribute to that burden. Furthermore, ECG is not 100% sensitive for ECG-detectable disorders, and the age at which cardiac conditions present varies. This raises questions regarding the timing of screenings and requirements for repeat screening. In addition, some cardiac conditions do not manifest as ECG abnormalities, or they show up sporadically and may not be present at the time the ECG is obtained, and, therefore, would not be identified via ECG screening. The optimal age and frequency to conduct CV screening of athletes are also not well established, but these screenings are generally conducted between the ages of 12 and 14 years and repeated every 1 to 3 years. They should be done well in advance of a sports season to be able to conduct secondary screening of abnormal screening results.

Currently, there is no consensus or clear evidence-based research advocating for a single universal screening strategy for all athletes. At this time, physicians should implement a CV screening strategy customized to their athlete population and local resources. The primary factors to consider when deciding to add ECG to screening include

1. Individual risk of SCA and SCD based on age, sex, race, sport, and level of play
2. Physician expertise, available infrastructure, and available cardiology resources to conduct an ECG screening program with high quality and accuracy
3. Physician assessment of risk-benefit analysis that use of ECG screening will optimize athletes' outcomes and minimize their harm

For example, a physician may choose to not use ECG for high school female athletes, but may choose to implement ECG screening for male African American college basketball players. It is also important to optimize strategies to ensure accurate ECG interpretation and provide cardiology resources to adequately follow up abnormal findings on ECGs. No screening program offers guaranteed safeguards against SCA and SCD; therefore, it is critical that an emergency action plan and access to an automatic external defibrillator are established to improve outcomes of potential SCA in athletes.

TAKE-HOME POINTS

▶ Cardiovascular disease is rare in young athletes.

▶ When cardiovascular incidents occur, they can be quite serious.

▶ Recognizing the warning signs for cardiovascular disease in young athletes is essential for safety.

▶ Preparation for cardiopulmonary events—including cardiopulmonary resuscitation training, appropriate protective equipment, and a plan of care—is essential.

Spine Injury Prevention

Case 6
Spondylolysis, a preventable overuse injury of the spine

Description

A 13-year-old female elite gymnast presents with lower back pain aggravated by activity (particularly hyperextension) for the past month. She reports no other neurologic symptoms and no known trauma. On physical examination, discomfort can be elicited with deep palpation just lateral to midline over the lumbar transverse processes. She does not experience pain with forward flexion but experiences discomfort with hyperextension. Pain is worsened with one-legged Stork test and extension, more so on the right leg than left.

The patient exhibits signs concerning for not only an overuse injury but spondylolysis. Workup for the patient typically begins with oblique lumbar radiographs, which may show the collar on a "Scottie dog" profile; however, plain radiographs are found to be only 32% sensitive. Lateral oblique radiographs should not be considered as the definitive investigation for spondylolysis. Many clinicians are forgoing the radiation exposure and proceeding straight to advanced imaging. Despite magnetic resonance imaging's decreased radiation exposure, it is not as accurate as CT in demonstrating bony detail. A CT scan at diagnosis is typically not necessary. A limited CT scan, focusing only on the affected level, may help provide more information for prognosis if the patient has had persistent pain for 6 to 8 weeks.

Workup and Management

With the rise in sport specialization, overuse injuries have become increasingly prevalent. Overuse injury is defined as repetitive submaximal loading of the musculoskeletal system, including microtrauma. In these instances, rest is not adequate to allow structural adaptation and repair to take place.

Similar to sport specialization (see Sport Specialization section), both intrinsic and extrinsic factors increase likelihood of overuse injuries.

Intrinsic risk factors include growth-related factors, previous injury, previous level of conditioning, anatomical factors (alignment and flexibility), menstrual dysfunction, and psychological and developmental factors. Growth-related factors include susceptibility of growth cartilage to repetitive stress and the adolescent growth spurt. During adolescence, patients develop tight thoracolumbar fascia and hamstrings and an anterior pelvic tilt with mild hyperlordosis. However, it has been shown that when corrected for growth, patients still experience overuse injuries when they specialize in one sport.

Extrinsic factors leading to overuse injury are sport specialization and high numbers of hours devoted to practicing a sport. Extrinsic risk factors include training workload (rate, intensity, and progression), training and competition schedules, equipment, environment, technique, and psychological factors, such as adult and peer influences.

Spondylolysis is the predominant injury to the spine that affects young athletes and is caused by overuse. Gymnasts, dancers, and tennis and volleyball players are more frequently injured because of increased prevalence of repeated lumbar spine hyperextension (Figure 2-4). Repeated hyperextension places stress to the posterior elements of the vertebral body, namely, the pars interarticularis, between the facet joints. Overtime, there is enough stress across the pars that a fracture occurs. The fracture can be unilateral or bilateral, but most often it is bilateral (80%). Bilateral involvement can result in spondylolisthesis, a slippage of one vertebrae anteriorly over the level below. Spondylolysis is most commonly seen at the fifth lumbar vertebrae (L5) (85%–95%), followed by L4 (5%–15%).

The key to optimal treatment is early recognition. Treatment for spondylolysis requires a period of relative rest, until the athlete is pain-free. Most

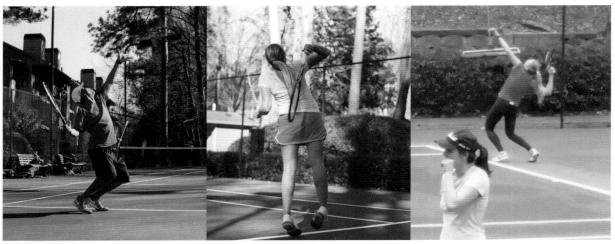

FIGURE 2-4

Examples of lumbar hyperextension in tennis players. The serve in tennis and volleyball is a common culprit of overuse injuries, including spondylolysis.

Photos by Margaux Boivin and Kishane Taylor.

treatment regimens recommend modification and removal from sport for 3 to 4 months. It is critical to focus on gradual strengthening and stabilization of the core and back muscles protecting the spine, optimizing hamstring flexibility, and gradual return to play. Rigid anti-lordotic bracing in a hard lumbosacral orthosis, the most common of these being a Boston brace, remains controversial. A study has not definitively demonstrated heeling with or without bracing. The bracing protocol has been recommended in cases of young athletes who have had 3 to 4 months of symptoms. Bracing would be combined with activity modification, especially decreased lumbar hyperextension, for roughly 4 to 6 weeks. Reintegration into a physical therapy program and physical activities can occur after pain has improved, which may be around 6 weeks after initiation of the rigid brace. The brace may be modified into a transitional rigid brace. The goal of most physical therapy programs will be peripelvic strengthening and core stabilization. Rehabilitation will be advanced as the participant gains strength and pain improves, to incorporate lumbar extensors while limiting hyperextension of the spine.

Return to play is typically seen between 3 and 6 months after the initiation of treatment, depending on the individual's symptoms. Surgical referral is indicated if the athlete has spondylolisthesis with a slip of greater than 50%, radicular or neurologic symptoms, or painful spondylolysis with nonunion after 6 months of nonoperative treatment and at least 9 to 12 months of symptoms. Prevention of recurrent spine injury is emphasized through continued strengthening of core and back muscles and modifying technique to protect the spine during competitive play.

TAKE-HOME POINTS

▶ Spondylolysis is an overuse injury to the posterior elements of the spine, typically caused by repetitive hyperextension.

▶ Early diagnosis and treatment to avoid prolongation of symptoms and progression to chronic fracture is crucial.

▶ Pars interarticularis stress injuries can be prevented with good core stabilization, attention to biomechanics, and avoidance of overuse.

ACL Injury Prevention

Case 7
ACL injury prevention in young athletes

Description
A 17-year-old high school soccer player presents with left knee pain and swelling after sustaining a lateral blow to her planted left leg by a player on the other team. She endorses a popping sensation that occurred at the time of the fall and afterward she experienced immediate pain, swelling, and instability. The pediatrician suspects a ligament injury and asks if she had been participating in any sort of structured ACL prevention program with her team.

Concerned about an ACL tear, the pediatrician conducts a proper examination and workup, leading up to a diagnosis of a tear. She likely would have benefited from an injury prevention program, integrating neuromuscular training into her soccer practice before her current season began. Rehabilitation will be essential after surgical reconstruction of her ACL to decrease risk of re-tear to her graft and to decrease risk of contralateral ACL tear.

Workup and Management
In recent years, there has been a 400% increase in ACL injuries reported in children and adolescents. It is estimated that 50% of all patients with an ACL tear are between the ages of 15 and 25 years. Most ACL injuries are sports related, and they occur most often in girl's and women's sports; gymnastics, soccer, and basketball have the highest rates of ACL injuries.

The function of the ACL is primarily knee stability in cutting and pivoting motions. Anterior cruciate ligament tears occur most frequently when an athlete is turning or changing direction on a plated foot, and most are noncontact injuries (80%). Risk factors include previous ACL injury, female sex, intensity of play, muscle and strength imbalances of the body, and genetics.

Advances in injury prevention regarding ACL tears are centered around preventive neuromuscular training interventions. Many physical therapy centers, injury prevention programs, and sports teams are starting to implement these across the country to decrease ACL injury rates. Anterior cruciate ligament prevention has been found effective; however, adherence is poor (Figure 2-5).

For girls and women, the most likely to experience an ACL tear, the peak age of injury is between 15 and 19 years. This timing is most likely related to completion of adolescent growth spurts, when patients get taller, but they have not yet developed motor control or strength to support their new height. This early age of injury compounds the difficulty with injury prevention programs. Current meta-analysis revealed an age-related association between neuromuscular training implementation and reduction of ACL injuries. It was also concluded that neuromuscular training preformed earlier by a younger population showed greater efficacy. On the basis of meta-analysis data, there was a 72% risk reduction for female athletes younger than 18 years, but only a 16% decrease in risk for female athletes older than 18 years. There seems to be a window of opportunity for ACL injury prevention programs during preadolescent years. Younger athletes may be more receptive to neuromuscular training, decreasing their future risk.

Prevention programs are on the rise to address this season-changing injury. The focus is primarily on optimizing neuromuscular control of the knee. These programs incorporate dynamic plyometrics, balance, and strengthening and stability exercises.

Plyometrics is a rapid, dynamic movement first capitalizing on the eccentric (lengthening) phase of a muscle, then followed by the concentric (shortening) phase. High-intensity plyometrics are thought to increase muscle power and may be an important component in reducing ACL injuries. They should be done more than once

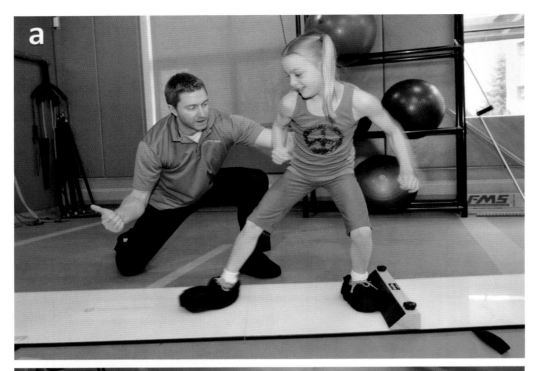

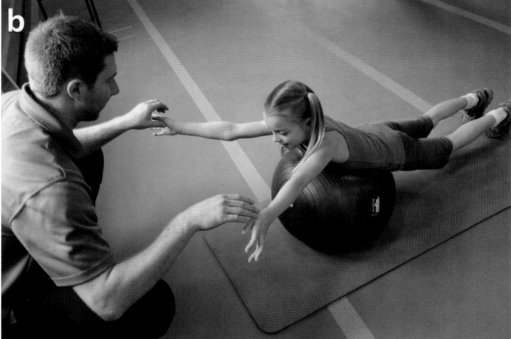

FIGURE 2-5

a) Training targeting improving hip muscle strength by using a slide board. b) Training for peri scapular and upper trunk muscles, and core muscle strength and stabilization.

per week for at least 6 weeks. Athletes should focus on proper technique, including landing on the balls of the foot with knees flexed and the chest upright in line with the knees.

Balance training often incorporates use of wobble, balance boards or the Bosu ball. Sport-specific dynamic exercises may include throwing a ball to a partner while balancing on one leg, on either dry land or more challenging surfaces.

Strength and stability exercises each include both dynamic exercises and closed chain exercises, such as jump landing training on a single leg and subsequently holding that position.

Many teams are adopting these exercises and incorporating them into their warm-up, during practices and competition. An example is a 15-minute prevention program integrated into warm-up of physical education class for second graders (age 7 years) 2 times a week. Ideally, these programs would be implemented before the season for the sport has begun.

Contemporary research details that athletes adhered to the interventions; nearly 90% of athletes performed more than two-thirds of the assigned neuromuscular training exercises. However, coaches had a harder time adhering. Coaches at the high school level were better than those at the middle school level. Unfortunately, earlier interventions, such as those attempted at the middle school level, may be the most important, because of the age of occurrence of ACL injuries, but also the hardest to perform.

TAKE-HOME POINTS

▶ Anterior cruciate ligament (ACL) injuries are becoming increasingly common among young athletes.

▶ These injuries can have devastating and lifelong consequences.

▶ Prevention of ACL injury should be an essential part of sport participation for all young athletes.

Bone Health and Energy Deficiency

Case 8
Bone health and young athletes— early recognition

Description

A 17-year-old female cross-country runner presents with persistent right lower leg pain. She has a history of a distal tibial stress fracture, which ended her junior year of track prematurely. She is currently reporting more proximal tibia pain that starts hurting 30 minutes into track practice and aches even when she is not running. She has been able to return to running after periods of rest. Despite previous interventions, her pain has not improved. She is a vegan.

The pediatrician determines that she has amenorrhea. Her estradiol is very low at intake, and she has stopped having her menstrual cycle. In addition, she is a vegan, raising concern for an eating disorder.

The patient is hospitalized for an eating disorder and afterward continues to see a therapist, nutritionist, and her primary care physician for follow-up treatment. Her coach was also included in the treatment process. As time passed from her inpatient treatment course, her estradiol level increased. She eventually restarted her menstrual cycle, roughly 9 months after inpatient treatment, and was able to integrate more weight-bearing exercise and running into her lifestyle again. Her path to recovery was a long one, and she had periods of regression.

Workup and Management

Stress fractures rarely occur in isolation. There are often metabolic abnormalities, past injuries, misdiagnoses, or nutritional deficiencies concurrent with the diagnosis. In 1992, an association was made between disordered eating, amenorrhea, and osteoporosis, and the association became recognized as the female athlete triad. This association has become more refined since 1992, with a position statement in both 2007 and 2014. The 2007 position statement extrapolated on findings that undernutrition or low energy availability impairs reproductive and skeletal health (Figure 2-6). Disordered eating, calorie restriction, or increased caloric expenditure occurs more often with conditions that emphasize leanness (performing arts, endurance events, or weight-class sports, to name a few). When energy put into the body does not meet the needs of the body for reproduction, amenorrhea or eumenorrhea results. Patients with amenorrhea or eumenorrhea, on average, have lower bone mineral densities. Menstrual irregularities and low bone mineral density (BMD) increase the risk of fracture. Even subtle menstrual changes (a delay in menarche, a history of oligomenorrhea [cycle >35 days], and amenorrhea [no cycle for 90 days] with or without low BMD) were significant risk factors for stress fractures and bone stress injury in athletes.

Frequency of all components of the triad (low BMD, low energy availability, and menstrual dysfunction) varies from 1.0% to 1.2% of high school girls with all 3 components to 70.0% of female college athletes with one component. Risk factors include "early age at sport specialization, family dysfunction, abuse and dieting." The triad is thought to be more common in players of sports emphasizing leanness or endurance, including, but not limited to, diving, volleyball, wrestling, light-weight rowing, gymnastics, dance, figure skating, cheerleading, long- and middle-distance running, and pole vaulting.

Preserving eumenorrhea and endogenous estrogen production inhibits bone reabsorption and assists in production of bone-stimulating hormones cortisol and leptin to form new bone. Estrogen deficiency is not the only contributor to abnormal bone remodeling. Abnormal pulsatility of gonadotropin-releasing hormone affects pulsatility of it and luteinizing hormone is suppressed; other hormone levels, including insulin, triiodothyronine, and insulinlike growth factor 1, may also decrease. Osteoporosis in adulthood may be caused by not accumulating optimal BMD in childhood and adolescence.

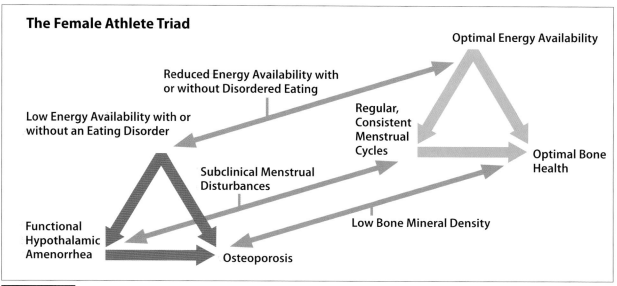

FIGURE 2-6

The continuum of the female athlete triad. As patients move toward health, they optimize their energy availability to meet total energy expenditure for reproductive and bone health needs. As energy availability decreases with or without disordered eating, bone mineral density decreases, as does menstrual regularity.

From Nattiv A, Loucks AB, Manore MM, Sanborn CF, Sundgot-Borgen J, Warren MP. American College of Sports Medicine position stand. The female athlete triad. *Med Sci Sports Exerc.* 2007;39(10):1868. Reproduced with permission.

The International Society for Clinical Densitometry recommended expressing BMD in Z scores. Z scores match individuals by age and sex to controls. An individual with a Z score less than −2.0 is considered to have "low bone mineral density" and a higher risk for fracture. Osteoporosis should be diagnosed only in these younger, athletic, and premenopausal populations when low BMD is associated with secondary risk factors (Nattiv). Secondary risk factors for low BMD are "chronic malnutrition, eating disorders, hypogonadism, glucocorticoid exposure, and previous fractures." Athletes in weight-bearing sports usually have 5% to 15% higher BMD than nonathletes. Therefore, a Z score less than −1.0 indicates low BMD in a weight-bearing athlete and is concerning for increased risk of fragility fracture. Stress fractures are 2 to 4 times more frequent in amenorrheic athletes.

The cause of the amenorrhea is important to deduce. Sustained low energy results in many health risks and poorer sport performance.

Hypoestrogenism can lead to musculoskeletal injuries as well as increased total cholesterol and low-density lipoprotein cholesterol levels. Endothelial dysfunction can negatively affect vasodilation of arteries in the heart, decreasing blood flow to muscles and impairing their productivity. Endothelial dysfunction and increased cholesterol level have been documented in amenorrheic athletes more so than eumenorrheic athletes, as frequently as 64% in professional dancers. Interestingly, folic acid was shown to correlate with improvements in brachial artery flow-mediated dilation.

If an eating disorder is diagnosed, treatment is paramount. The "prognosis for anorexia nervosa is grave with a six-fold increase in standard mortality rates compared to the public" (Nattiv). Disordered eating is extremely common in female athletes, especially in sports for which leanness is emphasized. With early sport specialization, there is an increased risk for early dieting, injury, stress, anxiety, and sudden increase in training volume, all of which have been thought to contribute to disordered eating behaviors. Inpatient and partial hospital programs have been offered to assist in treatment for eating disorders.

To change the trend, weight gain is found to improve BMD better than oral contraceptive pills. Increasing energy input can be achieved with high exercise loads. Pediatric and adolescent athletes should be given special attention to maximize bone mineral accrual by emphasizing nutritional requirements for their age, including calcium, vitamin D, and iron. Patients who experience primary amenorrhea or secondary amenorrhea should warrant a workup for causes, with importance placed on treatment. The younger the athlete, the more family involvement is helpful, along with nutritional counseling, psychotherapy, and coaches following medical recommendations for return to play. "By the end of adolescence, almost 90% of adult bone mass has been obtained"; therefore, prevention and early intervention are extremely important (Weiss Kelly).

Adolescent boys have demonstrated low BMD as well as low testosterone and estradiol levels. They were also found to have improvement of vascular function with folic acid supplementation. Bone health and bone remodeling are regulated by hormones including, but not limited to, parathyroid hormone, 1,25-dihydroxyvitamin D, insulinlike growth factor 1, and calcitonin. A controversial new syndrome called relative energy deficiency in sport is emerging (Figure 2-7). The concept includes that male athletes also have bone stress injuries if they are undernourished. The idea includes other systems of the body that are also affected by low energy availability, such as metabolism, the immune system, and psychological effects, to name a few.

Optimizing calcium and vitamin D intake of young athletes is important to decrease the risk of stress fractures. "Significantly more athletes with stress fractures have low calcium intakes than do athletes without stress fractures" was reported in 2016 (Weiss Kelly). The AAP recommends 1,300 mg of calcium daily for children

and youths aged 9 to 18 years. Calcium is better absorbed in smaller amounts (500 mg) 3 times a day. Routine calcium supplementation is not recommended for healthy children, secondary to decreased bioavailability of calcium from supplements. However, it is recommended to increase dietary intake to meet daily requirements. Milk has come in and out of favor over the years, but it is still estimated that 70% to 80% of dietary calcium intake comes from milk.

A glass of 237 mL (8 oz) of milk provides 300 mg of calcium, and skim milk contains no fat and only 80 kcal. Despite milk's benefits, only 14.9% of high school students drank 3 or more 8-oz servings of milk daily, with only 9.3% of girls (the high-risk population) drinking their serving amount. Other good sources of calcium are yogurt, natural cheese, green leafy vegetables, legumes, nuts, calcium-fortified breakfast cereals, and fruit juices (Table 2-5). Calcium supplementation is preferred through dietary changes.

Vitamin D is a fat-soluble vitamin, important for absorption of calcium and bone health. The AAP also recommends intake of 600 IU vitamin D daily for children and youths aged 1 to 18 years (Table 2-6). Other sources cite higher intake recommendations to maintain a goal 25-hydroxyvitamin D level between 32 and 50 ng/mL in athletes. One study reported vitamin D related most closely, over calcium or dietary intake, with reduced risk of stress fractures in 6,712 physically active female athletes. Dietary sources of vitamin D include cod liver oil, mushrooms, fatty fish (salmon, sardines, and tuna), fortified foods, formula, juices, and milk.

One article in *Pediatrics* reported, "bone mass attained in early life is thought to be the most important modifiable determinant of lifelong skeletal health" (Golden). Adolescent years, when patients are maturing and girls are starting their menstrual cycle, are responsible for 40% to 60% of adult bone mass accrual. The age of peak bone mass density lags behind peak height achievement by 6 to 12 months in both boys and girls. This period

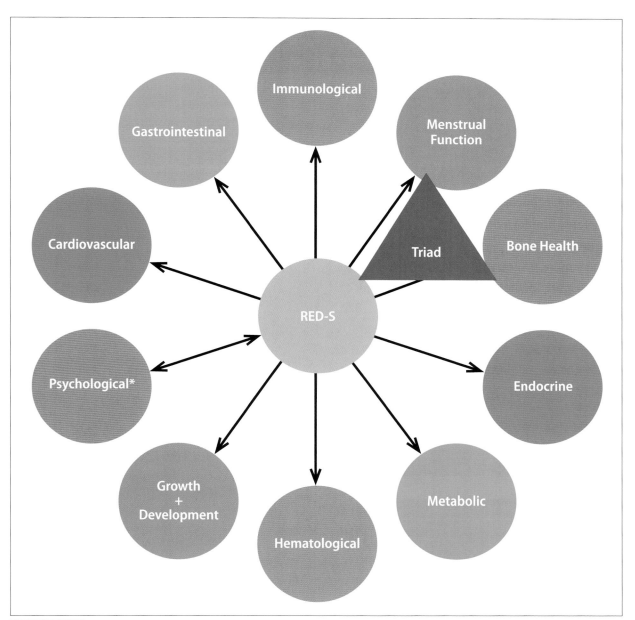

FIGURE 2-7

Health consequences of relative energy deficiency in sport showing an expanded concept of the female athlete triad (*psychological consequences can either precede relative energy deficiency in sport or be the result).

From Mountjoy M, Sundgot-Borgen J, Burke L, et al. The IOC consensus statement: beyond the female athlete triad—relative energy deficiency in sport (RED-S). *Br J Sports Med.* 2014;48(7):491–497.

Table 2-5. Dietary Sources of Calcium

Food	Serving Size	Calories per Portion	Calcium Content (mg)
Dairy Foods			
Milk			
Whole milk	8 oz.	149	276
Reduced-fat milk (2%)	8 oz.	122	293
Low-fat milk (1%)	8 oz.	102	305
Skim milk (nonfat)	8 oz.	83	299
Reduced-fat chocolate milk (2%)	8 oz.	190	275
Low-fat chocolate milk (1%)	8 oz.	158	290
Yogurt			
Plain yogurt, low-fat	8 oz.	143	415
Fruit yogurt, low-fat	8 oz.	232	345
Plain yogurt, nonfat	8 oz.	127	452
Cheese			
Romano cheese	1.5 oz.	165	452
Swiss cheese	1.5 oz.	162	336
Pasteurized processed American cheese	2 oz.	187	323
Mozzarella cheese, part skim	1.5 oz.	128	311
Cheddar cheese	1.5 oz.	171	307
Muenster cheese	1.5 oz.	156	305
Nondairy Foods			
Salmon	3 oz.	76	32
Sardines, canned	3 oz.	177	325
White beans, cooked	1 cup	307	191
Broccoli, cooked	1 cup	44	72
Broccoli, raw	1 cup	25	42
Collards, cooked	1 cup	49	226
Spinach, cooked	1 cup	41	249
Spinach, raw	1 cup	7	30
Baked beans, canned	1 cup	680	120
Tomatoes, canned	1 cup	71	84
Calcium-Fortified Food			
Orange juice	8 oz.	117	500
Breakfast cereals	1 cup	100–210	250–1000
Tofu, made with calcium	0.5 cup	94	434
Soy milk, calcium fortified[a]	8 oz.	104	299

[a] Not all soy beverages are fortified to this level.

From Golden NH, Abrams SA; American Academy of Pediatrics Committee on Nutrition. Optimizing bone health in children and adolescents. *Pediatrics.* 2014;143(4):e1229–e1243. Reproduced with permission.

Table 2-6. Daily Upper Limits of Vitamin D Intake for Young Athletes

Age	Maximum Vitamin D Intake Recommended (IU)
Infants <6 mo	1,000
Infants 6–12 mo	1,500
Children 1–3 y	2,500
Children 4–8 y	3,000
Children and youths 9–18 y	4,000

Adapted from Golden NH, Abrams SA; American Academy of Pediatrics Committee on Nutrition. Optimizing bone health in children and adolescents. *Pediatrics.* 2014;134(4):e1229–e1243, with permission.

of 6 to 12 months may be time of "increased vulnerability to bone fragility" and may contribute to frequency of fractures in boys aged 10 to 14 years and girls 8 to 12 years (Golden). Weight-bearing activities are preferable, over biking or swimming, to optimize bone health. Even non–weight-bearing activities are preferred, over a sedentary lifestyle, because lean-muscle mass is bone protective as well. For adult athletes, obesity, smoking, caffeine intake, and alcohol intake are all associated with reduced BMD.

Iron intake has been linked to low BMD. Among rats, bone reformation rate and resorption by osteoclast was significantly decreased in groups who were given an iron-deficient diet. The iron-deprived rats also had reduced bone mineral content, hemoglobin level, and hematocrit, in addition to low BMD. Similar findings have been found in human subjects, particularly females. Females are more likely to have anemia than males. Stress fractures have been linked to men and women in the military. However, a recent study focusing on anemia found female participants who sustained a stress fracture have significantly lower levels of serum iron and iron saturation. High incidence of anemia and iron deficiency was found among the female participants who sustained a stress fracture. Iron requirements for endurance athletes are increased by nearly 70%, and iron deficiency is very common in the endurance athlete population. Iron treatment has been found to reverse the diagnosis of anemia or low

serum ferritin level and improved maximum oxygen consumption of endurance athletes.

Special populations of athletes who prefer a vegetarian or vegan diet are at a greater risk of low energy intake and decreased macronutrients. Particularly, amounts of iron, calcium, vitamin D, riboflavin, zinc, and vitamin B_{12} can be low in these diets, and recommendations of a sports nutritionist are advised to avoid metabolic abnormalities in these adolescents. Vegetarian diets can typically provide good protein quality, if eating a variety of foods and an adequate amount (10% more than non-vegetarian diets). The greatest concern for these diets is the risk of iron deficiency. Vegan diets are more concerning for protein deficiency than vegetarian diets, and there are additional concerns of limited lysine, threonine, tryptophan, or methionine intake. Switching to a vegetarian or vegan diet may be a way of restricting energy intake or disordered eating, and it should capture the attention of practitioners.

B vitamins and folate are important for the production of red blood cells, and severe energy deficiencies in either vitamin B_{12} or folate may result in anemia and reduced endurance performance. Antioxidants and vitamin E may play a role in reducing inflammation and muscle soreness during recovery. Other performance-related minerals are zinc and magnesium. Studies have shown both to be involved in processes that contribute to performance and strength.

Other causes of metabolic abnormalities may be explained by endocrinopathies or disease. Osteogenesis imperfecta, idiopathic juvenile osteoporosis, Turner syndrome, cerebral palsy, connective tissue disorders, and conditions for which children are treated with corticosteroids are related to severe deficiencies in bone mass. Corticosteroid exposure or chemotherapeutic treatments are possible causes of low BMD. Thyroid dysfunction, hyperprolactinemia, primary ovarian insufficiency, hypothalamic and pituitary disorders (genetic or acquired), and hyperandrogenic conditions, including polycystic ovarian syndrome, tumors, and Cushing syndrome, are also associated with amenorrhea and therefore reduced bone health.

TAKE-HOME POINTS

▶ The importance of bone health is paramount to developing better bone mineral density and decreasing the risk of osteopenia and osteoporosis later in life.

▶ Identifying disordered eating early and intervening may be lifesaving.

▶ Calcium, vitamin D, iron, and other bone-aiding minerals should be asked about during pediatric history taking to ensure adequate diets and behaviors.

▶ Disordered eating is shockingly high among female athletes (about 1 out of 5) and among up to 70% of dancers.

Summary

In conclusion, pediatricians and health care providers who care for young athletes have a challenging and yet rewarding task at hand. The goal to increase athletic participation in a safe and healthy way is a difficult one. As the population becomes more overweight and more specialized, recommendations from this chapter may be applied to assist in keeping young athletes involved and injury-free. (Box 2-6)

Box 2-6
Actions Pediatricians Can Take to Reduce the Risk for Injury in Youth Sports

- Encourage general health maintenance and fitness year-round

- Suggest temporary reductions or restructuring in training load to allow for more adequate rest between training sessions during vulnerable periods of growth

- Educate young women athletes and their parents about neuromuscular training programs to reduce anterior cruciate ligament and other lower extremity injuries

- Encourage participation in neuromuscular training programs aimed at building hip and core strength especially for young prepubescent girl athletes (optimally before signs of injury)

- Encourage proper sleep hygiene including maximizing sleep quantity and quality each night

- Encourage plenty of time for free play, "cross training," and sport diversity early in childhood (delaying specialization in a single sport until late adolescence)

- Encourage proper sport-specific gear use and fit

- Enforce early recognition of sport-related concussion and removal from competition until medical evaluation, treatment, and clearance for return to sport criteria have been met

- Educate young athletes about the symptoms of concussions and encourage them to report symptoms promptly to coaches, trainers, and parents

- Support and advocate for policies that promote fair play and rule enforcement as well as youth sports schedules that do not compromise sleep

From Stracciolini A, Sugimoto D, Howell DR. Injury prevention in youth sports. *Pediatr Ann.* 2017;46(3):e99–e105. Reproduced with permission.

Bibliography

Ackerman KE, Davis B, Jacoby L, Misra M. DXA surrogates for visceral fat are inversely associated with bone density measures in adolescent athletes with menstrual dysfunction. *J Pediatr Endocrinol Metab*. 2011;24(7-8):497–504

American Academy of Family Physicians, American Academy of Pediatrics, American College of Sports Medicine, American Medical Society for Sports Medicine, American Orthopaedic Society for Sports Medicine, American Osteopathic Academy of Sports Medicine. *Preparticipation Physical Evaluation*. 4th ed. Elk Grove Village, IL: American Academy of Pediatrics; 2010

American Academy of Pediatrics. Committees, councils and sections: council on sports medicine and fitness; patient education. American Academy of Pediatrics Web site. https://www.aap.org/en-us/about-the-aap/Committees-Councils-Sections/Council-on-sports-medicine-and-fitness/Pages/Patient-Education.aspx. Accessed June 30, 2017

American Academy of Pediatrics. Safety & prevention: at play. HealthyChildren.org Web site. https://www.healthychildren.org/english/safety-prevention/at-play/pages/default.aspx. Accessed June 30, 2017

American Dietetic Association, Dietitians of Canada, American College of Sports Medicine. Nutrition and athletic performance. *Med Sci Sports Exerc*. 2009;41(3):709–731

Armstrong LE, Casa DJ, Millard-Stafford M, Moran DS, Pyne SW, Roberts WO. American College of Sports Medicine position stand: exertional heat illness during training and competition. *Med Sci Sports Exerc*. 2007;39(3):556–572

Bahr R, Holme I. Risk factors for sports injuries—a methodological approach. *Br J Sports Med*. 2003;37(5):384–392

Baren JM, Rothrock SG, Brennan JA, Brown L, eds. *Pediatric Emergency Medicine*. Philadelphia, PA: Saunders Elsevier; 2008:992

Bergeron MF. Exertional heat cramps: recovery and return to play. *J Sport Rehabil*. 2007;16(3):190–196

Boden BP, Dean GS, Feagin JA Jr, Garrett WE Jr. Mechanisms of anterior cruciate ligament injury. *Orthopedics*. 2000;23(6):573–578

Bouchama A, Knochel JP. Heat stroke. *N Engl J Med*. 2002;346(25):1978–1988

Brenner JS; American Academy of Pediatrics Council on Sports Medicine and Fitness. Sports specialization and intensive training in young athletes. *Pediatrics*. 2016:138(3):e20162148

Bross MH, Nash BT Jr, Carlton FB Jr. Heat emergencies. *Am Fam Physician*. 1994;50(2):389–396

Burden RJ, Morton K, Richards T, Whyte GP, Pedlar CR. Is iron treatment beneficial in, iron-deficient but non-anaemic (IDNA) endurance athletes? A systematic review and meta-analysis. *Br J Sports Med*. 2015;49(21):1389–1397

Bytomski JR, Squire DL. Heat illness in children. *Curr Sports Med Rep*. 2003;2(6):320–324

Casa DJ, Becker SM, Ganio MS, et al. Validity of devices that assess body temperature during outdoor exercise in the heat. *J Athl Train*. 2007;42(3):333–342

Casa DJ, Csillan D; Inter-Association Task Force for Preseason Secondary School Athletics Participants. Preseason heat-acclimatization guidelines for secondary school athletics. *J Athl Train*. 2009;44(3):332–333

Casa DJ, Kenny GP, Taylor NA. Immersion treatment for exertional hyperthermia: cold or temperate water? *Med Sci Sports Exerc*. 2010;42(7):1246–1252

Casa DJ, McDermott BP, Lee EC, Yeargin SW, Armstrong LE, Maresh CM. Cold water immersion: the gold standard for exertional heatstroke treatment. *Exerc Sport Sci Rev*. 2007;35(3):141–149

Centers for Disease Control and Prevention (CDC). Heat illness among high school athletes—United States, 2005-2009. *MMWR Morb Mortal Wkly Rep*. 2010;59(32):1009–1013

Centers for Disease Control and Prevention, National Center for Injury Prevention and Control, Division of Unintentional Injury Prevention. Heads Up to youth sports. CDC Heads Up Web site. https://www.cdc.gov/headsup/youthsports. Updated February 1, 2017. Accessed June 30, 2017

Corwin DJ, Zonfrillo MR, Master CL, et al. Characteristics of prolonged concussion recovery in a pediatric subspecialty referral population. *J Pediatr*. 2014;165(6):1207–1215

Côté J, Lidor R, Hackfort D. ISSP position stand: to sample or to specialize? Seven postulates about youth sport activities that lead to continued participation and elite performance. *Int J Sport Exerc Psychol*. 2009;7(1):7–17

De Souza MJ, Nattiv A, Joy E, et al; Expert Panel. 2014 female athlete triad coalition consensus statement on treatment and return to play of the female athlete triad: 1st International Conference held in San Francisco, California, May 2012 and 2nd International Conference held in Indianapolis, Indiana, May 2013. *Br J Sports Med*. 2014;48(4):289

De Souza MJ, Williams NI, Nattiv A, et al. Misunderstanding the female athlete triad: refuting the IOC consensus statement on relative energy deficiency in sport (RED-S). *Br J Sports Med*. 2014;48(20):1461–1465

d'Hemecourt PA, Gould LE, Bottino NM. Spondylolysis. In: Stein CJ, Stracciolini A, Ackerman KE, eds. *Contemporary Pediatric and Adolescent Sports Medicine: The Young Female Athlete*. Cham, Switzerland: Springer International Publishing Switzerland; 2016:87–99

DiFiori JP, Benjamin HJ, Brenner J, et al. Overuse injuries and burnout in youth sports: a position statement from the American Medical Society for Sports Medicine. *Clin J Sport Med*. 2014;24(1):3–20

DiFiori JP. Evaluation of overuse injuries in children and adolescents. *Curr Sports Med Rep*. 2010;9(6):372–378

Drezner JA, O'Connor FG, Harmon KG. AMSSM position statement on cardiovascular preparticipation screening in athletes: current evidence, knowledge gaps, recommendations, and future directions. *Clin J Sport Med.* 2016;26(5):347–361

Eckart RE, Shry EA, Burke AP, et al; Department of Defense Cardiovascular Death Registry Group. Sudden death in young adults: an autopsy-based series of a population undergoing active surveillance. *J Am Coll Cardiol.* 2011;58(12):1254–1261

Ellis MJ, Leiter J, Hall T, et al. Neuroimaging findings in pediatric sports-related concussion. *J Neurosurg Pediatr.* 2015;16(3):241–247

Faigenbaum AD, Myer GD, Farrell A, et al. Integrative neuromuscular training and sex-specific fitness performance in 7-year-old children: an exploratory investigation. *J Athl Train.* 2014;49(2):145–153

Finocchiaro G, Papadakis M, Robertus JL, et al. Etiology of sudden death in sports: insights from a United Kingdom regional registry. *J Am Coll Cardiol.* 2016;67(18):2108–2115

Fleisig GS, Andrews JR, Cutter GR, et al. Risk of serious injury for young baseball pitchers: a 10-year prospective study. *Am J Sports Med.* 2011;39(2):253–257

Fleisig GS, Andrews JR. Prevention of elbow injuries in youth baseball pitchers. *Sports Health.* 2012;4(5):419–424

Foley C, Gregory A, Solomon G. Young age as a modifying factor in sports concussion management: what is the evidence? *Curr Sports Med Rep.* 2014;13(6):390–394

Golden NH, Abrams SA; American Academy of Pediatrics Committee on Nutrition. Optimizing bone health in children and adolescents. *Pediatrics.* 2014;134(4):e1129–e1243

González-Alonso J, Mora-Rodríguez R, Below PR, Coyle EF. Dehydration markedly impairs cardiovascular function in hyperthermic endurance athletes during exercise. *J Appl Physiol.* 1997;82(4):1229–1236

Hainline B, Drezner JA, Baggish A, et al. Interassociation consensus statement on cardiovascular care of college student-athletes. *J Am Coll Cardiol.* 2016;67(25):2981–2995

Harmon KG, Asif IM, Maleszewski JJ, et al. Incidence, cause, and comparative frequency of sudden cardiac death in national collegiate athletic association athletes: a decade in review. *Circulation.* 2015;132(1):10–19

Harmon KG, Drezner JA, Wilson MG, Sharma S. Incidence of sudden cardiac death in athletes: a state-of-the-art review. *Br J Sports Med.* 2014;48(15):1185–1192

Hewett TE, Lindenfeld TN, Riccobene JV, Noyes FR. The effect of neuromuscular training on the incidence of knee injury in female athletes. A prospective study. *Am J Sports Med.* 1999;27(6):699–706

Huggins RA, Martschinske J, Applegate K, et al. Influence of hydration status on core body temperature changes during exercise in the heat: a meta-analysis. *Med Sci Sports Exerc.* In review

Jayanthi N, Pinkham C, Dugas L, Patrick B, Labella C. Sports specialization in young athletes: evidence-based recommendations. *Sports Health.* 2013;5(3):251–257

Jayanthi NA, LaBella CR, Fischer D, Pasulka J, Dugas LR. Sports-specialized intensive training and the risk of injury in young athletes: a clinical case-control study. *Am J Sports Med.* 2015;43(4):794–801

Katsumata S, Katsumata-Tsuboi R, Uehara M, Suzuki K. Severe iron deficiency decreases both bone formation and bone resorption in rats. *J Nutr.* 2009;139(2):238–243

Kurd MF, Patel D, Norton R, Picetti G, Friel B, Vaccaro AR. Nonoperative treatment of symptomatic spondylolysis. *J Spinal Disord Tech.* 2007;20(8):560–564

Lee YM, Wu A, Zuckerman SL, et al. Obesity and neurocognitive recovery after sports-related concussion in athletes: a match cohort study. *Phys Sportsmed.* 2016;44(3):217–222

Lee-Chiong TL Jr, Stitt JT. Heatstroke and other heat-related illnesses. The maladies of summer. *Postgrad Med.* 1995;98(1):26–36

Ljungqvist A, Jenoure P, Engebretsen L, et al. The International Olympic Committee (IOC) consensus statement on periodic health evaluation of elite athletes March 2009. *Br J Sports Med.* 2009;43(9):631–643

Malina RM. Early sport specialization: roots, effectiveness, risks. *Curr Sports Med Rep.* 2010;9(6):364–371

Malina RM. Physical activity and training: effects on stature and the adolescent growth spurt. *Med Sci Sports Exerc.* 1994;26(6):759–766

Mandelbaum BR, Silvers HJ, Watanabe DS, et al. Effectiveness of a neuromuscular and proprioceptive training program in preventing anterior cruciate ligament injuries in female athletes: 2-year follow-up. *Am J Sports Med.* 2005;33(7):1003–1010

Mannix R, Berkner J, Mei Z, et al. Adolescent mice demonstrate a distinct pattern of injury after repetitive mild traumatic brain injury. *J Neurotrauma.* 2017;34(2):495–504

Maron BJ, Doerer JJ, Haas TS, Tierney DM, Mueller FO. Sudden deaths in young competitive athletes: analysis of 1866 deaths in the United States, 1980-2006. *Circulation.* 2009;119(8):1085–1092

Maron BJ, Friedman RA, Kligfield P, et al. Assessment of the 12-lead electrocardiogram as a screening test for detection of cardiovascular disease in healthy general populations of young people (12-25 years of age): a scientific statement from the American Heart Association and the American College of Cardiology. *J Am Coll Cardiol.* 2014;64(14):1479–1514

Maron BJ, Haas TS, Murphy CJ, Ahluwalia A, Rutten-Ramos S. Incidence and causes of sudden death in U.S. college athletes. *J Am Coll Cardiol.* 2014;63(16):1636–1643

Maron BJ, Levine BD, Washington RL, Baggish AL, Kovacs RJ, Maron MS. Eligibility and disqualification recommendations for competitive athletes with cardiovascular abnormalities: task force 2; preparticipation screening for cardiovascular disease in competitive athletes: a scientific statement from the American Heart Association and American College of Cardiology. *J Am Coll Cardiol.* 2015;66(21):2356–2361

Maron BJ, Thompson PD, Ackerman MJ, et al. Recommendations and considerations related to preparticipation screening for cardiovascular abnormalities in competitive athletes: 2007 update; a scientific statement from the American Heart Association Council on Nutrition, Physical Activity, and Metabolism: endorsed by the American College of Cardiology Foundation. *Circulation.* 2007;115(12):1643–1655

Maron BJ. Sudden death in young athletes. *N Engl J Med.* 2003;349(11):1064–1075

McDermott BP, Casa DJ, Ganio MS, et al. Acute whole-body cooling for exercise-induced hyperthermia: a systematic review. *J Athl Train.* 2009;44(1):84–93

McLendon LA, Kralik SF, Grayson PA, Golomb MR. The controversial second impact syndrome: a review of the literature. *Pediatr Neurol.* 2016;62:9–17

Merkel DG, Moran DS, Yanovich R, et al. The association between hematological and inflammatory factors and stress fractures among female military recruits. *Med Sci Sports Exerc.* 2008;40(11)(suppl):S691–S697

Micheli LJ, Wood R. Back pain in youth athletes. Significant difference from adults in causes and patterns. *Arch Pediatr Adolesc Med.* 1995;149(1):15–18

Mountjoy M, Sundgot-Borgen J, Burke L, et al. The IOC consensus statement: beyond the female athlete triad—relative energy deficiency in sport (RED-S). *Br J Sports Med.* 2014;48(7):491–497

Mueller FO, Cantu RC. *Catastrophic Sports Injury Research: Twenty-sixth Annual Report.* University of North Carolina at Chapel Hill; 2008

Murphy M, McCutcheon BA, Kerezoudis P, et al. 199 multiple concussions in young athletes: identifying patients at risk for repeat injury. *Neurosurgery.* 2016;63(suppl 1):178

Myer GD, Jayanthi N, DiFiori JP, et al. Sports specialization, part II: alternative solutions to early sports specialization in youth athletes. *Sports Health.* 2016;8(1):65–73

Myer GD, Sugimoto D, Thomas S, Hewett TE. The influence of age on the effectiveness of neuromuscular training to reduce anterior cruciate ligament injury in female athletes: a meta-analysis. *Am J Sports Med.* 2013;41(1):203–215

National Collegiate Athletic Association. Estimated probability of competing in athletics beyond the high school interscholastic level. NCAA Web site. http://www.ncaa.org about/resources/research/probability-competing-beyond-high-school. Accessed July 17, 2017

National Council of Youth Sports. *Report on Trends and Participation in Organized Youth Sports.* Stuart, FL: National Council of Youth Sports; 2008. http://www.ncys.org/pdfs/2008/2008-ncys-market-research-report.pdf. Accessed July 2, 2017

Nattiv A, Loucks AB, Manore MM, Sanborn CF, Sundgot-Borgen J, Warren MP. American College of Sports Medicine position stand. The female athlete triad. *Med Sci Sports Exerc.* 2007;39(10):1867–1882

Naughton GA, Carlson JS. Reducing the risk of heat-related decrements to physical activity in young people. *J Sci Med Sport.* 2008;11(1):58–65

Ono KE, Burns TG, Bearden DJ, McManus SM, King H, Reisner A. Sex-based differences as a predictor of recovery trajectories in young athletes after a sports-related concussion. *Am J Sports Med.* 2016;44(3):748–752

Papa L, Ramia MM, Edwards D, Johnson BD, Slobounov SM. Systematic review of clinical studies examining biomarkers of brain injury in athletes after sports-related concussion. *J Neurotrauma.* 2015;32(10):661–673

Pringle RG, McNair P, Stanley S. Incidence of sporting injury in New Zealand youths aged 6-15 years. *Br J Sports Med.* 1998;32(1):49–52

Proffen BL, Murray MM. ACL injuries in the female athlete. In: Stein CJ, Stracciolini A, Ackerman KE, eds. *Contemporary Pediatric and Adolescent Sports Medicine: The Young Female Athlete.* Cham, Switzerland: Springer International Publishing Switzerland; 2016:121–133

Radcliff KE, Kalantar SB, Reitman CA. Surgical management of spondylolysis and spondylolisthesis in athletes: indications and return to play. *Curr Sports Med Rep.* 2009;8(1):35–40

Roberts WO. Determining a "do not start" temperature for a marathon on the basis of adverse outcomes. *Med Sci Sports Exerc.* 2010;42(2):226–232

Rose MS, Emery CA, Meeuwisse WH. Sociodemographic predictors of sport injury in adolescents. *Med Sci Sports Exerc.* 2008;40(3):444–450

Rowland T. Thermoregulation during exercise in the heat in children: old concepts revisited. *J Appl Physiol (1985).* 2008;105(2):718–724

Saifuddin A, White J, Tucker S, Taylor BA. Orientation of lumbar pars defects: implications for radiological detection and surgical management. *J Bone Joint Surg Br.* 1998;80(2):208–211

Schneider KJ, Iverson GL, Emery CA, McCrory P, Herring SA, Meeuwisse WH. The effects of rest and treatment following sport-related concussion: a systematic review of literature. *Br J Sports Med.* 2013;47(5):304–307

Seto CK, Way D, O'Connor N. Environmental illness in athletes. *Clin Sports Med.* 2005;24(3):695–718, x

Simon HB. Hyperthermia. *N Engl J Med.* 1993;329(7):483–487

Sone JY, Kondziolka D, Huang JH, Samadani U. Helmet efficacy against concussion and traumatic brain injury: a review. *J Neurosurg*. 2017;126(3):768–781

Sonneville KR, Gordon CM, Kocher MS, Pierce LM, Ramappa A, Field AE. Vitamin D, calcium, and dairy intakes and stress fractures among female adolescents. *Arch Pediatr Adolesc Med*. 2012;166(7):595–600

Sport for Life Society. Physical literacy. Physical Literacy for Life Web site. http://physicalliteracy.ca/physical-literacy. Accessed June 30, 2017

Stein CJ, MacDougall R, Quatman-Yates CC, et al. Young athletes' concerns about sport-related concussion: the patient's perspective. *Clin J Sports Med*. 2016;26(5):386–390

Stracciolini A, Sugimoto D, Howell DR. Injury prevention in youth sports. *Pediatr Ann*. 2017;46(3):e99–e105

Sugimoto D, Mattacola CG, Bush HM, et al. Preventive neuromuscular training for young female athletes: comparison of coach and athlete compliance rates. *J Athl Train*. 2017;52(1):58–64

US Department of Health and Human Services. *2008 Physical Activity Guidelines of Americans*. Washington, DC: Office of Disease Prevention and Health Promotion; 2008. ODPHP publication U0036. https://health.gov/paguidelines/pdf/paguide.pdf. Published October 2008. Accessed June 30, 2017

Van Camp SP, Bloor CM, Mueller FO, Cantu RC, Olson HG. Nontraumatic sports death in high school and college athletes. *Med Sci Sports Exerc*. 1995;27(5):641–647

Wegmann M, Faude O, Poppendieck W, Hecksteden A, Fröhlich M, Meyer T. Pre-cooling and sports performance: a meta-analytical review. *Sports Med*. 2012;42(7):545–564

Weiss Kelly AK, Hecht S; American Academy of Pediatrics Council on Sports Medicine and Fitness. The female athlete triad. *Pediatrics*. 2016;138(2):e20160922

Part ➋
Injuries

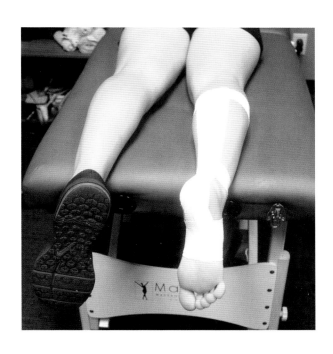

CHAPTER 3
Ankle and Foot Injuries in the Young Athlete

Joshua A. Metzl, MD

Anatomical Overview

1. Ankle

The distal tibia and fibula compose the roof of the ankle joint. The dome of the talus fits firmly into the distal tibia and fibula. The subtalar joint contains the anterior, middle, and posterior articulations between the talus and the calcaneus. They are separated laterally by the sinus tarsi and medially by the tarsal canal.

Several important ligamentous structures connect the bones of the ankle. The anterior talofibular ligament (ATFL) connects the talus and distal fibula anteriorly. The calcaneofibular ligament (CFL) connects the calcaneus and distal fibula directly inferior to the medial malleolus. The posterior talofibular ligament connects the talus and fibula posteriorly. The deltoid ligament, located on the medial side of the ankle, is a broad band of connective tissue that has 4 separate divisions that connect the distal tibia with the talus, calcaneus, and navicular bones. Figure 3-1 demonstrates this anatomy.

The muscles of the foot and ankle can be divided into those that originate above the ankle (extrinsic causes) and within the foot (intrinsic causes). The anterior (extensor) compartment of the leg includes the tibialis anterior, extensor hallucis longus, and extensor digitorum longus. The peroneus tertius inserts on the base of the fifth metatarsal bone and acts in a minor role in dorsiflexion and eversion of the foot. The lateral compartment of the leg contains the peroneus longus and peroneus brevis. The superficial posterior compartment of the leg contains the gastrocnemius and soleus complex, which inserts via the Achilles tendon into the posterior surface of the calcaneus. The deep posterior compartment of the leg contains the tibialis posterior, flexor digitorum longus, and flexor hallucis longus (FHL).

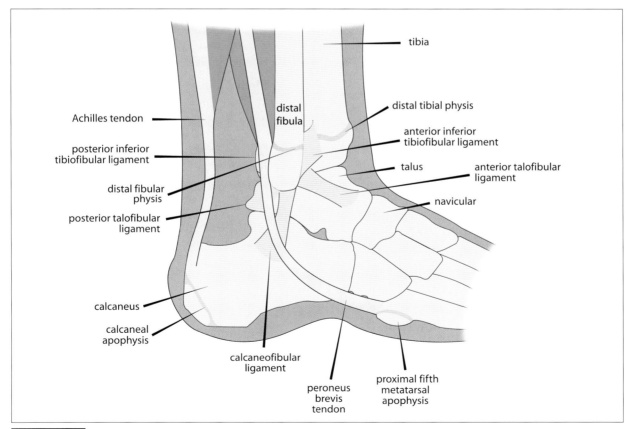

FIGURE 3-1

Lateral view of foot and ankle showing important anatomical landmarks.

The common peroneal and tibial nerves are the 2 major divisions of the sciatic nerve that branch just above the knee. The common peroneal nerve splits into superficial and deep branches just distal to the fibular head. The superficial branch provides sensation to the lateral aspect of the dorsum of the foot and innervates the peroneal muscles. The deep branch provides sensation to the interdigital space between the first and second toe and is responsible for dorsiflexing the ankle and toes.

The dorsalis pedis artery is a continuation of the anterior tibial artery that crosses the anterior joint line of the ankle, just deep to the extensor hallucis longus. As the artery proceeds down the long axis of the foot to the proximal first intermetatarsal space, it divides into a deep plantar artery and an arcuate artery that sends off branches to each of the toes.

2. Foot

The foot is best described in 3 functional parts: the hindfoot, midfoot, and forefoot. The hindfoot, which consists of the talus and the calcaneus, connects to the midfoot at the midtarsal (Chopart) joint. The midfoot contains the navicular, the cuboid, and the 3 cuneiform bones; it connects to the forefoot at the Lisfranc joint. The forefoot comprises everything distal of the Lisfranc joint, including the metatarsals, sesamoids, and pha-langes. The foot has 4 joints: the ankle (mortise), subtalar (talocalcaneal), midtarsal (Chopart), and midfoot (Lisfranc). The talonavicular and calca-neocuboid articulations compose the midtarsal joint and divide the hindfoot from the midfoot. The midfoot, or Lisfranc, joint is the articulation between the cuneiform bones and the proximal second metatarsal. Lastly, the plantar fascia is the primary aponeurosis that originates on the plantar aspect of the calcaneus and fans out to attach to the base of each of the 5 metatarsal heads.

Physical Examination

Please view video clip: "Physical Examination of the Ankle and Foot."

1. Ankle
- **Mechanism of injury:** inversion, eversion, or axial-load injury
- **Patient presentation**
  - **Gait**
  - **Visible swelling, discoloration, or deformity**
- **Palpation of important landmarks**
  - **Lateral ankle**
    1. Fibular head
    2. Fibular shaft
    3. Distal fibular physis
    4. Anterior talofibular ligament
    5. Calcaneofibular ligament
    6. Posterior talofibular ligament
    7. Syndesmosis ligament
    8. Proximal fifth metatarsal
  - **Medial ankle**
    1. Tibial physis
    2. Deltoid ligament
- **Strength testing**
  - **Inversion**
  - **Eversion**
- **Special tests**
  - **Ligamentous stability**
    1. Anterior drawer test (ATFL laxity)
    2. Talar tilt test (CFL laxity)

2. Foot
- **Mechanism of injury**
- **Identification of foot type:** cavus, pronated, or pes planus
- **Palpation of calcaneal apophysis:** patients younger than 13 years
- **Identification of specific injury sites**

Radiographs

Please view video clip:
"Radiographic Evaluation of the Ankle."

1. Ankle

The anteroposterior (AP), lateral, and mortise views (figures 3-2–3-4) are the radiographic views that can give the most information about the most common ankle injuries.

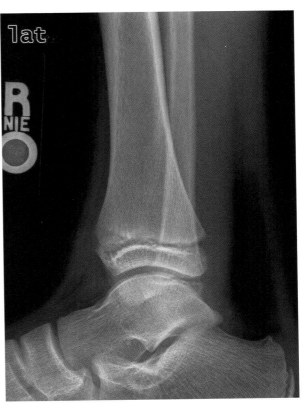

FIGURE 3-3
Lateral view of ankle.

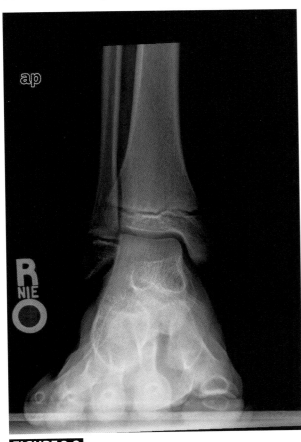

FIGURE 3-2
AP view of ankle.

Abbreviation: AP, anteroposterior.

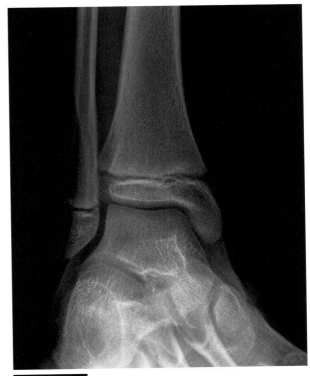

FIGURE 3-4
Mortise view of ankle.

Please view video clip:
"Radiographic Evaluation of
the Foot."

2. Foot

The common radiographic views for most
foot injuries are AP, lateral, and oblique views
(figures 3-5–3-7).

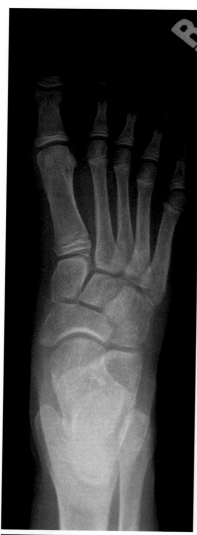

FIGURE 3-5
AP view of foot.

Abbreviation: AP, anteroposterior.

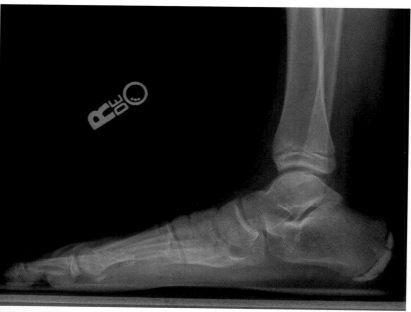

FIGURE 3-6
Lateral view of foot.

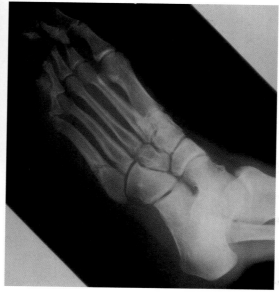

FIGURE 3-7
Oblique view of foot.

Case Files: Ankle and Foot Injuries

1. Acute Trauma

Case 1

Inversion injury with anterior talofibular ligament sprain in 17-year-old basketball player

Description

A 17-year-old basketball player comes into the office after "rolling" her ankle. Inversion injury, rolling inward of the ankle, is by far the most common mechanism with ankle injury, and it generally results in a lateral injury to the foot or ankle. As is mentioned in the Physical Examination section, examination of the lateral ankle is essential with this type of mechanism.

Please view video clip:
"Case 1: Inversion Injury to the Ankle With Closed Physis."

Ankle injuries are among the most common injuries that present to primary care offices and emergency departments. Sprained ankles have been estimated to comprise approximately 15% of all sports-related injuries. Ankle sprains result from forces around the ankle that exceed the tensile limits of the supportive ligaments of the ankle, but these forces are less than the forces necessary to break the ankle bones. The most common type of ankle injury involves inversion of the plantar-flexed foot, with resultant injury to the

lateral ligamentous complex (ATFL, talofibular ligament, CFL, and posterior talofibular ligament).

The most important feature of physical examination of the injured ankle is differentiation between ankle fractures and ankle sprains. A sprain often presents with pain over the affected ligament, with the ankle resting in its normal anatomical position. In comparison, ankle fractures, as discussed in the next case, present with an area of maximal tenderness on the bony anatomy, generally the distal fibula or fifth metatarsal when the mechanism of injury is inversion. In comparison, eversion injuries require much stronger force, and they generally produce both medial injury (including deltoid ligament injury) and lateral injury (generally a mid-shaft or proximal fibular fracture).

Workup and Management

The ATFL is the first, or only, ligament to be injured in most ankle sprains. With ankle sprains, local swelling and bruising depends on the severity of the injury. In general, ATFL injuries are diagnosed with pain to palpation of the ligament (Figure 3-8). A positive anterior drawer test result is also indicative of an ATFL sprain, and it helps grade the severity of the injury: the more laxity that is present with an anterior drawer test, the higher the grade of injury, and, generally speaking, the longer time to return to play.

The anterior drawer test is performed with the patient dangling his or her leg over the edge of the examination table (Figure 3-9). The physician should cup one hand over the heel and place the other hand over the front of the tibia, to provide counterpressure. The degree of movement should be

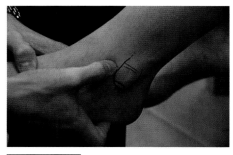

FIGURE 3-8
Palpation of ATFL.

Abbreviation: ATFL, anterior talofibular ligament.

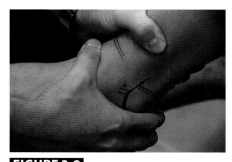

FIGURE 3-9
Anterior drawer test for ATFL laxity.

Abbreviation: ATFL, anterior talofibular ligament.

compared between both ankles. A positive ankle drawer test result simply finds a difference of movements between the injured and uninjured side, with the injured side having more movement than the uninjured side. The CFL runs from the tip of the fibula to the calcaneus. It can be injured during severe inversion injuries as well. To test the CFL, the examiner should hold the ankle in a neutral position while applying an inversion force to the talus. Increased laxity on inversion stress suggests incompetence of the CFL.

If the diagnosis of a sprain or fracture is unclear, a plain radiograph should be obtained to confirm the diagnosis. If indicated, AP, lateral, and mortise radiographic views should be performed. The Ottawa ankle rules were developed to help determine which patients with acute ankle injuries need radiographic evaluation. The Ottawa ankle rules, however, were not developed specifically for pediatric and adolescent patients, so, if ever there is a question of physeal involvement, specifically point tenderness on the bone, it is important to obtain radiographs.

Most lateral ankle ligament sprains can be managed in a similar fashion. Initial management goals are to limit inflammation and swelling and to maintain range of motion. Early treatment includes RICE (rest, ice, compression, and elevation) and early mobilization. From the beginning, exercises, including plantar flexion, dorsiflexion, and foot circles, should be done to maintain range of motion. Ankle splints or braces can limit extremes of joint motion and allow early weight bearing. The most effective means of managing ankle injuries involves rehabilitation and also good ankle strengthening, to prevent reinjury and chronic ankle instability.

The video section of the book shows effective ways to splint an ankle, as well as how to properly use crutches (figures 3-10 and 3-11). The physical therapy section will show several exercises that can be used to start prevention programs for children or adolescents who have had this injury (Figure 3-12). Referral to a sports-minded physical therapist, however, can help athletes who have had this injury, both through initial treatment and with prevention going forward.

Please view video clip:
"Icing, Compression, and Splinting Technique for the Injured Ankle."

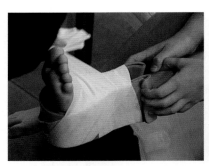

FIGURE 3-10
Ankle splinting.

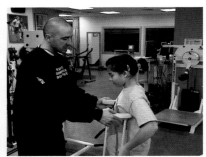

FIGURE 3-11
Fitting for crutches.

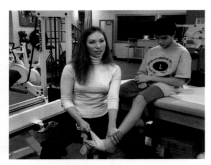

FIGURE 3-12
Preventive ankle strengthening.

Rehabilitation and Prevention Exercises

For the initial management of an ankle sprain, minimizing the swelling is essential to restoring the range of motion, strength, and proprioception. Progressive non-painful strengthening can begin in open chain exercises, to isolate muscle groups (dorsiflexors, eversion muscles, inversion muscles, and plantar flexors). The athlete will graduate to closed chain exercises that demand coactivation around the ankle, as well as kinesthetic and proprioceptive awareness. Ankle sprains might be the result of weakness in other areas higher up in the kinetic chain. These athletes may benefit from global hip, knee, and core strengthening.

The following exercises are helpful for the prevention of lateral ankle sprains:

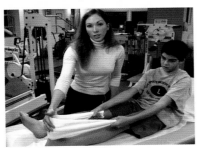

Heel Cord Towel Stretch (targets stretching the gastrocnemius and soleus complex)

Please view video clip: **"Gastrocnemius and Soleus Complex Exercises (Towel Stretch)."**

1. Begin sitting with a towel placed around the ball of the foot.
2. Pull on ends of towel toward the upper body, dorsiflexing the foot.
3. A stretch is felt in the calf.
4. Hold this position for 30 seconds.
5. Repeat 5 times on each leg.

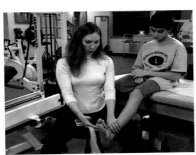

Ankle Dorsiflexion (targets tibialis anterior)

Please view video clip: **"Tibialis Anterior Exercises."**

1. Begin with a supported leg and relaxed ankle.
2. Flex the ankle, bringing the toes up toward the shin.
3. Hold this position for 2 to 5 seconds.
4. Return slowly to resting position.
5. Perform 10 repetitions; do 2 to 3 sets.

To advance: Use resistance band.

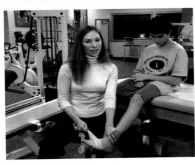

Ankle Eversion (targets peroneus brevis and longus)

Please view video clip: **"Peroneus Brevis and Longus Exercises."**

1. Begin with a supported leg and relaxed ankle.
2. Bring toes away from midline, only moving from the ankle.
3. Hold this position for 2 to 5 seconds.
4. Return slowly to resting position.
5. Perform 10 repetitions; do 2 to 3 sets.

To advance: Use resistance band.

Ankle Inversion (targets tibialis posterior)

1. Begin with a supported leg and relaxed ankle.
2. Bring toes toward midline, only moving from the ankle.
3. Hold this position for 2 to 5 seconds.
4. Return slowly to resting position.
5. Perform 10 repetitions; do 2 to 3 sets.

To advance: Use resistance band.

continued

Rehabilitation and Prevention Exercises, *continued*

Ankle Alphabets (targets rotational and kinesthetic awareness)

Using the toes, "draw" the uppercase alphabet A through Z.

To advance: Draw the lowercase alphabet (which is more rounded and therefore more difficult).

Bilateral Heel Raises (targets plantar flexors, using body weight as resistance)

1. Begin standing erect with toes pointing forward.
2. Raise heels off the floor.
3. Hold this position for 2 to 5 seconds.
4. Return to starting position.
5. Perform 10 repetitions; do 2 to 3 sets.

To advance: Stand on one leg and perform heel raises.

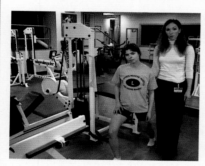

Contralateral Hip Abduction (targets ankle proprioception, balance reactions, and coactivation of the entire stance leg, with the opposite hip abductor muscles targeted as well)

Please view video clip: "Hip Abductor Muscle Exercises."

1. Begin standing erect with toes pointing forward.
2. Bring one leg out to the side while maintaining erect posture.
3. Hold the leg out to the side for 2 to 5 seconds.
4. Return to beginning posture without putting lifted foot on the floor.
5. Perform 10 repetitions; do 2 to 3 sets.

To advance: Add resistance band (wrapped around the ankles).

TAKE-HOME POINTS

Anterior Talofibular Ligament Sprain

▶ Anterior talofibular ligament (ATFL) sprains are the most common lateral ankle injury, and they are characterized by an inversion mechanism. Generally, the athlete will present with lateral pain and swelling, and the area of maximal tenderness is in the ATFL, not the fibula or fifth metatarsal. Anterior talofibular ligament injuries tend to occur mainly in athletes who are skeletally mature (age generally >14 years), when the fibular physis is closed, thus making the ligament the weakest area of the lateral ankle joint. Radiographs are essential in the presence of bone pain because of the risk of a possible fracture. The RICE (rest, ice, compression, and elevation) protocol is essential for initial management, as are splinting and crutch use if weight is difficult to bear. Rehabilitation exercises are helpful to prevent further injury.

▶ Finally, return to play can be considered only when the ankle is non-tender to palpation, strength is equal in both ankles, and the athlete can stand with his or her eyes closed and balance on the previously injured side for 30 seconds. The rough time period to expect these results is within 2 weeks' post-injury, but it can be longer, if the ligament injury is more significant.

Case 2
Inversion injury with Salter-Harris fracture of the distal fibular physis in 12-year-old soccer player

 Please view video clip:
"Case 2: Inversion Injury to the Ankle With Open Physis."

Description

A 12-year-old soccer player comes into the office with a similar mechanism of inversion injury to that in case 1. The difference here is that this patient is 12 years of age. He is skeletally immature; his growth plates, including epiphyses and apophyses, are still cartilaginous, or "open."

Workup and Management

Unlike in case 1, in which the distal fibular physis is closed, in this case, with the same mechanism of injury, the physis is open. The result is pain and swelling with palpation of the lateral malleolus, specifically at the distal fibular physis. This is a physeal, or growth plate, fracture, and it needs to be recognized and managed appropriately. Because of the risk of further injury and potential growth arrest, these injuries are splinted or casted, and they require follow-up, including possible repeat radiographic evaluation 5 to 6 months after the initial injury, to ensure a growth arrest has not occurred. If plain radiographs suggest physeal arrest, referral to a pediatric orthopedic surgeon is indicated for appropriate management. Unrecognized physeal arrest can cause angular growth deformity of the lower extremity.

Figure 3-13 shows the area of maximal tenderness when fibular physeal (growth plate) fracture has occurred.

Pediatric and adolescent ankle fractures are most common between ages 10 and 15 years, as the growth plates begin to fuse. These ankle fractures account for about 5% of pediatric and adolescent fractures and 15% of physeal injuries. Because ligaments generally are stronger than open physes, low-energy trauma (eg, an inversion injury) that might result in a ligament injury in an adult often results in a physeal fracture in an athlete who is skeletally immature. It is important to correlate physical and radiographic findings, because accessory ossification centers may be misread as fractures.

The Salter-Harris classification system of epiphyseal fractures is the most commonly used anatomical system to describe pediatric and adolescent ankle fractures (Figure 3-14). The Salter-Harris scheme also provides prognostic significance. In general, more severe Salter-Harris fractures pose an increased risk for damage to the physis. Type I and II injuries have lower risks of physeal arrest than do injuries classified as types III, IV, and V.

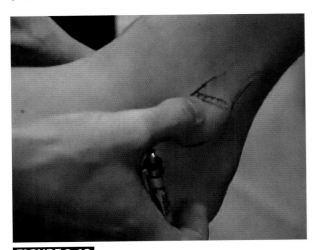

FIGURE 3-13
Palpation of distal fibular physis.

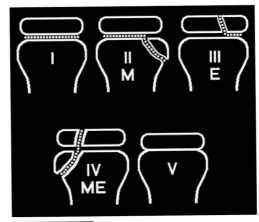

FIGURE 3-14
Salter-Harris classification system for epiphyseal fractures.

Typically, patients will report what seems to be localized joint pain, often following a traumatic event (eg, fall or collision). Swelling near a joint with focal tenderness over the physis is usually present. The patient will usually be unable to bear weight on the affected side. A careful neurovascular examination of the extremity should be performed, although a precise motor and sensory examination may be difficult with a frightened child. A thorough evaluation can provide insight into the mechanism of injury and can aid in planning the reduction.

Three radiographic views should be performed in the evaluation of pediatric ankle injuries. For subtler injuries, such as the Salter-Harris type I, the only radiographic abnormal finding visible may be soft-tissue swelling adjacent to the physis or minimal widening of the physis (Figure 3-15). We stress that, in cases of Salter-Harris type I fractures, which are the most common, radiographs are often not helpful in diagnosis, and physical examination is the essential tool in diagnosis.

Salter-Harris type I and II physeal injuries with displacement can usually be managed adequately with closed manipulative reduction. If there is no displacement of the physis, no reduction is required. Upon reduction, these injuries are typically stable, and casting suffices. Growth arrest may occur with these fractures, because significant compression may have occurred at the time of injury. Injuries to the physis generally should be referred from the primary care office because of the risk of growth arrest in the future. In general, this risk increases with higher severity of Salter-Harris fractures.

Initial management of a suspected growth plate fracture in the ankle is similar to that of all lateral ankle injuries: RICE. In this case, however, crutches and referral are generally indicated.

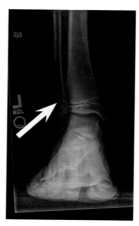

FIGURE 3-15
Skeletally immature ankle with Salter-Harris type I fibular fracture, diagnosed by physical examination. Arrow points to distal fibular physis, the area of maximal tenderness.

TAKE-HOME POINTS

Distal Fibular Physeal Fracture (Salter-Harris Type I)

▶ Case 2 is a Salter-Harris type I fracture. The mechanism of injury is inversion, but, unlike in case 1, the patient is skeletally immature (ie, the epiphyses are still open). The result is that the inversion mechanism produces a fracture through the distal fibular physis. Radiographic evaluation is important, to rule out a more significant injury, but, in this case, the radiographic findings are normal. This injury is initially treated with splinting and RICE (rest, ice, compression, and elevation), and casting can be considered, depending on the amount of pain and swelling. Stirrup splinting generally is sufficient for most patients after the swelling reduces. These injuries generally heal in 4 to 6 weeks, and a period of rehabilitation is essential, as described in case 1, before sending an athlete back onto the field.

▶ Follow-up radiographic evaluation at 6 months can be performed if there is concern regarding growth arrest. In general, most suspected Salter-Harris fractures are referred.

Case 3

Inversion injury with osteochondritis dissecans of the talus in 16-year-old softball player

Description

A 16-year-old softball player comes into the office with a similar mechanism of inversion injury to that in cases 1 and 2. In this case, the patient reports pain over the anteromedial aspect of the ankle joint. On examination, it becomes apparent that the pain is over the medial talar dome.

Workup and Management

The broad group of osteochondral lesions of the talus includes a variety of different pathologies with confusing nomenclature. Acute transchondral fractures are true fractures of the talar dome, usually anterolateral, sustained with an ankle injury. They can occur with malleolar fracture, or independently, and are easy to miss. Treatment is always surgical, either excision or reduction and fixation. Chronic osteochondral lesions are common in adults or older adolescents, and they probably result from chronic trauma or multiple episodes of ankle instability. These injuries will have some combination of cartilage injury and subchondral bone edema or cysts. They are not commonly seen in young children.

Osteochondritis dissecans (OCD) is a disease of abnormal ossification. Osteochondritis dissecans was first described by Konig in 1888, when he identified a disease process that involved loose body formation in the setting of articular cartilage and subchondral bone fracture in the knee, and he coined the phrase "osteochondritis dissecans." In 1922, Kappis applied the phrase to similar pathology within the ankle. The exact etiology of OCD is still unknown, but it is likely a combination of trauma, vascular compromise, and genetic predisposition. Lesions of the lateral dome, which are usually shallow compared with medial lesions, have been associated with a history of trauma. Deeper medial lesions have not typically been preceded by trauma. The medial dome is more frequently involved. In

our practice, the most common presentation of OCD of the talus is incidental; a patient with a new ankle injury (and no previous ankle problem) is noted to have an OCD lesion on the ankle radiograph. If the physician obtains a radiograph of the opposite ankle, the lesion may be seen there as well, suggesting the OCD lesion is not related to the new injury. A short period of rest and rehabilitation usually leads to normal function, because many patients with incidental discovery of an OCD lesion will have no symptoms. Although the natural history of these lesions is not known, it probably is benign.

In contrast, some patients with OCD of the talus will present with chronic ankle pain with or without injury. The typical clinical presentation for a symptomatic OCD lesion of the talus is chronic and vague, with reports of persistent pain and swelling that are not responsive to activity modification and rest. Physical examination findings are relatively benign, with some tenderness over the anteromedial or anterolateral ankle, or both.

The typical radiographic appearance is a well-circumscribed osteochondral fragment demarcated from the adjacent bone by a radiolucent line, as shown in Figure 3-16. Anteroposterior, lateral, and mortise radiographic views should be performed.

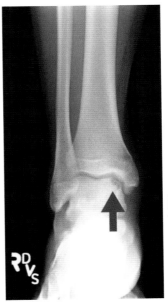

FIGURE 3-16

Typical radiographic appearance of chronic medial talar dome OCD.

Abbreviation: OCD, osteochondritis dissecans.

In the past, clinicians relied on multiple plain radiographic views to identify OCD, but magnetic resonance images (MRIs) should now be obtained when there is reasonable suspicion. On MRI, a thin, abnormal hyperintensity line at the base of the fragment on T2-weighted images (shown in Figure 3-17) has been characteristic of partially attached fragments, while completely detached fragments have been demonstrated by a smooth hyperintensity line surrounding the fragment.

Initial treatment for OCD lesions of the talus in adolescents is nonsurgical, with restrictive weight bearing, boot or cast immobilization, and possibly a corticosteroid injection. Indications for operative intervention for OCD in children include an unsuccessful course of nonoperative treatment or further displacement of the osteochondral

fragment. A surgical procedure begins with ankle arthroscopy; then loose cartilage is debrided. If the overlying cartilage is damaged and the lesion is less than 1.5 cm in size, the base of the lesion is drilled in multiple areas, introducing healing tissue into the lesion (microfracture) as shown in Figure 3-18. For large lesions (>15 mm), it is worth considering an osteochondral transfer. With arthroscopic debridements, we generally keep the patient on crutches for 1 month, and then we begin an ankle rehabilitation program.

In the case of the 16-year-old girl with likely a chronic medial talar dome OCD, she was treated with 6 weeks of boot immobilization, followed by physical therapy, and was able to return to play pain-free.

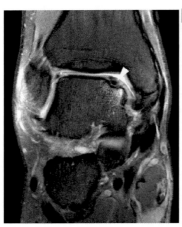

FIGURE 3-17

MRI appearance of medial talar dome OCD.

Abbreviations: MRI, magnetic resonance image; OCD, osteochondritis dissecans.

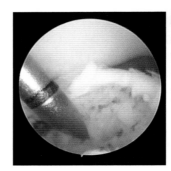

FIGURE 3-18

Arthroscopic appearance of talar OCD after microfracture.

Abbreviation: OCD, osteochondritis dissecans.

TAKE-HOME POINTS

▶ Osteochondritis dissecans of the talus is a cause of ankle pain in adolescents.

▶ History, physical examination, standing radiographs, and a magnetic resonance image are all part of a complete workup.

▶ Initial treatment is almost always conservative, using immobilization, rest, and possibly an injection. If this treatment fails, surgery may alleviate symptoms.

Case 4
Compression injury to the ankle with triplane ankle fracture in 15-year-old football player

Description

A 15-year-old athlete comes crashing down directly on his ankle (the axial-loading mechanism). In this case, the mechanism of acute injury is not a "roll" but rather a direct compression injury to the ankle. Chronologically, this patient is at an age during which his muscular strength is increasing, but his epiphyses are still open. The result is that the high force generated at the ankle from this type of injury is often tolerated poorly. He hobbles into the office with a significant injury.

 Please view video clip:
"Case 4: Compression and Axial-Load Injury to the Ankle."

Triplane fractures of the distal tibia generally occur during adolescence, before complete closure of the distal tibial physis. This unique fracture occurs because a partially open distal lateral tibial growth plate creates a plane of weakness when a shearing force is applied to the ankle. More specifically, an external rotation (eversion) of the foot on the tibia creates a stress along the open distal lateral tibial growth plate. The fracture pattern extends through the transverse (growth plate), sagittal (epiphysis), and coronal (distal tibial metaphysis) anatomical planes, disrupting the tibial plafond intra-articularly.

The distal tibial epiphysis begins to close with a centrally located epiphyseal hump and proceeds medially. Adolescents are susceptible to the triplane fracture following medial physeal closure and before lateral physeal closure. The 3 types of triplane fractures are 2-part triplane fractures, 3-part triplane fractures, and 4-part triplane fractures. Each type may have a coexisting fibular fracture as well, but only tibial fragments are counted as part of the triplane fracture.

Workup and Management

Patients with triplane ankle fractures can present with pain, ecchymosis, swelling, ankle deformity, and the inability to bear weight on the affected limb. A complete neurovascular examination is necessary. It is also important to look for any lacerations or abrasions that may be indicative of an open fracture. Because fibular fractures are commonly associated with triplane fractures, the fibula should be inspected and palpated along its entire length. Other areas at high risk for fracture include the calcaneus and the base of the fifth metatarsal.

In this case, radiographic evaluation should be performed, including AP, lateral, and ankle mortise views, with the foot in 15° of internal rotation (figures 3-19–3-21). Triplane and other ankle fractures are frequently associated with fibular fractures. Spiral stresses, in particular, may result in a Maisonneuve fracture of the proximal fibula. If pain or tenderness is elicited anywhere on the length of the fibula, obtain a fibular radiograph.

Any triplane fracture should be splinted and immediately referred to a pediatric orthopedic surgeon. Closed reduction, which results in adequate fracture reduction in all planes, can be achieved in approximately 30% to 50% of cases of triplane fractures. Generally, reversing the motion that produced the injury, along with axial distraction, will produce acceptable realignment. Adequate closed reduction is followed by 4 to 6 weeks of above-the-knee casting. The cast is then replaced with a below-the-knee cast, to allow limited weight bearing with crutches for an additional 4 weeks. Gradual return to play should follow. Any triplane fracture that demonstrates 2 mm or greater of displacement after closed reduction needs operative management. These injuries should always be referred to an orthopedic surgeon for management.

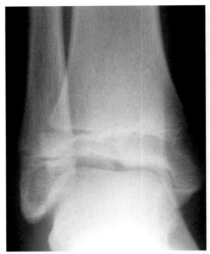

FIGURE 3-19

AP view of triplane ankle fracture.

Abbreviation: AP, anteroposterior.

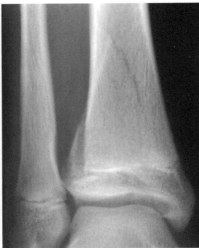

FIGURE 3-20

Lateral view of triplane ankle fracture.

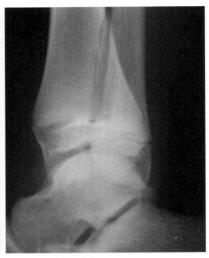

FIGURE 3-21

Mortise view of triplane ankle fracture.

TAKE-HOME POINT

Triplane Fracture

▶ The most serious of all the described ankle injuries, case 4 involves a direct compression to the ankle. The key to appropriately diagnosing this injury is a good patient history, physical examination, and high index of suspicion. Initial management includes splinting and crutch use, and rapid orthopedic surgical consultation is warranted.

2. Overuse Injury

Case 5
Heel pain (Sever apophysitis) in 12-year-old soccer player

Description

A 12-year-old soccer player comes into the office reporting heel pain with running. This is a common scenario in the pediatric office.

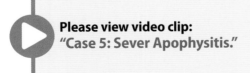

▶ **Please view video clip:**
"Case 5: Sever Apophysitis."

Sever apophysitis, also called Sever disease, was originally described by James W. Sever in 1912 as a condition characterized by inflammation of the

calcaneal apophysis, a normal bony projection or outgrowth found on the posterior aspect of the os calcis, or calcaneus. The condition, which is generally self-limited, is more common in boys than girls and usually affects children and adolescents between the ages of 9 and 14 years who participate in running and jumping sports, peaking in incidence between ages 10 and 12 years. Approximately 60% of the time, it is a bilateral condition, in which patients present with diffuse pain and swelling of the heels that worsens with activity and may cause difficulty ambulating. It is thought to occur by a process of repetitive microtrauma, caused by the pull of the Achilles tendon on its bony insertion. Because the apophysis does not undergo bony fusion with the rest of the calcaneus until around age 17 years, it is weaker than the attached tendon and becomes inflamed.

Workup and Management

On physical examination, patients will demonstrate focal bony tenderness when the heel is palpated at the insertion of the Achilles tendon (Figure 3-22). Unlike plantar fasciitis, in which the underside of the heel is most often tender, Sever apophysitis is usually localized to the posterior aspect of the heel. Pain may also be induced at the site when the ankle is brought into maximal dorsiflexion and generally is relieved with plantar flexion or equinus positioning of the foot. The ankle joint itself, the surrounding ligamentous structures, and the medial and lateral malleoli should not be tender. Even when a patient's concerns are limited to one side, the contralateral heel should be examined because of the high incidence of bilateral inflammation.

Radiographs of the ankle and foot may be obtained to rule out other entities (Figure 3-23), but the findings are often negative in cases of Sever apophysitis, the diagnosis of which is clinical. Sclerosis and fragmentation of the calcaneal apophysis may be observed with the lateral radiographic view, but such findings may also be seen in patients without the condition.

Like most overuse injuries in active children and adolescent athletes, the criterion standard of treatment is rest, activity modification, and judicious use of nonsteroidal anti-inflammatory drugs (NSAIDs). Physical therapy, focusing on stretching exercises

for the heel cord, or Achilles tendon, should also be pursued, and icing the heel may provide some relief to patients. In one large study, approximately 85% of affected children and adolescents returned to athletic participation within 2 months of treatment. If Sever apophysitis is left untreated, it can worsen to limitation of even normal activity. For mild cases in which the desire to continue with sports is strong, heel lifts or orthotic inserts may be inserted into casual and athletic shoes or cleats, which may decrease symptoms of the condition. In rare severe cases, a brief (<1 month) period of casting may be used, but referral to a pediatric sports specialist is strongly encouraged. There is no role for steroid or other injection therapy. Parents may be reassured that the condition is self-limited, and no long-term adverse sequelae have been identified for Sever apophysitis.

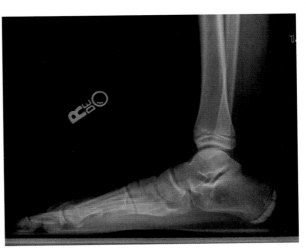

FIGURE 3-23
Lateral view of foot in patient with Sever apophysitis.

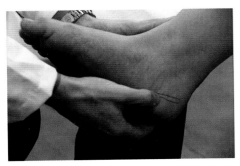

FIGURE 3-22
Palpation of the calcaneal apophysis.

Rehabilitation and Prevention Exercises

The following exercises are helpful for the patient with Sever apophysitis. They should be performed by the adolescent only when there is not an active inflammation or pain at rest in the calcaneus. The stretches should be prolonged and gentle, to prevent aggravation of the symptoms.

The adolescent may find pain relief by icing after the stretches.

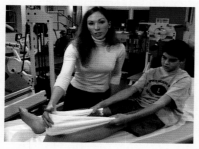

Heel Cord Towel Stretch (targets stretching the gastrocnemius and soleus complex)

Please view video clip: "Gastrocnemius and Soleus Complex Exercises (Towel Stretch)."

1. Begin sitting with a towel placed around the ball of the foot.
2. Pull on ends of towel toward the upper body, dorsiflexing the foot.
3. A stretch is felt in the calf.
4. Hold this position for 30 seconds.
5. Repeat 5 times on each leg.

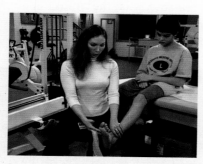

Ankle Dorsiflexion (targets tibialis anterior)

Please view video clip: "Tibialis Anterior Exercises."

1. Begin with a supported leg and relaxed ankle.
2. Flex the ankle, bringing the toes up toward the shin.
3. Hold this position for 2 to 5 seconds.
4. Return slowly to resting position.
5. Perform 10 repetitions; do 2 to 3 sets.

To advance: Use resistance band.

Long-Sitting Hamstring Muscle Stretch (targets hamstring muscles)

1. Sit erect on the edge of a table or bed, with one leg outstretched on the table.
2. Lean forward from the hips, without flexing your back, until a stretch is felt in the back of the thigh.
3. Hold this position 30 seconds, and repeat 5 times on each leg.

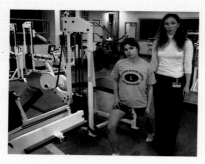

Runner's Stretch (targets gastrocnemius and soleus complex)

Please view video clip: "Gastrocnemius and Soleus Complex Exercises (Runner's Stretch)."

1. Stand with legs staggered.
2. The front knee should be bent, and the back knee should be straight.
3. Keep both heels on the ground, and lean into the front leg until a stretch is felt in the back calf muscle.
4. Hold this position for 30 seconds.
5. Perform 5 repetitions on each leg.

TAKE-HOME POINT

Sever Apophysitis

▶ Sever apophysitis is a common overuse injury in adolescent athletes, characterized by heel pain with running. Symptoms generally are worse with exercise. Initial management includes stretching, icing, and consideration of orthotic use. Physical therapy can aid in the control of symptoms.

Case 6
Posterior ankle impingement in 14-year-old dancer

Description

A 16-year-old ballet dancer comes to the office reporting posterior ankle pain while dancing. The more she dances *en pointe* (on point), the more it hurts. Participation is becoming difficult. Appropriately, you recognize this as a red flag.

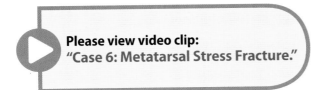

Please view video clip:
"Case 6: Metatarsal Stress Fracture."

Although anyone can develop posterior ankle problems, the ballet dancer is most at risk for it. Going en pointe brings the calcaneus against the posterior tibia, compressing the back of the ankle joint in the process. These athletes are prone to injure structures in that area, including the posterior process of the talus, the FHL, or both.

Young ballerinas are more prone to injuries after they go en pointe. The ideal age for starting en pointe has been a topic of debate in the dance community. Most dance teachers and physicians have chosen age 13 years, on the grounds that skeletal maturity, which girls attain about that age, reduces the chance of injury. This may be a false assumption. The increasing intensity of ballet as a child grows, the variable physique of dancers, and the strain on the body of dancing en pointe probably do more than skeletal immaturity to account for the high incidence of injury after ballerinas go en pointe. Most physicians agree that the decision to go en pointe should be made on the basis of dancing experience, physical maturity, and the successful completion of a pre-pointe strengthening program.

Workup and Management

Posterior ankle pain has many causes. Achilles tendon injuries are the most common problem in adults, but they are less common in adolescents. Posterior heel pain in preadolescent children (Sever apophysitis) is also common and, like Achilles tendinitis, is evident by tenderness over the affected structure. However, FHL or posterior talar pathologies are subtler; the patient may report pain at the back of the ankle, but the examiner cannot palpate these structures. Maximal ankle plantar flexion may reproduce the pain. This can be done by asking the patient to rise en pointe or by passively plantar flexing the patient's ankle. The FHL can be provoked by passively dorsiflexing the patient's first toe through the interphalangeal and metatarsophalangeal joints or by resisting the patient's active toe flexion.

The posterior process of the talus protrudes posteriorly and medially from the talus, and it is further divided into a posteromedial and posterolateral process. Between the processes is a groove in which the FHL tendon lies. The posterolateral process is often called the trigonal process, and when it does not fuse, it is called an os trigonum. The os trigonum appears between the ages of 8 and 11 years as a secondary center of ossification and usually fuses to the talus within 1 year after its appearance. The os trigonum is typically asymptomatic. However, in adolescents who participate in sports with repetitive plantar flexion, such as soccer or ballet dancing, the os trigonum can impinge between the posterior aspect of the tibia and the calcaneus and become a source of chronic discomfort. In patients older than 11 or 12, the fused trigonal process may fracture after forceful plantar flexion and become a source of pain as well. Plain radiographs will show the presence of an os trigonum (Figure 3-24). If the diagnosis is still in doubt, MRI (Figure 3-25) may show edema and hyperintensity in the region of the os trigonum. A computed tomography scan can be useful if operative intervention is planned.

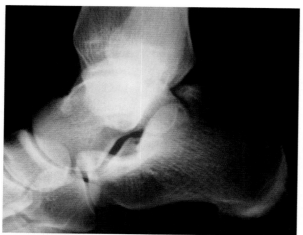

FIGURE 3-24
Radiographic appearance of os trigonum.

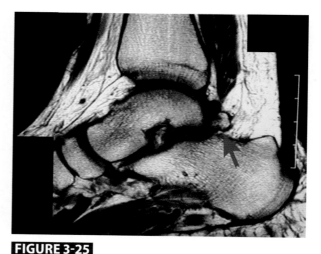

FIGURE 3-25
MRI appearance of os trigonum (green arrow).
Abbreviation: MRI, magnetic resonance image.

First-line therapy of the symptomatic os trigonum should consist of activity modification, rest, and NSAIDs. A persistently symptomatic os trigonum can be resected. Many surgeons advocate a posterolateral approach, with the patient prone, but the incision often injures the sural nerve. A posteromedial approach is safe and provides good visualization of the FHL and the back of the ankle. Arthroscopic excision of an os trigonum is also possible and provides a minimally invasive approach to treat this problem.

The FHL tendon is also a source of posterior ankle pain. Repetitive plantar flexion in activities such as ballet, distance running, or soccer can cause repetitive microtrauma to the tendon, with resultant FHL tendinitis or tenosynovitis. Flexor hallucis longus tendinitis is so common in these athletes that it is sometimes called "dancer's tendinitis." Patients present with activity-related pain at the posteromedial aspect of the ankle, sometimes with radicular symptoms into the medial plantar arch. Resisted plantar flexion of the great toe should reproduce the symptoms in most cases.

Flexor hallucis longus tendinitis is usually responsive to a short course of rest, activity modification, and NSAIDs. Surgery is required when severe stenosis of the fibro-osseous tunnel is present, accompanied by pain, triggering, and tendon contracture or tendon tears. The typical procedure involves release of the constrictive flexor retinaculum to free the FHL tendon. This can be done both arthroscopically and open, as discussed previously (Figure 3-26).

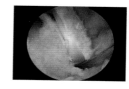

FIGURE 3-26
Arthroscopic visualization of the FHL tendon.
Abbreviation: FHL, flexor hallucis longus.

TAKE-HOME POINTS

▶ Os trigonum and flexor hallucis longus tenosynovitis are common causes of posterior ankle pain in athletic patients.

▶ A careful physical examination, along with standing radiographs and a magnetic resonance image, can help confirm the diagnosis.

▶ Rest and possibly an injection are the best initial treatment options.

▶ If symptoms persist, surgery can help to alleviate pain and facilitate return to play.

CHAPTER 4

Knee and Lower Leg Injuries in the Young Athlete

Robert G. Marx, MD, MSc, FRCSC

Anatomical Overview

Knee

The knee (Figure 4-1) is a complex, tri-compartmental joint, in which the medial and lateral condyles of the distal femur articulate with the medial and lateral condyles of the proximal tibia to form the medial and lateral compartments. These compartments are separated by the tibial eminence, comprising the medial and lateral tibial spines, which, along with the cruciate ligaments, occupy the space of the intercondylar notch of the distal femur. The third compartment of the knee, the patellofemoral compartment, is formed by the articulation of the cartilaginous undersurface of the patella with the femoral trochlea, the large cartilaginous groove between the femoral condyles. These compartments are contiguous with each other, and the synovial fluid of the joint moves freely between them, bathing the hyaline cartilage surfaces and aiding in the biomechanical cushioning, nutrition, and metabolism of the joint tissues. The patella serves as a pulley and a lever to increase the moment arm of the quadriceps or extensor mechanism, while the femorotibial articulation functions as the major load-bearing component of the hinge joint of the knee.

The lateral and medial menisci (crescent-shaped fibrocartilaginous structures attached to the tibial condyles) have many functions, including enhancing knee stability by deepening the articular surfaces of the tibia, absorbing some of the load transmitted through the joint, guiding the motion of the femoral condyles as the knee flexes, and helping distribute the synovial fluid throughout the joint. Two of the 4 major stabilizing ligaments of the knee are cruciate ligaments (they are located in a crossing pattern near the center of the joint), while the collateral ligaments are located on either side of the joint. The anterior cruciate ligament (ACL) prevents forward displacement of the tibia, while the posterior cruciate ligament (PCL) prevents backward displacement of the tibia, relative to the femur. The ACL originates on the tibial plateau, just medial and anterior to the tibial eminence, and inserts on the posteromedial wall of the lateral femoral condyle, in the intercondylar notch. The PCL, which also runs in the notch, originates at the posterior aspect of the tibial plateau, just lateral to its center point, and inserts on the middle of the lateral wall of the medial femoral condyle. The lateral collateral ligament (LCL) prevents varus displacement of the knee, while the medial collateral ligament (MCL) prevents valgus displacement of the knee. While most of the major neurovascular structures of the lower extremity run behind the joint in the popliteal fossa, the important common peroneal nerve branches forward on the lateral side of the knee, just distal to the superior end, or head, of the fibula.

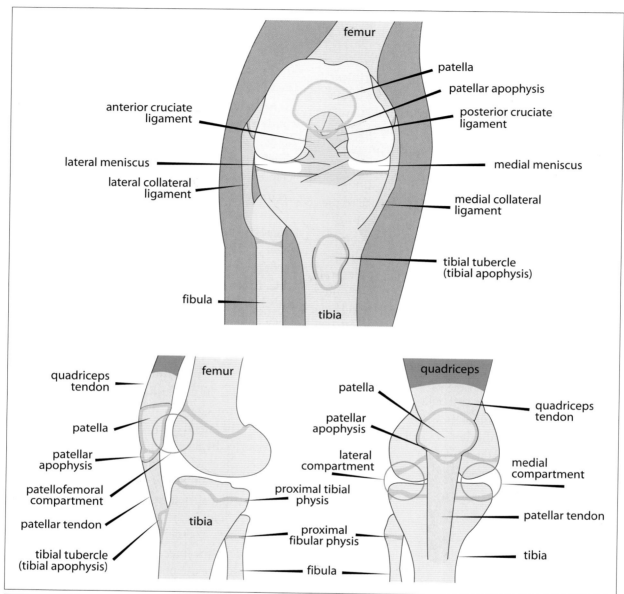

FIGURE 4-1
Knee anatomy.

Physical Examination

1. Knee: Position-Based Examination

Please view video clip: "Physical Examination of the Knee."

- **Seated position:** knee bent in 90° over the table
  - **Joint line tenderness:** palpation of medial and lateral joint space
  - **Palpation of distal pole of patella:** origin of patellar tendon (apophysis)
  - **Palpation of tibial tuberosity:** insertion of patellar tendon (apophysis)
  - **Evaluation of patellar tracking**
- **Thirty degrees of flexion:** isolation of knee ligaments, ACL, PCL, MCL, and LCL
  - **Valgus stress test:** laxity and pain (MCL stress test to assess for MCL injury)
  - **Varus stress test:** laxity and pain (LCL stress test to assess for LCL injury)
  - **Lachman test:** used to assess for ACL injury
  - **Reverse Lachman test:** used to assess for PCL injury
- **Full extension:** knee straight
  - **Presence of knee effusion:** optimal position to evaluate for effusion
  - **Palpation of medial patellar facet:** often tender in cases of medial patellar facet overload and entity of patellofemoral pain
  - **Medial quadriceps femoris strength:** muscular factor that influences patellofemoral joint
  - **Hip flexor strength:** muscular factor that affects patellofemoral joint
  - **Hamstring muscle flexibility (popliteal angle):** muscular factor that influences pelvic tilt angle and stress on patellofemoral joint
  - **Quadriceps femoris flexibility (Thomas test):** muscular factor that shows quadriceps femoris flexibility and stress on patellofemoral joint

- **Assessment for multi-ligament instability:** knees that are unstable in full extension, to valgus and varus stress, and have multi-ligament damage, including a collateral (LCL or MCL) and a cruciate (ACL or PCL)
- **Full flexion**
  - **McMurray test:** full flexion and rotation of the knee to assess for underlying meniscal injury

2. Lower Leg

Please view video clip: "Physical Examination of the Lower Leg."

- **Evaluation of foot mechanics:** Foot types include pronated, cavus, and pes planus.
- **Palpation of posterior medial tibia:** Tender in presence of medial tibial stress syndrome (MTSS) and posterior medial tibial stress fracture.
- **Palpation of anterior tibial spine:** Tender in presence of anterior tibial stress injury and, when pain is focal and severe, anterior tibial stress fracture.
- **Palpation of the anterior compartment:** Tender in presence of exertional compartment syndrome (ECS) of the anterior compartment.

Radiographs

Please view video clip:
"Radiographic Evaluation of the Knee."

1. Knee

Knee radiographs are essential for the diagnosis of many conditions in the knee. In the adolescent patient, 4 views of the knee are generally suggested: anteroposterior (AP), lateral, Merchant (patellar), and tunnel (figures 4-2–4-5). Each view provides different information. Anteroposterior and lateral views provide a 90° assessment of the joint, and they are essential for visualization of the relationship among the 3 compartments of the knee, as well as excellent visualization of the tibial and distal patellar apophyses with the lateral view. Merchant views show the orientation of the patella in the femoral trochlea, and tunnel views show the full anatomical relationship of the femoral condyles to the tibia.

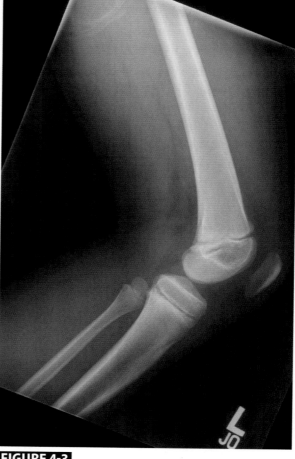

FIGURE 4-3
Lateral view of the knee.

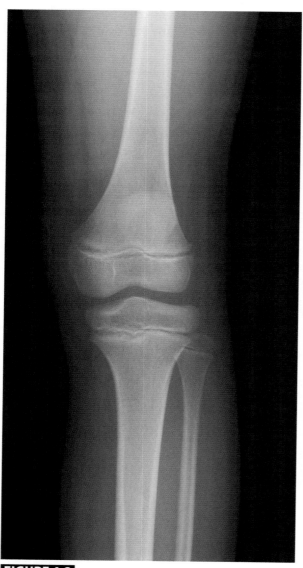

FIGURE 4-2
AP view of the knee.

Abbreviation: AP, anteroposterior.

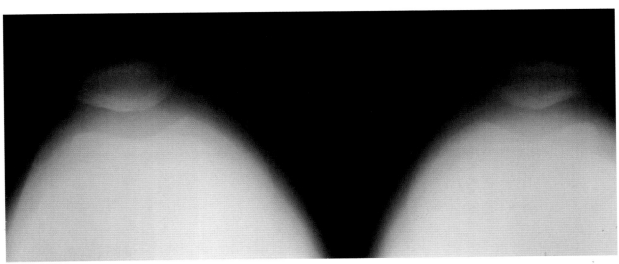

FIGURE 4-4
Merchant (patellar) view of the knee.

FIGURE 4-5
Tunnel view of the knee.

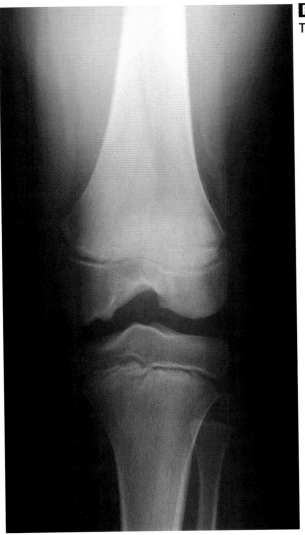

2. Tibia and Fibula

Please view video clip:
"Radiographic Evaluation of the Lower Leg."

Patients with suspected fractures and stress fractures in the tibia and fibula require radiographic evaluation. For the lower leg, these radiographs include AP and lateral views (figures 4-6 and 4-7).

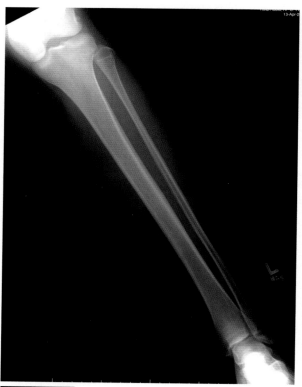

FIGURE 4-6

AP view of anterior tibial stress fracture.

Abbreviation: AP, anteroposterior.

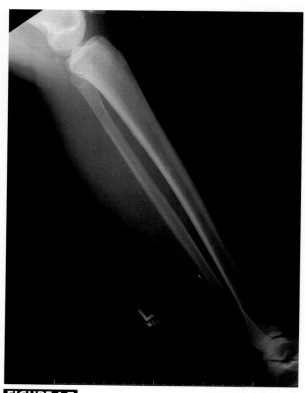

FIGURE 4-7

Lateral view of anterior tibial stress fracture.

Case Files: Knee and Lower Leg Injuries

1. Acute Trauma

Case 1
Twisting injury with planted foot (anterior cruciate ligament rupture or patellar dislocation) in 16-year-old soccer player

Description

The typical patient who injures the ACL or dislocates the patella is someone who experiences a planting, twisting, noncontact injury. In this case, a 16-year-old soccer player comes in after twisting her knee. The knee is swollen. The 2 most common causes (ACL rupture and patellar dislocation) are examined in this vignette. The key issues are the mechanism of injury and onset of swelling. The patient experiences a noncontact, twisting injury to the knee and has a knee that swells rapidly.

Please view video clip:
"Case 1: Anterior Cruciate Ligament Rupture or Patellar Dislocation."

Anterior Cruciate Ligament Rupture

Patients with rupture of the ACL sustained while playing sports will often report that they landed awkwardly following a jump or lunge or, more commonly, having cut or twisted on a planted foot. Many times, a patient will describe having heard or felt a snap or pop, followed by pain and difficulty bearing weight on the knee. While typically a noncontact injury, about 30% of ACL ruptures occur because of direct contact with another player or object. In addition to pain, the patient may report a feeling of instability when attempting to walk or simply bear weight. A knee effusion secondary to an acute hemarthrosis is also typical in the initial days following injury.

Workup and Management of Anterior Cruciate Ligament Rupture

In addition to the standard features of the knee examination, particular attention should be paid toward the Lachman test (Figure 4-8), anterior drawer test, and pivot shift test, one or more of which should have positive results in cases of ACL rupture. These results are most easily assessed within 1 hour of injury, before swelling has ensued. As such, sideline knee examination is an important consideration. While these tests may not always be well tolerated by patients in the early period following the injury, they can be an essential part of the diagnostic workup. In the age of magnetic resonance imaging (MRI), confirmation of the presence of ACL injury has been helped considerably.

It is essential for the examiner to recognize that the following clues in the history are often consistent with an ACL injury:

- Twisting, noncontact injury
- Presence of a "pop" with injury
- Sensation of the femur and tibia "slipping" in the knee
- Swelling in the knee (within 24 hours)

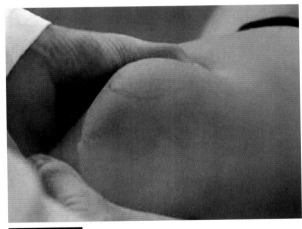
FIGURE 4-8
Lachman test.

Following physical examination, the first step should be obtaining a knee radiograph, which should include AP, lateral, Merchant, and tunnel views, specifically to rule out patellar dislocation or fracture (figures 4-9–4-12). Please note that the radiographic finding of a small bony fragment above the lateral edge of the tibial plateau represents an avulsion fracture (Segond fracture or lateral capsule fracture) as the lateral capsule tears off the plateau, and this finding is highly suggestive of ACL rupture. Radiographic evaluation of the knee is essential for any case involving swelling in the knee. In unison,

the 4 recommended views provide a complete evaluation of the bony anatomy of the knee.

If no other bony abnormalities are seen on radiograph, MRI can be considered (especially if there is swelling in the pediatric or adolescent knee), but it may be undergone subsequently, as an outpatient. In addition to showing injury to the ACL, an MRI should pick up any pathology in the other soft tissues of the joint, including meniscus tears (Figure 4-13).

Management considerations related to ACL injury may be divided into acute (short-term) and subacute

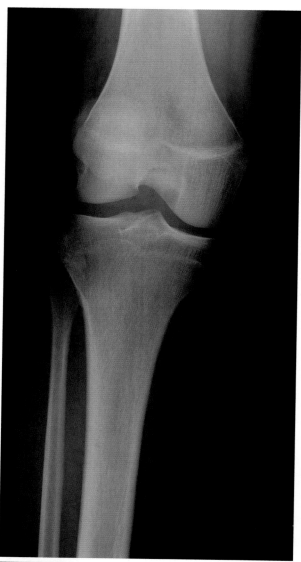

FIGURE 4-9

AP view of the knee with ACL injury.

Abbreviations: ACL, anterior cruciate ligament; AP, anteroposterior.

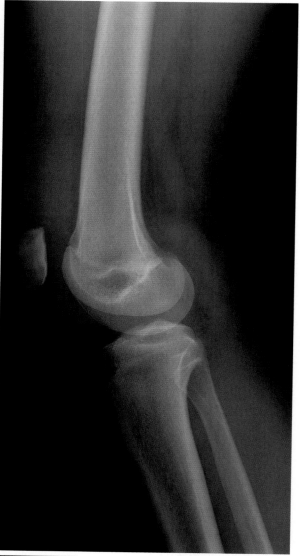

FIGURE 4-10

Lateral view of the knee with ACL injury.

Abbreviation: ACL, anterior cruciate ligament.

or chronic (long-term) considerations. Because flexing the knee is often extremely painful immediately following the injury, patients should use crutches to avoid limping. Gentle range of motion should begin within a week or so following the injury, provided there is no associated meniscus tear, as demonstrated by an MRI. Nonsteroidal anti-inflammatory drugs will help control inflammation in the days following the injury, but they may be inadequate for analgesia, so a simultaneous dose of acetaminophen can accompany nonsteroidal anti-inflammatory drug use and can alleviate symptoms. Low-dose opiate analgesia is generally avoided, if possible, in pediatric patients. Referral to a sports medicine clinic or sports medicine orthopedic

FIGURE 4-11

Merchant view of the knee with ACL injury.

Abbreviation: ACL, anterior cruciate ligament.

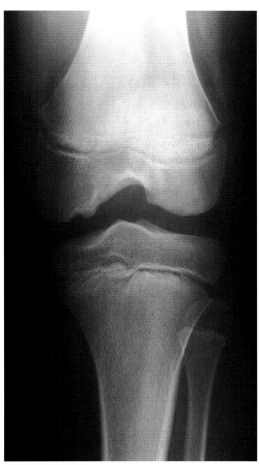

FIGURE 4-12

Tunnel view of the knee with ACL injury.

Abbreviation: ACL, anterior cruciate ligament.

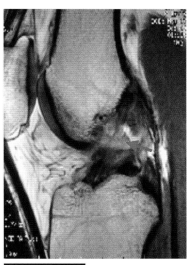

FIGURE 4-13

Sagittal MRI showing ACL rupture (red arrow).

Abbreviations: ACL, anterior cruciate ligament; MRI, magnetic resonance image.

surgeon is warranted within several days of injury, particularly in the setting of a combined ACL injury and meniscus tear.

Because of the increased risk of ongoing knee instability in active adolescents, surgical management of ACL injury is the current standard of care. Preferably, this is done before ongoing episodes of knee instability, which, if untreated, can lead to an increased risk of joint damage. Controversy still exists about treatment of the skeletally immature, pediatric patient with an ACL rupture, regarding the timing of surgical reconstruction. Some experts advocate early fixation, while others attempt a period of conservative treatment, including bracing, as the initial course of treatment.

In general, return to play, particularly to cutting sports, such as basketball, soccer, and football, is contraindicated for pediatric and adolescent patients without an ACL reconstruction, particularly if episodes of knee instability are ongoing. Surgery is generally performed when inflammation in the knee has resolved, full range of motion has returned, and the risk of developing postsurgical arthrofibrosis is diminished. Therefore, part of the physician's role is managing the expectations of young athletes eager to return to play.

Studies that investigated gender disparities in the incidence of adolescent ACL injury have revealed several interesting trends and provide clues for prevention strategies as well. Girls are 2 to 9 times more likely than boys to experience the injury, which is felt to be caused by a combination of different factors, including limb alignment differences (secondary to having naturally wider hips), greater ligamentous and joint laxity (at least in part because of hormonal differences), a narrower femoral intercondylar notch, and differences in proprioceptive and strength training. Encouraging lower-extremity strength training in young female athletes, particularly toward a goal of balanced hamstring muscle and quadriceps femoris strength and flexibility, is important for primary care professionals. There are several ways to implement these ACL injury prevention programs, including coordinating with Web-based programs and physical therapists and certified athletic trainers who are familiar with ACL injury prevention programming.[1]

Patellar Dislocation

Another common injury pattern with the same mechanism of injury is the patellar dislocation. Most of these injuries occur with the noncontact, twisting mechanism, as is the case with ACL injury. Also, as is the case with ACL injury, the spectrum of patellar instability, from the subluxing (slipping) patella to the dislocating patella, are more common in female athletes. In some cases, the patella will reduce spontaneously, back into the trochlear groove, when the patient straightens his or her knee. If it remains dislocated on presentation, however, the diagnosis is usually made easily on the basis of the gross subcutaneous appearance of the displaced patella, either medial or, much more commonly, lateral to its usual location. A soft defect may also be palpated under the skin where the patella normally lies anterior to the trochlea.

Workup and Management of Patellar Dislocation

While radiographic confirmation of a diagnosis of patellar dislocation is often sought, some clinicians advocate that reduction or relocation of the patella can be performed without radiographic confirmation. A gentle medial-to-lateral push with the thumbs may be all that is needed to reduce the patella, but, if any difficulty is encountered, conscious sedation should be considered to relax the quadriceps femoris and prevent any potential damage to the patellar articular cartilage with the reduction.

If the patient presents with the patella already reduced, or a question exists whether the patella actually was dislocated during an injury, the apprehension test should be performed.

During an apprehension test with results that are positive, when medial-to-lateral pressure is applied to the patella, the patient will report a feeling of instability, or apprehension, that the patella is going to dislocate. In all cases, radiographs should be obtained following patellar reduction to rule out any concomitant fractures or anatomical variations that may have predisposed the patient to dislocation, such as lateral patellar subluxation or a hypoplastic lateral femoral condyle (Figure 4-14). Magnetic resonance imaging is also important in evaluation of patellar dislocation, specifically in evaluating the articular cartilage for the presence of a cartilage shear injury, which can produce an osteochondral loose body that can benefit from early surgery to repair it.

Subacute or chronic patellar dislocation can be a difficult problem to manage, but management generally involves quadriceps femoris and hip strengthening. Surgical management is rarely pursued as the initial form of treatment. Instead, a long-term physical therapy regimen, designed to strengthen the medial stabilizers of the patella, primarily the vastus medialis portion of the quadriceps femoris, represents first-line therapy. Patients and their families should be informed that recurrence of patellar dislocation is fairly common and makes operative management more likely as a necessary definitive measure. Surgeries range from soft-tissue procedures to more invasive bony realignment techniques. There is still discussion regarding the surgical versus nonsurgical treatment for the first-time patellar dislocation, but the chronic patellar dislocation is generally managed surgically, because patients are highly likely to continue experiencing instability without surgery. The following are clinical signs that indicate patellar instability:

- Presence of a pop
- Immediate swelling
- Sensation of the patella slipping
- Tenderness along the medial border of the patella

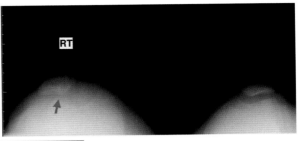

FIGURE 4-14

Lateral subluxation of the patella, as seen with the Merchant view (noted by the arrow).

Many cases of acute injuries to the knee do not involve acute hemarthrosis. Of these cases, collateral ligament injuries are the most common. These often involve a valgus or varus stress to the knee. Unlike ACL injuries or patellar dislocations, collateral ligament injuries do not swell appreciably. As such, they can be managed with gradual strengthening and return to play.

Box 4-1
Initial Management of Suspected Anterior Cruciate Ligament Injury or Patellar Dislocation

1. Crutches for non–weight bearing
2. RICE (rest, ice, compression, and elevation)
3. Radiographs of the knee (4 views: AP, lateral, Merchant, and tunnel)
4. Referral to sports medicine center

Abbreviation: AP, anteroposterior.

TAKE-HOME POINT

Anterior Cruciate Ligament Tear and Patellar Dislocation

▶ For the primary care professional, these are cases to refer to a specialist (Box 4-1). The key in the primary care office is to recognize these injuries when they occur, characterized by a twisting injury, a "pop," swelling, and a sense of instability in the knee. Treatment initially includes RICE (rest, ice, compression, and elevation), crutches, radiographic evaluation, and referral. Athletic teens who report their knee giving out with twisting can sometimes present with chronic symptoms. These patients can often have a previously undiagnosed anterior cruciate ligament tear. These injuries generally are characterized by a Lachman and pivot shift test with positive results.

84

Sports Medicine in the Pediatric Office—2nd Edition

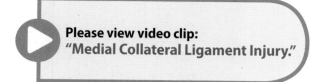

Please view video clip:
"Medial Collateral Ligament Injury."

2. Overuse Injury

Cases of knee overuse are to be distinguished from cases of acute knee injury, in which patients come in with a concern of knee pain. In comparison, ACL and patellar instability cases often present with a concern of the knee giving out, while overuse injury is characterized by pain in the knee that worsens with activity.

Case 2

Knee pain (Osgood-Schlatter and Sinding-Larsen–Johansson diseases) in 13-year-old basketball player

Description

A 13-year-old basketball player comes into the office reporting pain just below the knee that worsens with jumping. This vignette explores 2 possible causes.

Please view video clip:
"Case 2: Osgood-Schlatter and Sinding-Larsen–Johansson Diseases."

Osgood-Schlatter Disease

The patient with classic Osgood-Schlatter disease presents with pain with jumping, at the insertion site of the patellar tendon into the tibia. Osgood-Schlatter disease, first described in 1903, is an avulsion of the developing ossification center of the tibial tuberosity, the prominent portion of the proximal tibia at which the patellar tendon inserts. Primarily, it affects children and adolescents between the ages of 10 and 15 years. Boys are more commonly affected than girls. Some authors state that up to 15% of teenaged boys and 10% of teenaged girls may be affected; the symptoms worsen during periods of rapid

skeletal growth, when the rate of bone elongation exceeds the concomitant gains in muscle flexibility. This percentage increases with teenagers who are more physically active. Osgood-Schlatter disease may be bilateral in up to one-half of boys and one-fourth of girls. Patient concerns are exacerbated during running and jumping activities, when stresses across the knee are high.

Workup of Osgood-Schlatter Disease

Physical examination reveals pain localized to the tibial tubercle, to which the patellar tendon attaches (Figure 4-15). Local swelling and erythema may also be present. The knee joint itself is spared and should be free of pain or swelling. Lower-extremity alignment should be evaluated as possible contributors to this entity, including femoral anteversion, valgus knees, foot overpronation, and increased quadriceps femoris, or Q, angle. If the patient reports an acute onset of pain with trauma, a tibial tubercle fracture should be considered in the differential diagnosis.

Radiographic studies include AP, lateral, and oblique knee views as part of the initial workup, although they are not absolutely necessary to make the diagnosis. The lateral view provides the most useful information (Figure 4-16). Most commonly, the tibial tubercle is prominent and one or more ossicles may be visible adjacent to it.

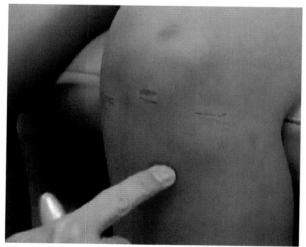

FIGURE 4-15
Tibial tuberosity test.

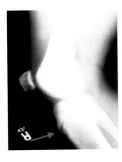

FIGURE 4-16
Lateral view of the knee showing Osgood-Schlatter disease with widening (red arrow) at the tibial apophysis.

Treatment is primarily supportive, and reassurance is key for the teen and the parents. It is important to emphasize the benign course of this disease process to them. Most patients have complete resolution of symptoms as the physis closes. Mild discomfort with activity may persist until this time. Few patients experience persistent pain, and they should be referred to a sports medicine physician for further evaluation. Activity restriction is not necessary unless severe pain exists. Because adolescents lose flexibility with growth, the symptoms of Osgood-Schlatter disease worsen during peak growth periods. Often, referral to a sports-oriented physical therapist can help alleviate symptoms, with improved flexibility and strength. Physical therapy includes stretching and strengthening. Countertraction straps, applied just proximal to the site of tenderness, can alleviate symptoms.

Outlined below are treatment options for Osgood-Schlatter disease.

- Pain relief medication.
- Hamstring muscle stretching and progressive conservative quadriceps femoris strengthening.
- Icing for 15 minutes after activity.
- Countertraction knee straps that rest between the distal pole of the patella and the tibial tuberosity.
- *Do not* administer steroid injections.

Rehabilitation and Prevention Exercises

Restoring flexibility will normalize the torque about the knee, thus decreasing the stress on the tibial tubercle. The patient diagnosed as having Osgood-Schlatter disease will often have significant improvement of symptoms with aggressive hamstring muscle stretching and gentle quadriceps femoris strengthening.

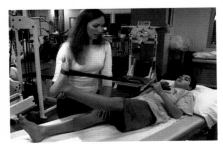

Hamstring Muscle Stretch (targets hamstring muscles)
Please view video clip: "Hamstring Muscle Exercises."
1. Begin lying on your back with a towel or strap wrapped around one foot.
2. Raise the leg (with knee straight) with the towel or strap until a stretch is felt in the back of the thigh.
3. Hold this position for 30 seconds, and repeat 5 times on each leg.

Long-Sitting Hamstring Muscle Stretch (targets hamstring muscles)
1. Sit erect on the edge of a table or bed, with one leg outstretched on the table.
2. Lean forward from the hips, without flexing your back, until a stretch is felt in the back of the thigh.
3. Hold this position 30 seconds, and repeat 5 times on each leg.

continued

Rehabilitation and Prevention Exercises, *continued*

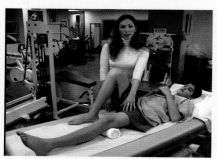

Quadriceps Femoris Sets With Towel Roll (targets quadriceps femoris)

Please view video clip: "Quadriceps Femoris Exercises."

1. Begin lying on your back with one leg bent and with the other straight with a small towel roll under the knee.
2. Tighten the quadriceps femoris so the back of the knee presses into the towel.
3. Hold the contraction for 5 seconds; then relax.
4. Perform 10 repetitions; do 3 sets.

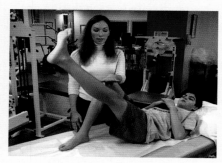

Straight-Leg Raises (targets knee extensors and hip flexors)

Please view video clip: "Knee Extensor and Hip Flexor Exercises."

1. Begin lying on your back with one leg bent and the other straight.
2. Tighten the quadriceps femoris while lifting the straight leg to the height of the bent knee.
3. Slowly return it to starting position.
4. Perform 10 repetitions; do 2 to 3 sets.

To advance: **Cuff weights may be used to add resistance.**

Note: This exercise should be done only when a straight knee is maintained while lifting. If the knee bends while lifting, decrease the weights until there is no lag or return to quadriceps femoris sets.

The patient may benefit from the following additional exercises: Thomas test, heel cord towel stretching, clamshells, prone hip extension, side-lying hip abduction, side-lying hip adduction, heel raises, contralateral hip abduction, and wall slides (only if patient is asymptomatic).

Sinding-Larsen–Johansson Disease

Sinding-Larsen–Johansson (SLJ) disease is a similar entity to Osgood-Schlatter disease, but it involves traction on the growing inferior pole of the patella, with ossicle formation and fragmentation. First described in 1921 by Sinding-Larsen, Johannson, and Smillie, this condition, sometimes referred to as "jumper's knee" in the adult patient, is actually an apophyseal injury to the distal pole of the patella in children and young teens. Because growth velocity and subsequent loss of flexibility is greater in boys than in girls, boys develop SLJ disease more commonly. Symptoms typically occur in active adolescents during running, jumping, stair-climbing, or kneeling and are localized to the inferior border of the patella. In general, these cases are more recalcitrant than Osgood-Schlatter disease, are often more difficult to treat, and are often a source of frustration for adolescent athletes.

Workup of Sinding-Larsen–Johansson Disease

Physical examination reveals tenderness at the inferior pole of the patella (Figure 4-17). No other knee findings typically exist, except for muscular inflexibility and weakness. Pain can be more specifically elicited with the knee flexed at 90°.

Radiographic workup includes AP, lateral, and oblique knee views (figures 4-18 and 4-19). The lateral view confirms the presence of calcification at the inferior patella pole.

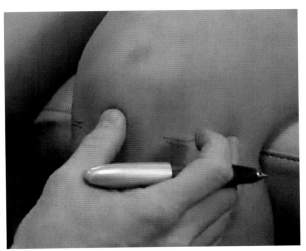

FIGURE 4-17
Palpation of distal pole of the patella.

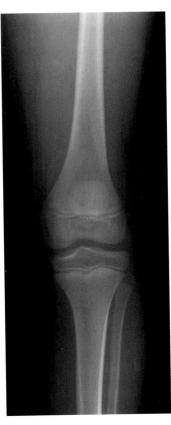

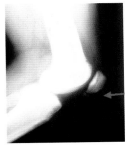

FIGURE 4-19
Lateral view of the knee showing chronic avulsion (red arrow) of the distal pole of the patella, consistent with SLJ disease.

Abbreviation: SLJ, Sinding-Larsen–Johansson.

FIGURE 4-18
AP view of the knee with SLJ disease.

Abbreviations: AP, anteroposterior; SLJ, Sinding-Larsen–Johansson.

Treatment for Sinding-Larsen–Johansson Disease

Treatment involves reassurance to the patient and parents. A more cautious approach than with Osgood-Schlatter disease is warranted, because of the more prolonged, recalcitrant nature of SLJ disease. Although absolute activity restriction is not necessary, activity modification is often needed, especially in the early stages of SLJ disease. Many practitioners find that referral of SLJ disease to a pediatric sports medicine specialist is helpful, because these cases often involve familial tension regarding appropriate levels of activity when considering return to play.

Sinding-Larsen–Johansson disease is an overuse injury (ie, it occurs over time). Similar to the avulsion injury at the insertion of the patellar tendon, which is an avulsion fracture (not Osgood-Schlatter disease), a patellar sleeve fracture is an acute fracture and partial avulsion of the patellar tendon from the distal pole of the patella. The key is that Osgood-Schlatter disease and SLJ disease are chronic injuries. If these happen acutely, fracture is more likely and referral is indicated.

Outlined below are treatment options for SLJ disease.

- Pain control
- Activity modification
- Referral to sports medicine physical therapist
- Icing for 15 minutes after activity

Rehabilitation and Prevention Exercises

Long-Sitting Hamstring Muscle Stretch (targets hamstring muscles)

1. Sit erect on the edge of a table or bed, with one leg outstretched on the table.
2. Lean forward from the hips, without flexing your back, until a stretch is felt in the back of the thigh.
3. Hold this position 30 seconds, and repeat 5 times on each leg.

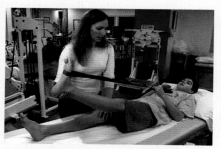

Hamstring Muscle Stretch (targets hamstring muscles)

Please view video clip: "Hamstring Muscle Exercises."

1. Begin lying on your back with a towel or strap wrapped around one foot.
2. Raise the leg (with knee straight) with the towel or strap until a stretch is felt in the back of the thigh.
3. Hold this position for 30 seconds, and repeat 5 times on each leg.

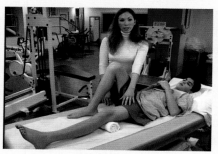

Quadriceps Femoris Sets With Towel Roll (targets quadriceps femoris)

Please view video clip: "Quadriceps Femoris Exercises."

1. Begin lying on your back with one leg bent and with the other straight with a small towel roll under the knee.
2. Tighten the quadriceps femoris so the back of the knee presses into the towel.
3. Hold the contraction for 5 seconds; then relax.
4. Perform 10 repetitions; do 3 sets.

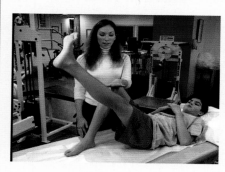

Straight-Leg Raises (targets knee extensors and hip flexors)

Please view video clip: "Knee Extensor and Hip Flexor Exercises."

1. Begin lying on your back with one leg bent and the other straight.
2. Tighten the quadriceps femoris while lifting the straight leg to the height of the bent knee.
3. Slowly return it to starting position.
4. Perform 10 repetitions; do 2 to 3 sets.

***To advance:* Cuff weights may be used to add resistance.**

Note: This exercise should be done only when a straight knee is maintained while lifting. If the knee bends while lifting, decrease the weights until there is no lag or return to quadriceps femoris sets.

The following therapeutic exercises are suggested: heel cord towel stretching, clamshells, prone hip extension, side-lying hip abduction, side-lying hip adduction, contralateral hip abduction, Thomas test, and wall slides (only if patient is asymptomatic).

TAKE-HOME POINTS

Osgood-Schlatter Disease and Sinding-Larsen–Johansson Disease

▶ Overuse injuries of the extensor mechanism, the group of muscles that extend the knee, often cause 1 of 2 problems (Osgood-Schlatter disease and Sinding-Larsen–Johansson [SLJ] disease) in the athlete who is skeletally immature. Osgood-Schlatter disease is usually the less serious of the two. These are overuse injuries, generally characterized by focal pain with palpation of the tibial tuberosity or the distal pole of the patella, and occur over time. Symptoms worsen with activity. Generally, the causative factor is the loss of quadriceps femoris flexibility during rapid skeletal growth; the rate of femoral growth far exceeds the associated quadriceps femoris growth. The treatment for Osgood-Schlatter disease includes good stretching and the use of a countertraction strap. The treatment for SLJ disease also includes stretching, but a period of relative rest is also indicated.

▶ Acute trauma at both of these sites (avulsion fractures at the tibial tuberosity and patellar sleeve fractures at the distal pole of the patella) also occur. These injuries have similar focal, acute pain, but the difference is that these are acute injuries (caused by an acute, eccentric loading force to a flexed knee [eg, sliding into a base or landing a jump from a hurdle]). Acute fractures should be referred.

Case 3
Anterior knee pain (patellofemoral pain) in 16-year-old soccer player

Description

A 16-year-old soccer player comes into the office reporting patellar pain that worsens during and after running, as well as when using stairs.

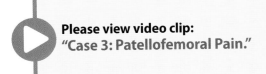

▶ **Please view video clip:**
"Case 3: Patellofemoral Pain."

The patient with classic patellofemoral knee pain comes into the office reporting pain "underneath the kneecap" during and after running. Often, this is associated with pain walking up and down stairs, as well as after prolonged sitting. In general, there is no swelling in the knee with patients who have patellofemoral pain.

Like with patellar instability, patellofemoral pain syndrome (PFPS) primarily affects adolescent girls, but, in some cases, it can affect boys. Generally, pain results from excessive force loaded onto the patella, which, in turn, causes a chronic inflammatory reaction in the cartilage and bony undersurface

of the patella. Patellofemoral pain syndrome may result from malalignment of the leg caused by anteversion of the femoral neck, external rotation of the tibia, or overpronation of the foot. The result is an increase in the Q angle of the knee, "knock-kneed angle," and irritation of the underlying cartilage. The Q angle is a measure of the tendency of the patella to move laterally when the quadriceps femoris is contracted. When the Q angle is increased, stress increases in the patellofemoral joint. Other causative factors of PFPS result from rapid bone growth and resultant loss of muscle flexibility during peak adolescent growth velocity, and these factors can include a tight patellar retinaculum, the supporting fibrous tissue on the medial and lateral patella, and underlying loss of quadriceps femoris, hamstring muscle, and hip muscle flexibility.

Patients with PFPS report anterior knee pain in the patella that worsens with squatting, stair-climbing, or sitting for long periods of time.

Workup of Anterior Knee Pain

Physical examination findings may be benign in mild cases. Patients point to the front of their knee as the problem area, often saying "it hurts here," as they grab their patella. Pain is elicited with direct palpation of the undersurface of the patella. Medial or lateral translation forces to the patella may reveal a tight, nonmobile patella or an extremely mobile patella (figures 4-20 and 4-21). Patients with a tight patella may report greater pain on the lateral side of the patella. Patients with a mobile patella may report that the patella feels unstable or is slipping.

Complete evaluation for PFPS includes examination of the feet, knees, and hips. Overpronation of the foot is associated with PFPS, and it generally causes medial facet pain. Sometimes, cases with medial overload can be managed with a corrective orthotic device, if the foot is overpronated. In the muscles about the knee, PFPS is associated with tight quadriceps femoris, tested by the Thomas test, and tight hamstring muscles, tested by assessing the popliteal angle. (Note: During the Thomas test, the

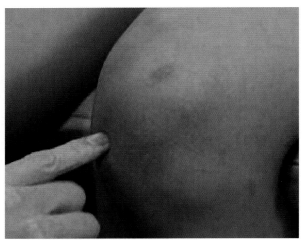

FIGURE 4-20
Palpation of medial joint space.

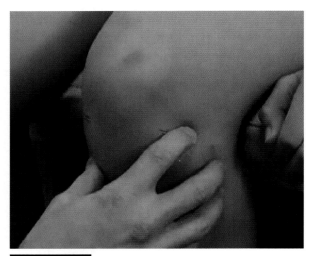

FIGURE 4-21
Palpation of lateral joint space.

patient is lying flat on his or her back and the hip is flexed. A positive test result is when the opposite quadriceps femoris flexes before the full flexion of the hip is obtained, thus indicating muscular tightness in the quadriceps femoris.) Finally, hip structure and strength are associated with PFPS. In addition to femoral anteversion, tested by assessing the amount of internal rotation of the femur once the foot and tibia are placed in neutral, hip muscle strength is an essential issue to consider. Hip strength affects the valgus stress placed at the knee; a stronger hip results in a more neutral dynamic alignment of the knee. This can be tested by having the patient extend the leg against resistance while lying supine or by using the Trendelenburg test, to assess hip orientation with single-leg squatting. Weaker hip musculature results in a "falling," unsteady pelvis with single-leg squatting.

Radiographic workup includes the standard 4-view knee series, including the Merchant view. The Merchant view allows one to look at the axial alignment of the patella and evaluate the tilt of the patella and its relationship to the groove of the femur on which the patella rests. Radiographs generally are recommended for patellofemoral pain if any swelling is in the joint, if the pain has persisted for more than 6 weeks, or if pain worsens during the night. The distal femur is the most common site of bone-related tumor in the adolescent boy, so attention to history is important with this type of concern.

Outlined below are treatment options for PFPS.

- Pain relief
- Hip strengthening and quadriceps femoris and hamstring stretching
- Shoe orthotic inserts
- Patellar taping
- Icing for 15 minutes after activity

Treatment for PFPS is centered on strengthening of the quadriceps femoris, specifically the vastus medialis obliquus. Stretching of the hip flexors, quadriceps femoris, iliotibial band, hamstring muscles, and gastrocnemius is also beneficial. Formal physical therapy provides observation of treatment and assurance of safe and effective strengthening of the proper muscles. Patient education consists of teaching patients to take breaks to straighten the knee when sitting for long periods and to avoid full squats.

In addition to strengthening and stretching, other modalities have been shown to provide pain relief, such as taping, to correct patellar alignment, and biofeedback, to improve quadriceps femoris timing with specific activities. Taping of the patella, otherwise known as McConnell taping, can be taught by a certified physical therapist or sports medicine physician. Orthotic inserts into shoes for patients with overpronation of the feet have been shown to decrease symptoms by decreasing the valgus stress at the knee.

Surgical intervention for patellofemoral pain in adolescent athletes should be considered only after a prolonged course of nonoperative management and careful discussion of the outcome measures of the surgical procedures used to manage PFPS.

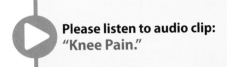

Please listen to audio clip: "Knee Pain."

Rehabilitation and Prevention Exercises

There is much controversy on the best therapeutic program for patients with patellofemoral knee pain. This may be, in part, caused by how each patient presents with patellofemoral pain syndrome, from the patient with instability of the patella (presenting with patella alta and lateral tracking with extension) to the patient with global patellar pressure syndrome (tight medial and lateral retinacular structures). A thorough assessment of the patient to identify flexibility limitations, the mechanics of the patient's patellar tracking during open- and closed-chain activity (eg, descending a stair), and muscle strength is necessary for patients with chronic knee pain.

Some therapeutic guidelines for the patient include limiting stair negotiation and avoiding deep squats, running, or other activities that recreate the pain. Improving the athlete's flexibility of the hip flexors, rectus femoris, hamstring muscles, iliotibial band (ITB), and gastrocnemius and soleus complex will decrease the load on the patellofemoral joint. For example, for a patient with a tight ITB, the fibers connect with the lateral retinaculum, which may tilt the patella laterally and put more stress on the lateral femoral condyle. Patients with tight hamstring muscles may take shorter strides and may walk with a flexed knee, which puts greater demands on the quadriceps femoris and more pressure on the patellofemoral joint. In either scenario, improving the flexibility will decrease the symptoms.

The following exercises are helpful for the management and prevention of PFPS:

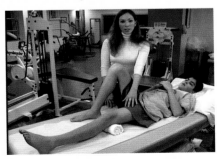

Quadriceps Femoris Sets With Towel Roll (targets quadriceps femoris)

Please view video clip: "Quadriceps Femoris Exercises."

1. Begin lying on your back with one leg bent and with the other straight with a small towel roll under the knee.
2. Tighten the quadriceps femoris so the back of the knee presses into the towel.
3. Hold the contraction for 5 seconds; then relax.
4. Perform 10 repetitions; do 3 sets.

continued

Rehabilitation and Prevention Exercises, *continued*

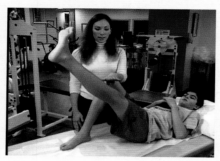

Straight-Leg Raises (targets knee extensors and hip flexors)

Please view video clip: **"Knee Extensor and Hip Flexor Exercises."**

1. Begin lying on your back with one leg bent and the other straight.
2. Tighten the quadriceps femoris while lifting the straight leg to the height of the bent knee.
3. Slowly return it to starting position.
4. Perform 10 repetitions; do 2 to 3 sets.

To advance: **Cuff weights may be used to add resistance.**

Note: This exercise should be done only when a straight knee is maintained while lifting. If the knee bends while lifting, decrease the weights until there is no lag or return to quadriceps femoris sets.

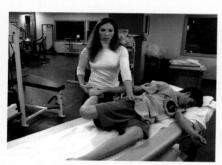

Thomas Test (targets hip flexors, rectus femoris, and ITB)

Please view video clip: **"Hip Flexor, Rectus Femoris, and Iliotibial Band Exercises."**

1. Begin lying with both knees pulled into the chest.
2. Release one leg so it extends off the supporting surface.
3. Maintain the extended leg in neutral rotation, in line with your body.
4. A stretch should be felt across the hip and thigh.
5. Hold this position for 30 seconds.
6. Return to the starting position.
7. Repeat 5 times on each leg.

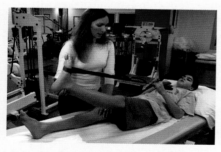

Hamstring Muscle Stretch (targets hamstring muscles)

Please view video clip: **"Hamstring Muscle Exercises."**

1. Begin lying on your back with a towel or strap wrapped around one foot.
2. Raise the leg (with knee straight) with the towel or strap until a stretch is felt in the back of the thigh.
3. Hold this position for 30 seconds, and repeat 5 times on each leg.

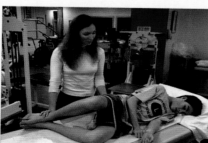

Clamshells (targets hip external rotators)

Please view video clip: **"Hip External Rotator Exercises."**

1. Begin side lying with both hips and knees bent, stacked on top of one another.
2. Raise the top knee away from the bottom knee, maintaining feet together and not rocking at the hips.
3. Hold the open-knee position for 2 to 5 seconds, and slowly return to the starting position.
4. Perform 10 repetitions; do 2 to 3 sets.

To advance: **Wrap resistance bands above the knees. Increase band resistance to up the challenge.**

continued

Rehabilitation and Prevention Exercises, *continued*

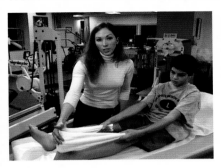

Heel Cord Towel Stretch (targets stretching the gastrocnemius and soleus complex)

Please view video clip: "Gastrocnemius and Soleus Complex Exercises (Towel Stretch)."

1. Begin sitting with a towel placed around the ball of the foot.
2. Pull on ends of towel toward the upper body, dorsiflexing the foot.
3. A stretch is felt in the calf.
4. Hold this position for 30 seconds.
5. Repeat 5 times on each leg.

The patient may progress to the following additional exercises: prone hip extension, side-lying hip adduction, contralateral hip abduction, contralateral hip extension, and wall slides (only if patient is asymptomatic).

TAKE-HOME POINT

Patellofemoral Pain Syndrome

▶ Patellofemoral pain syndrome (PFPS) is a multifactorial problem that generally presents with an adolescent patient reporting pain underneath the patella (with stair-climbing and bending). Swelling or trauma is generally uncharacteristic of PFPS, and presence of these issues should prompt consideration of another entity. In general, patients with PFPS have several underlying issues that contribute to the problem, including anatomical considerations such as foot type and rotational anatomy of the tibia and femur. Soft-tissue causes, such as a tight patellar retinaculum, as well as tight muscles around the knee, can also cause PFPS. Treatment includes activity modification while pain persists, maintaining fitness with activities that do not worsen this condition. A physical therapist or a school-based certified athletic trainer, or both, can aid in the treatment for PFPS through the use of the exercises mentioned above. When symptoms do not improve after 6 weeks, magnetic resonance imaging can be considered to rule out articular cartilage lesion beneath the patella.

Case 4

Shin pain (medial tibial stress syndrome and exertional compartment syndrome) in 16-year-old track star

Description

A 16-year-old runner comes into the office reporting shin pain. (This vignette explores the possible causes of this problem and the several causes of shin splints pain.)

Please view video clip:
"Case 4: Medial Tibial Stress Syndrome and Exertional Compartment Syndrome."

The athlete who comes into the office with shin splints can be a frustrating, and often recurrent, situation. However, most adolescents with shin problems do well with accurate diagnosis and treatment. Exercise-induced pain in the lower leg is a common concern in the recreational and competitive adolescent and teen runner. Causes can range from simple conditions requiring rest and activity modification to serious conditions requiring surgery.

It is important to obtain an accurate history and physical examination, to provide clues to the diagnosis. Several important questions to ask include

- "What are the intensity, location, and duration of symptoms?"
- "Do symptoms continue after exercise has stopped?"
- "Do you have pain at night?"

Pain during exercise that is relieved by rest suggests MTSS. Pain that persists when exercise has stopped is associated with ECS. Night pain may be associated with infection or tumor. Increases in exercise intensity, muscle tightness in the posterior compartment of the leg, changes in shoe wear, and type of running surface are all significant contributors to pain.

Medial Tibial Stress Syndrome

Medial tibial stress syndrome, also known as shin splints, is an overuse syndrome of pain in the posteromedial portion of the distal tibia, found most commonly in runners. This is the most common form of shin pain, characterized by medial shin pain during, and especially after, running. The syndrome consists of inflammation of the periosteum surrounding the tibia. The causes are multifactorial. The powerful ankle flexors, such as the soleus and flexor digitorum longus, have origins along the medial tibia and create high stresses during running, which contribute to irritation of the periosteum. Shin splints are exacerbated by prolonged periods of exercise and by overpronation of the feet during the running motion. In severe cases, a stress fracture may occur when forces overcome the body's ability to maintain the integrity of the bone.

Patients with MTSS describe the pain as dull, aching, and located in the middle to distal third of the tibia. Pain is worse during activity and is relieved by rest. Eventually, performance is negatively affected, with patients describing a decrease in the speed and intensity at which they are able to run. Symptoms classically occur during changes in the intensity of training. On examination, diffuse tenderness is found on the medial border of the distal tibia, with palpation, and swelling may be present. In cases of a true stress fracture, pain is located in a more discrete area of point tenderness. Knee, ankle, and foot range of motion are typically unaffected and not painful. Symptoms may be one-sided or bilateral. Observation of the foot may reveal a flat arch or an overpronated foot with weight bearing.

Workup and Management of Medial Tibial Stress Syndrome

Radiographic findings of the tibia are typically negative, but they may show periosteal reaction and scalloping of the distal tibia. In cases of stress fracture, a lucent line (known as the "dreaded black line") may be visible (figures 4-22 and 4-23). Computed tomography scans are not of diagnostic assistance. Magnetic resonance imaging is often of value, particularly because it shows areas of edema inside bone well before any changes are apparent on radiograph.

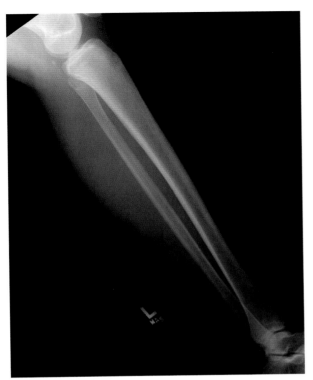

FIGURE 4-22

AP view of the tibia and fibula showing anterior tibial stress fracture with callous formation in the anterior tibial cortex, demonstrating healing.

Abbreviation: AP, anteroposterior.

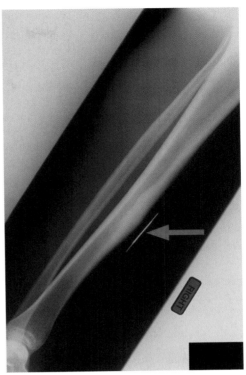

FIGURE 4-23

Lateral view of the tibia and fibula showing anterior tibial stress fracture with callous formation in the anterior tibial cortex, demonstrating healing (see arrow).

Management of MTSS centers on relative rest, ice, and nonsteroidal anti-inflammatory drugs that are the staples for overuse injuries. Symptoms may take several months to fully resolve. During that time, adolescents are encouraged to cross-train by alternating activities of less impact, such as swimming and biking, in place of running. Proper shoe wear and training surface are paramount in injury prevention. Heel cord stretching can also provide preventive benefit. For patients who have overpronation of the foot, orthotic inserts or motion control shoes that limit pronation, or both, may provide mechanical stability to the extremity.

Medial tibial stress syndrome is often a precursor on the spectrum of overuse injury to bone. The more serious portion of this spectrum is stress fracture, a clinical entity composed of focal pain that is often so severe that it can cause patients to limp. Initially, the workup for suspected tibial stress

fracture is the same for that of MTSS. However, if the diagnosis is made, often through both clinical history and physical examination, and sometimes with confirmatory radiographs or MRIs, the treatment is different. Tibial stress fracture requires a 4- to 6-week cessation from sports participation, with appropriate cross-training, such as swimming, to maintain fitness. In addition, as was described in the patient with metatarsal stress fracture, tibial stress fracture should prompt consideration of causative factors, including loading activity, foot mechanics, and bone density. As discussed in Chapter 3, Ankle and Foot Injuries in the Young Athlete, stress fracture should prompt consideration of the underlying issues of bone health.

A more serious entity, the anterior tibial stress fracture, presents with pain on palpation of the anterior tibial cortex. Patients with this stress fracture present with pain with running, and they have tenderness to palpation on the anterior spine of the tibia. The difference between anterior and posterior medial shin pain is that the anterior surface of the tibia is the tension side of the bone (ie, the area of the tibia that is under tension when the bone is loaded). The result is that stress injury and stress fracture to the anterior portion of the tibia is much more serious and is classified as a high-risk stress fracture. Concern regarding anterior tibial stress fracture should result in a total cessation of loading activity (crutches are indicated for suspected stress fractures), and evaluation should include both radiographs and MRIs. In general, anterior stress injuries to the tibia are best managed with patient referral.

Exertional Compartment Syndrome

Chronic ECS is another overuse syndrome seen in adolescent runners. Unlike bone pain, which hurts during and especially after running and is characterized by pain to palpation of the bony anatomy, ECS results from elevated pressures in the compartments in the lower leg. Patients with chronic ECS often report a "tightening" pain in the lower leg that worsens with exercise. Exertional compartment syndrome can occur in any of the 4 compartments of the lower leg, the anterior, lateral, superficial posterior, and deep posterior. The most common cases, accounting for roughly 70% of cases, occur in the anterior compartment.

The pain from ECS is thought to result from muscle ischemia as pressure builds inside the compartments, each of which is wrapped by a separate fascial lining. Increased compartment pressures occur during exercise and can remain elevated after exercise ceases, although, generally, patients report a tightening pain that worsens with exertion and abates when exercise is stopped. Patients may describe paresthesia in the dorsum or plantar aspect of the foot and, sometimes, symptoms such as foot drop, depending on which compartment is more affected. Many patients have the symptoms of ECS for quite some time before diagnosis is made, because of failure to recognize the pattern of pain during and after exercise. During the off-season, many patients are often asymptomatic.

Workup and Management of Exertional Compartment Syndrome

The findings from physical examination with ECS may be negative, with intact pulses and sensation in the foot. Patients may have localized pain in the tibia. Unlike patients with bone overuse, patients with ECS have little or no pain on palpation of the tibia. Also, unlike bone-related shin pain, the symptoms of ECS tend to abate almost immediately after exercise, unlike in bone, where they persist.

Although patient history and physical examination may raise suspicion of chronic ECS, definitive diagnosis requires measuring intracompartmental pressures (ICPs) before and after exercise. These ICP measurements generally are performed at a sports medicine clinic. Measuring ICPs involves inserting a needle that is connected to a pressure transducer into the compartments of the leg and obtaining a pressure reading before and after exercise. This should be performed only by a sports medicine or orthopedic physician trained in performing and interpreting the results. Pre-exercise measurements greater than 15 mm Hg, 1-minute postexercise pressure greater than 30 mm Hg, or 5-minute postexercise compartment pressures greater than 20 mm Hg are diagnostic of chronic ECS.

Nonsurgical treatment for chronic ECS can be successful if initiated soon after the symptoms of ECS begin. However, if the symptoms have been ongoing for more than 6 to 12 months, conservative treatment is rarely successful. Some studies have shown that prolonged, strict rest (with complete activity avoidance) may provide relief.

When conservative treatment fails, ECS can be managed surgically, with a fasciotomy of the affected compartments. Minimally invasive techniques to release the fascia have shown to be effective.

TAKE-HOME POINTS

Shin Pain

▶ Shin splints are sometimes a confusing diagnosis for the practitioner and generally fall into one of several categories, including bone-related and muscular shin pain. Bone-related shin pain can be medial tibial stress syndrome (pain along the medial border of the tibia) or a focal, posterior medial, tibial stress fracture. The latter is more serious. In both cases, the keys to treatment include relative rest until bone pain subsides and the underlying issues that caused the injury are corrected. These issues can include the mechanics of the body, such as foot type and muscle strength; the amount of activity a patient is doing; and consideration to the underlying bone health, which might be low in patients with tibial stress injury and stress fracture. Dual-energy x-ray absorptiometry studies can be used to assess bone density.

▶ Anterior tibial stress injury is a more serious type of shin splint pain caused by the pressure that is distributed along the anterior aspect of the tibia, called the tension side of the bone. Anterior stress injury can quickly progress to anterior tibial stress fracture, which can sometimes require surgical rod fixation, if it is allowed to progress. Rapid evaluation of patients with anterior tibial pain should be the standard of care, including both radiographs and magnetic resonance images. These cases generally are best referred.

▶ Finally, exertional compartment syndrome (ECS) is also a cause of shin pain. Different than bone-related pain, muscular shin pain is characterized by pain that worsens with exertion and often produces a "tightening" sensation. If caught early, ECS can sometimes be managed effectively with physical therapy. If ECS is chronic, surgical treatment through a fasciotomy has been proven to be the most effective treatment thus far. Current studies with botulinum toxin (Botox) are underway to assess if this might give preferential results using a less invasive approach.

Reference

1. Marx RG, Myklebust G, Boyle BW, eds. *The ACL Solution: Prevention and Recovery From Sports' Most Devastating Knee Injury.* New York, NY: Demos Health; 2012

Bibliography

LaBella C, Hennrikus W, Hewett T, American Academy of Pediatrics Council on Sports Medicine and Fitness, American Academy of Pediatrics Section on Orthopaedics. *Pediatrics.* 2014;133(5):e1437-e1450

CHAPTER 5

Shoulder Injuries in the Young Athlete

Derrick M. Knapik, MD, and James E. Voos, MD

Anatomical Overview

Shoulder

To manage injuries of the shoulder in developing adolescents, a good overview and knowledge of anatomy is imperative in understanding each injury process. The extreme range of motion in the shoulder (ie, 180° of abduction and 90° of both internal and external rotation) comes at the cost of instability to stresses across the glenohumeral (GH) joint. Because this is the most unstable joint in the body, GH instability, including both subluxation ("slipping") and dislocation, is a common problem in adolescents.

The bony anatomy of the shoulder (Figure 5-1) consists of the proximal humerus, made up of the greater tuberosity, lesser tuberosity, and humeral head, which articulates with the glenoid fossa of the scapula. The greater and lesser tuberosity serve as attachment points for the rotator cuff muscles, which function to stabilize the shoulder within the GH joint. The scapula also articulates with the distal clavicle at the acromioclavicular (AC) joint, at the superior margin of the shoulder, providing a restraint against superior migration of the humeral head. The scapula also glides over the posterior chest wall cavity to allow abduction of the arm. The coracoid process of the scapula serves as an anchor for the short head of the biceps brachii, coracobrachialis, and pectoralis minor. The medial clavicle is anchored to the sternum at the sternoclavicular (SC) joint. Glenohumeral to scapulothoracic (ST) motion in arm elevation occurs in a 2:1 ratio contribution to flexion and abduction motion of the shoulder.

Shoulder stability is provided by the bony, capsular-ligamentous, and surrounding muscle structures. The glenoid labrum is surrounded by a connective tissue labrum, which adds surface area to the shallow glenoid, effectively increasing the depth and stability of the GH joint. The labrum, GH capsule, and GH ligaments provide static stability to the shoulder. Dynamic stabilizers of the shoulder include the rotator cuff muscles, long head of the biceps brachii, deltoid muscle (which provides bulk to the lateral shoulder), and scapular stabilizers. The static stabilizers provide stability to the shoulder at the extremes of range of motion, whereas the dynamic stabilizers guide stability during the active mid-ranges of motion.

The neurovascular structures innervating the shoulder and upper extremity, brachial plexus, and axillary artery pass in close proximity to the shoulder joint, just beneath the coracoid process and anteroinferior to the capsule. This relationship accounts for the high number of neuropraxias that accompany shoulder injuries, commonly known as "stingers" or "burners."

Of special consideration in young athletes are the developing growth plates, or physes, that are vulnerable to both acute and chronic shoulder injuries, especially during the throwing motion. Eighty percent of the growth of the humerus occurs at the proximal growth plate, providing the proximal humeral physis with incredible growth and remodeling potential. The proximal humeral physis is divided into 3 parts (the aforementioned greater tuberosity, lesser tuberosity, and humeral head) that coalesce between ages 5 and 7 years. Subsequently, the physis closes at approximately 14 to 17 years in adolescent girls and 16 to 18 years in adolescent boys and young men. These ages, however, are based on stage of skeletal maturation, not chronological age.

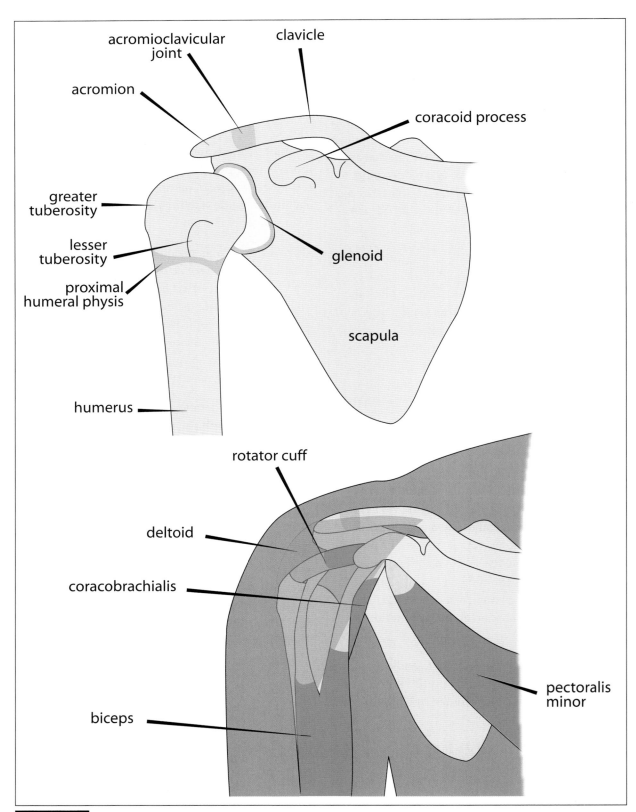

FIGURE 5-1
Shoulder anatomy with and without muscular anatomy.

Physical Examination

 Please view video clip: "Physical Examination of the Shoulder."

- **Neck examination**
  - **Range of motion:** rotational and flexion and extension evaluation to rule out injury
  - **Spurling test:** head rotated to 45°, with ipsilateral extension, to rule out cervical impingement
  - **Pain to palpation:** palpation of bony landmarks to rule out cervical spine injury
- **Range of motion (active motion):** active motion of GH joint to evaluate for muscle-tendon unit injuries
- **Palpation of major anatomical landmarks of shoulder with provocative testing**
  - **Acromioclavicular joint with cross-arm adduction test:** palpation of AC joint with subsequent cross-arm adduction to rule out AC joint injury
  - **Sternoclavicular joint with forward arm elevation test:** forward arm flexion and palpation of SC joint to rule out SC joint injury
  - **Glenohumeral joint:** range of motion of GH joint to rule out GH instability and palpation of greater tuberosity to rule out insertional tendinitis of the supraspinatus tendon
  - **Proximal humeral physis:** palpation of proximal humeral physis to rule out traction epiphyseal injury called Little League shoulder
  - **Scapulothoracic joint with palmar compression test:** evaluation of ST joint with palmar compression to rule out ST joint injury and ST joint weakness
- **Muscle strength**
  - **Rotator cuff strength testing**

- **External rotation:** external rotation of the shoulder at 90° of flexion to assess for injury or weakness, or both, to infraspinatus and teres minor
- **Internal rotation:** internal rotation of the shoulder at 90° of flexion to assess for injury or weakness, or both, to the subscapularis
- **Supraspinatus testing:** testing of the supraspinatus
- **Ligamentous examination**
  - **Modified Marshall test for generalized ligamentous laxity:** Volar flexion of thumb in direction of radius with wrist flexed to 90°. Positive results mean thumb touches radius. Used to grade generalized ligamentous laxity.
  - **Sulcus sign:** Traction on the humerus with the downward force, causing the presence of a sulcus "gap" in the GH joint to form. Indicative of ligamentous laxity in GH joint.
  - **Apprehension and relocation testing (for anterior GH instability):** Used to define anterior instability in shoulder. Patient lies supine on table with his or her arm abducted to 90° and externally rotated. A positive result occurs when the patient feels a slipping sensation, with motion, that is minimized when a posterior force is applied to the GH joint. The positive result here means that the humerus is slipping anteriorly, and the posterior force is what relocates it into position.

Radiographs

Radiographs of the shoulder are vital in the diagnosis of injuries to the shoulder. Evaluation of the major growth centers and the GH joint can generally be achieved with anteroposterior (AP) and axillary views; however, other views are available to assist in the diagnosis of specific pathologies affecting the adolescent shoulder (figures 5-2 and 5-3).

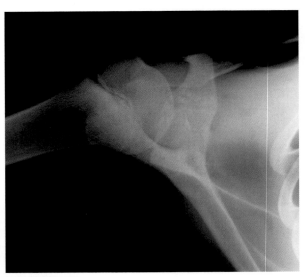

FIGURE 5-3
Axillary view of the shoulder.

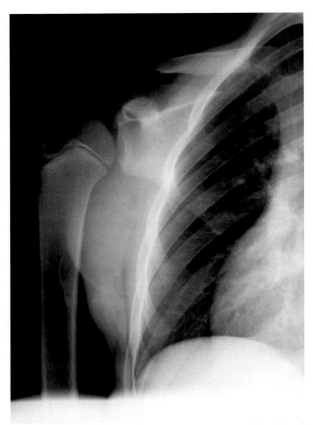

FIGURE 5-2
AP view of the shoulder.
Abbreviation: AP, anteroposterior.

Case Files: Shoulder Injuries

1. Acute Trauma

Case 1

Fall onto lateral shoulder (acromioclavicular joint injury and clavicular fracture) in 17-year-old football player

Description

In this case, the patient is a 17-year-old football player who has landed directly on the lateral shoulder. On the basis of the mechanism of injury, the lateral force from the blow of the shoulder against the hard ground drives force through the humeral head and up the clavicle. This is known as a fall in the lateral decubitus position.

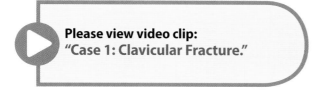

Please view video clip:
"Case 1: Clavicular Fracture."

The AC joint and clavicle are susceptible to injury because of their subcutaneous position in the shoulder girdle. Most AC joint and clavicle injuries occur from a direct blow to the shoulder, classically from a fall on the lateral shoulder. This injury commonly presents in players of football, hockey, and wrestling after being tackled or checked, or during takedowns. More recently, snowboarders have been reported to present after similar types of falls (with the rapid growth in the popularity of the sport). Indirect injury to the AC joint and clavicle has also been described from a fall on an outstretched hand as the humeral head is driven upward into the shoulder girdle, where energy is dissipated. The extent of injury to the ligaments supporting the shoulder girdle, including the AC ligament and coracoclavicular ligaments, depends on the severity of the force placed on the shoulder. In cases of severe injury, fractures of the distal clavicle may occur. Fractures to the mid-shaft of the clavicle, one of the most common fractures occurring in the active young athlete, result from a direct blow to the shoulder or a fall on the outstretched hand.

Workup and Management

On examination, patients with less severe AC joint sprains generally report pain on the top of the shoulder, directly over the AC joint. Meanwhile, clavicular fractures typically present with pain and a palpable deformity over the mid-clavicle. Shoulder range of motion is painful in both injuries (figures 5-4 and 5-5). With more severe injuries, the clavicle may be prominent under the skin. Comparison should be made to the opposite shoulder if the examiner is unsure of an anatomical disturbance.

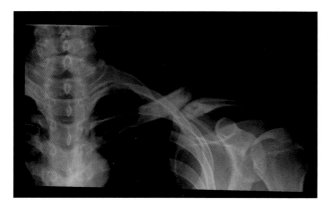

FIGURE 5-4
AP view of the shoulder with clavicular fracture.
Abbreviation: AP, anteroposterior.

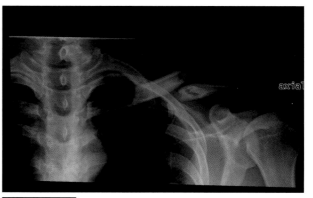

FIGURE 5-5
10° tilt view of the shoulder with clavicular fracture.

A thorough neurovascular examination of the affected extremity is essential to ensure that a neuropraxia or vascular injury has not occurred in patients with AC joint or clavicular injuries. Inspection of the overlying skin is important to determine if tenting is present, signifying risk for an open injury that is a surgical emergency. The cervical spine should also be examined as part of a complete evaluation.

The most sensitive view to diagnose AC joint pathology on radiographs is the Zanca view, in which a 15° cephalic tilt is used to evaluate the joint. Separation of the acromion from the clavicle signifies a more serious injury, resulting from disruption of the surrounding ligaments (Figure 5-6). Meanwhile, radiographic evaluation of the clavicle is best achieved through AP views and AP radiographs with a 10° cephalad tilt, to better assess the clavicle.

Treatment for minor AC joint sprains, in which the AC ligament is intact and the clavicle is not fractured or displaced, is conservative. A sling, ice, and nonsteroidal anti-inflammatory drugs (NSAIDs) provide pain relief, while gradual range-of-motion exercises for the shoulder, over the next week or two, will allow return to play within 2 weeks.

Athletes can be cleared to return to play with painless range of motion and full strength in the shoulder. Further care should be taken in the overhead athlete (eg, pitcher, quarterback, tennis player) to prevent chronic irritation of the shoulder girdle. Football players may wish to wear additional padding underneath the shoulder pads.

Treatment for more severe AC joint injuries, in which the clavicle is subluxated and the AC ligaments are disrupted, is more aggressive, with surgery possibly being indicated. Referral to a sports medicine physician or orthopedic surgeon should be made in a timely manner for further evaluation. Immobilization, ice, and NSAIDs are recommended for initial management. Fractures of the distal end of the clavicle require similar referral because of the high association of ligament injury and tendency toward nonunion.

Treatment for clavicle fractures is generally conservative. A sling, or sling and swathe, for 4 to 6 weeks provides sufficient treatment. Patients should be counseled that a residual bump in the shoulder may be present for some time after the injury, representing fracture callus. Surgical correction is considered

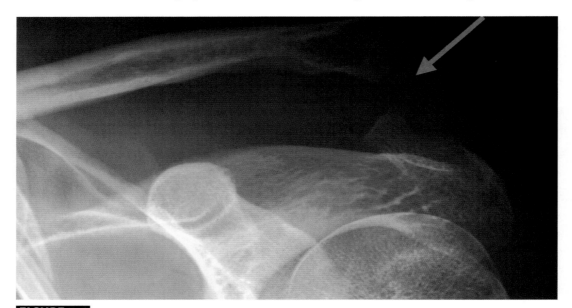

FIGURE 5-6

AP view of shoulder with grade 3 AC joint separation. Note the separation between the clavicle and acromion (see red arrow). In general, these injuries are managed nonsurgically when grades 1, 2, and usually 3 and surgically when grades 4 and 5.

Abbreviations: AC, acromioclavicular; AP, anteroposterior.

for open fractures, fractures with significant shortening, fractures with significant comminution, or fractures causing neurovascular symptoms.

Case 2
Fall onto outstretched arm (anterior shoulder instability) in 16-year-old basketball player

Description

In this case, the patient is a 16-year-old basketball player who fell during a basketball game and landed with his arm out to the side. The result is that this patient feels a "slip" in the shoulder.

 Please view video clip: "Case 2: Anterior Shoulder Instability."

Glenohumeral instability in the shoulder, including both GH subluxation and dislocation, is a common injury seen in young athletes, primarily those involved in collision sports. As such, hockey, football, and basketball are some of the sports for which shoulder dislocation is well described. The shoulder's extensive range of motion comes at the cost of instability, primarily anteriorly and inferiorly (Figure 5-7). Nearly half of all shoulder dislocations occur in patients younger than 22 years. Dislocation may occur from a fall on the outstretched hand or when additional stress on a fully abducted and externally rotated arm is applied.

When the shoulder dislocates, 3 concomitant injuries classically occur. The first is a disruption of the anterior glenoid labrum known as a Bankart lesion (Figure 5-8). When an associated fracture of the glenoid rim occurs, this is known as a "bony Bankart." The other entity is known as a Hill-Sachs lesion, which is a traumatic osteochondral defect created on the humeral head when the humeral head impacts the rim of the glenoid during dislocation. Additionally, the anterior capsule of the shoulder joint may be torn as the humeral head is anteriorly pushed with great force.

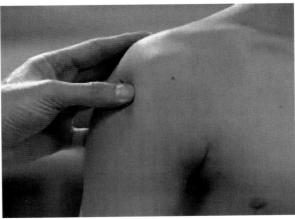
FIGURE 5-7
Palpation of the proximal humeral physis.

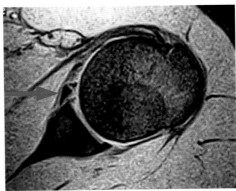
FIGURE 5-8
MRI of shoulder with red arrow pointing to Bankart lesion of the glenoid labrum.

Abbreviation: MRI, magnetic resonance image.

Workup and Management

On presentation, patients generally report pain and decreased motion in the shoulder. A specific traumatic event has almost always occurred, unless the patient recurrently dislocates his or her shoulder. Fullness in the front of the shoulder and feeling of instability are often described. Physical examination may reveal a flattening, or emptiness, of the lateral deltoid when compared with the contralateral side. The humeral head can be palpated in the axilla or anterior chest wall. The arm is usually held close to the side because of the feeling of instability. Because of the high incidence of axillary nerve palsy following shoulder dislocations, it is important to perform a thorough neurovascular examination. The presence of numbness over the skin over the deltoid or lateral shoulder and weakness in the deltoid muscle are suggestive of a nerve palsy. In the older teen, a rotator cuff tear may be confused with axillary nerve palsy.

Ligamentous laxity should be assessed, especially in female athletes with shoulder instability. Hyperextension of the elbows, metacarpophalangeal joints, knees, and hyper-dorsiflexion of the ankles are good indicators of ligamentous laxity. These findings are part of the modified Marshall test (named for John Marshall, MD, the former head of sports medicine at New York's Hospital for Special Surgery), an easy and effective screening test for generalized ligamentous laxity. Occasionally, shoulder instability is the first presenting symptom in patients with underlying connective tissue disorders, such as Marfan or Ehlers-Danlos syndrome.

Radiographic workup includes AP, lateral, and axillary views of the affected shoulder. The axillary view is the most sensitive in determining the presence and direction of shoulder dislocation. To confirm reduction, shoulder radiographic study must be repeated after reduction.

Computed tomography scan and magnetic resonance imaging (MRI) are not indicated in the acute setting of a shoulder dislocation, but they may assist in determining the extent of injury to the soft tissue and skeletal anatomy. If an associated fracture of the humerus or shoulder girdle is suspected and not clearly delineated on radiograph, a computed tomography scan may reveal additional bony injury. Magnetic resonance imaging is best at evaluating the integrity of the glenoid labrum, capsule, and articular cartilage that may be injured following subluxation or dislocation, and it is recommended following reduction to aid in formulating a rehabilitation plan.

In the acute setting, reduction of a dislocated shoulder should be performed only by a practitioner trained in safe, effective reduction methods. Reduction should not be attempted until acceptable

radiographs have been obtained to rule out potential fracture to the proximal humerus and minimize the risk of iatrogenic injury.

Initial management following shoulder dislocation differs on the basis of the degree of skeletal maturity in the patient. Associated capsular-labral or bony injuries following dislocation have been shown to be less common in skeletally immature patients aged 14 and younger because of the increased elasticity of the capsular structures, decreasing the risk for recurrent dislocation and injury to the capsular-labral complex. Moreover, when compared with older adolescent patients, skeletally immature patients possess a significantly lower rate of recurrent instability than has been reported in the past. Because of the low rate of recurrent instability in patients younger than 14, these patients may be treated with a short period of immobilization in a sling. Afterward, gradual shoulder range of motion and strengthening exercises should begin, with a focus on rotator cuff muscles and scapular stabilizers.

In patients between 14 and 17 years of age at the time of initial dislocation, the rate of recurrent instability has been documented at greater than 90% 7 years following initial dislocation. In addition, almost all patients have been shown to possess a concurrent Bankart lesion requiring eventual surgical intervention. To decrease the risk of recurrent instability and additional injuries to the GH joint, multiple authors advocate for surgical treatment following first-time dislocation of the shoulder because of the high failure rate following conservative treatment. Arthroscopic techniques have advanced greatly and provide patients with excellent results while being minimally invasive, involving less soft-tissue disruption and quicker recovery times. Thus, surgical consideration is recommended early for skeletally mature patients with any evidence of recurrent instability.

Rehabilitation and Prevention Exercises

Oftentimes, shoulder instability is greater in the overhead athlete. The ligaments may have greater laxity, compromising the static restraints of the shoulder. When the static stabilizers are less effective, the demands on the dynamic stabilizers increase. In addition, proprioception may also become diminished. Demands also become higher on the shoulder muscles if the scapular stabilizers are weak (as seen in patients with postural kyphosis). As such, it is important to address not only the rotator cuff muscles when guiding the adolescent athlete in preventive exercises but also the scapular stabilizers and deltoids. These athletes should work to improve their shoulder proprioception and reaction time (with plyometrics). (Note that training is sport specific and beyond the scope of this workbook.)

The following exercises are helpful in reducing instability in the glenohumeral joint of the adolescent athlete. These exercises are intended as prophylaxis in the overhead athlete and should not be performed if pain is experienced.

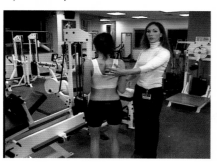

Scapular Retraction (targets middle trapezius and rhomboid muscles)

Please view video clip: **"Middle Trapezius and Rhomboid Muscle Exercises."**

1. Stand erect, holding therapeutic band lax in each hand with arms outstretched.
2. Squeeze the scapula together while bringing elbows next to the trunk.
3. Hold the position for 2 to 5 seconds, and slowly bring arms back to the starting position.
4. Perform 10 repetitions; do 2 to 3 sets.

Prone Shoulder Elevation (targets lower trapezius and shoulder musculature)

1. Lie on the stomach on a raised surface, with one arm hanging over it.
2. Raise the arm with a straight elbow and thumbs up, toward the sky, until arm is parallel with the ear. Focus on squeezing the scapula closer to your spine and downward.
3. Hold the position for 2 to 5 seconds, and slowly bring the arm back to the starting position.
4. Perform 10 repetitions; do 2 to 3 sets.

To advance: **Do exercise with both arms simultaneously.**

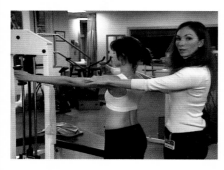

Scaption (targets synchronization of the scapular stabilizers with shoulder muscles)

Please view video clip: **"Scapular Stabilizer Exercises."**

1. Stand erect with shoulders back.
2. Elevate the arms in a V formation (as depicted) to shoulder height, with thumbs up, toward the ceiling.
3. Hold the position for 2 to 5 seconds, and slowly bring the arms back to the starting position.
4. Perform 10 repetitions; do 2 to 3 sets.

To advance: **Add 0.5 to 1 lb at a time. Do not exceed 4 lb unless you are under medical supervision.**

continued

Rehabilitation and Prevention Exercises, *continued*

External Rotation to Neutral (targets infraspinatus and teres minor)

1. Place a towel between the trunk and shoulder, and hold it in place. This helps activate the scapular muscles.
2. With the elbow bent to 90° and your arm across the stomach, bring the hand away from the body, while keeping the shoulder in place.
3. Hold the position for 2 to 5 seconds, and slowly return to the starting position.
4. Perform 10 repetitions; do 2 to 3 sets.

***To advance:* Increase the resistance with the use of therapy bands.**

Internal Rotation From Neutral (targets supraspinatus)

1. Place a towel between the trunk and shoulder, and hold it in place. This helps activate the scapular muscles.
2. With the elbow bent to 90° and your hand away from the body, pull the hand and forearm toward your stomach, while keeping the shoulder in place.
3. Hold the position for 2 to 5 seconds, and slowly return to the starting position.
4. Perform 10 repetitions; do 2 to 3 sets.

***To advance:* Increase the resistance with the use of therapy bands.**

Wall Push-ups With a Plus (targets serratus anterior and provides proprioception while engaging scapular and rotator cuff muscles)

1. Place both hands on the wall at least shoulder width apart, and gradually walk both feet away from the wall.
2. Maintain the trunk and body in a straight line, with tight abdominal muscles.
3. Bend your elbows for the push-up.
4. For the "plus," straighten the elbows and push away from the wall.
5. Perform 10 repetitions; do 2 to 3 sets.

TAKE-HOME POINTS

Glenohumeral Instability

▶ Glenohumeral (GH) instability in the adolescent athlete is a spectrum, from subluxation to dislocation. Subluxation, or "slipping," in the GH joint is characterized by the sensation of the GH joint sliding. Patients will often describe a "slip" when throwing a baseball or swimming. Most often, there are no associated neurologic findings from traction on the brachial plexus, particularly the axillary nerve, which can be seen in higher grades of instability. The treatment of GH subluxation is rehabilitation, with exercises designed to strengthen the dynamic stabilizers of the GH joint, providing stability to the adolescent athlete with GH subluxation. For patients with GH subluxation, the hope is that these episodes will not turn into a formal dislocation scenario.

▶ Further along the continuum, GH dislocation is the complete slip of the humeral head from the glenoid, often resulting in injury to the GH joint and a traction injury to the brachial plexus. In general, the adolescent athlete with full-blown GH dislocation is treated surgically, because recurrent instability rates approach 100% in adolescent athletes treated conservatively. Advancements in arthroscopic techniques have lessened the morbidity associated with open surgical techniques for the adolescent athlete with GH instability secondary to dislocation.

2. Overuse Injury

Case 3
Shoulder pain (rotator cuff overuse) in 15-year-old swimmer

Description
In this case, a 15-year-old swimmer comes into the office reporting worsening shoulder pain with swimming. This is a classic overuse injury (ie, worsening pain with activity). Sports such as swimming are classic for this type of presentation; worsening pain is a hallmark with increasing amounts of repetitive motion.

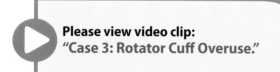

Please view video clip:
"Case 3: Rotator Cuff Overuse."

The most common overuse injury to the soft tissues in the shoulder is rotator cuff overuse, in which the supportive musculotendinous sleeve surrounding the GH joint undergoes chronic changes leading to inflammation of the tendons, known as tendinitis. The supraspinatus tendon, which runs over the top of the joint, just underneath the acromion, and inserts on the greater tuberosity of the humerus, is particularly vulnerable to such changes. When the humerus is placed in extremes of abduction and forward elevation, the area between the underside of the acromion and humeral head is reduced, impinging on the supraspinatus tendon, causing pain and inflammation.

This condition is seen in players of sports such as swimming, which requires repetitive overhead motions, as well as throwing sports, such as baseball, tennis, and football (in which quarterbacks are at risk). Instability of the GH joint, which may be secondary to physiologic ligamentous or capsular laxity, is a risk factor for rotator cuff overuse, as the muscles must work harder to stabilize the joint throughout its overhead motion.

Workup and Management
Physical examination is focused on assessment of bony tenderness, shoulder stability, range of motion, and provocative maneuvers (Figure 5-9). Standard tests of the shoulder examination, such as apprehension, Neer, Hawkins, supraspinatus, infraspinatus, cross-body adduction, O'Brien, Speed, and Yerguson tests, assist in differentiating rotator cuff pathology from biceps brachii tendon or AC joint pathology. Glenohumeral instability may be a concomitant finding or may suggest an alternative diagnosis.

Radiographs should be used to rule out stress fractures of the proximal humeral epiphysis, also known as Little League shoulder (see case 4), marked by sclerosis, widening, or displacement at the physis on radiograph. Negative findings on plain radiographs should raise the index of suspicion for rotator cuff overuse, the diagnosis of which should be confirmed with an MRI showing high signal intensity in the rotator cuff tendon, suggesting edema and inflammation.

Treatment for rotator cuff overuse injury includes cessation of the activity that precipitates the symptoms, as well as ice, NSAIDs, and physical therapy for multiple weeks. Return to play should be delayed until patients are symptom-free. Resumption of training and throwing activities must be gradual. Baseball and softball pitchers should pitch no more than 6 innings per week when they return to play, and vigilant post-competition cold therapy and NSAIDs should be used.

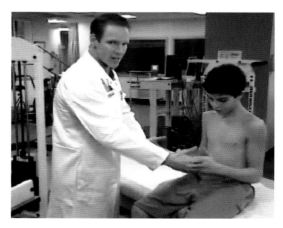

FIGURE 5-9
External rotation test.

Rehabilitation and Prevention Exercises

Physical therapy exercises of the shoulder are important to provide dynamic stability. These exercises are important to build stability around the glenohumeral joint. In cases of rotator cuff overuse (common in swimmers), there is tremendous importance in strengthening the scapulothoracic joint and rotator cuff muscles. The scapula and muscles that support the scapulothoracic joint are an integral part of the function of the shoulder joint. As such, muscular stability around the scapula is essential in treating most cases of rotator cuff overuse.

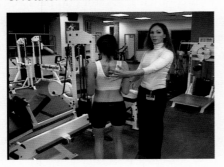

Scapular Retraction (targets middle trapezius and rhomboid muscles)

Please view video clip: "Middle Trapezius and Rhomboid Muscle Exercises."

1. Stand erect, holding the therapeutic band lax in each hand with arms outstretched.
2. Squeeze the scapula together while bringing elbows next to the trunk.
3. Hold the position for 2 to 5 seconds, and slowly bring arms back to the starting position.
4. Perform 10 repetitions; do 2 to 3 sets.

To advance: Increase the band resistance.

Prone Shoulder Elevation (targets lower trapezius and shoulder musculature)

1. Lie on the stomach on a raised surface, with one arm hanging over it.
2. Raise the arm with a straight elbow and thumbs up, toward the sky, until arm is parallel with the ear. Focus on squeezing the scapula closer to your spine and downward.
3. Hold the position for 2 to 5 seconds, and slowly bring the arm back to the starting position.
4. Perform 10 repetitions; do 2 to 3 sets.

To advance: Do exercise with both arms simultaneously.

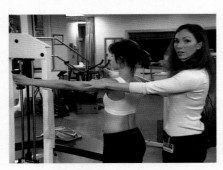

Scaption (targets synchronization of the scapular stabilizers with shoulder muscles)

Please view video clip: "Scapular Stabilizer Exercises."

1. Stand erect with shoulders back.
2. Elevate the arms in a V formation (as depicted) to shoulder height, with thumbs up, toward the ceiling.
3. Hold the position for 2 to 5 seconds, and slowly bring the arms back to the starting position.
4. Perform 10 repetitions; do 2 to 3 sets.

To advance: Add 0.5 to 1 lb at a time. Do not exceed 4 lb unless you are under medical supervision.

continued

Rehabilitation and Prevention Exercises, *continued*

External Rotation to Neutral (targets infraspinatus and teres minor)

1. Place a towel between the trunk and shoulder, and hold it in place. This helps activate the scapular muscles.
2. With the elbow bent to 90° and your arm across the stomach, bring the hand away from the body, while keeping the shoulder in place.
3. Hold the position for 2 to 5 seconds, and slowly return to the starting position.
4. Perform 10 repetitions; do 2 to 3 sets.

To advance: **Increase the resistance with the use of therapy bands.**

Internal Rotation From Neutral (targets supraspinatus)

1. Place a towel between the trunk and shoulder, and hold it in place. This helps activate the scapular muscles.
2. With the elbow bent to 90° and your hand away from the body, pull the hand and forearm toward your stomach, while keeping the shoulder in place.
3. Hold the position for 2 to 5 seconds, and slowly return to the starting position.
4. Perform 10 repetitions; do 2 to 3 sets.

To advance: **Increase the resistance with the use of therapy bands.**

Wall Push-ups With a Plus (targets serratus anterior and provides proprioception while engaging scapular and rotator cuff muscles)

1. Place both hands on the wall at least shoulder width apart, and gradually walk both feet away from the wall.
2. Maintain the trunk and body in a straight line, with tight abdominal muscles.
3. Bend your elbows for the push-up.
4. For the "plus," straighten the elbows and push away from the wall.
5. Perform 10 repetitions; do 2 to 3 sets.

TAKE-HOME POINTS

Muscular Overuse Injury

▶ Muscular overuse of the shoulder, most commonly affecting the rotator cuff, occurs when the demand placed on the shoulder is greater than the underlying strength provided from muscular support in the shoulder. When the offending activity, such as swimming or serving a tennis ball, is done repeatedly, gradual pain develops. In many cases, this is known as shoulder impingement syndrome, a "pinching" sensation when the shoulder is abducted beyond 90°.

▶ In many cases, shoulder impingement results from a combination of poor mechanics (eg, poor swim technique or poor serving technique) and insufficient strength. As such, technique and strength must be corrected and improved, as rest will only delay repeat symptoms and injury.

▶ The key to properly managing muscular overuse injuries in the shoulder includes keeping athletes active. If the shoulder is injured, keeping athletes running for fitness is important. Prompt referral to a sports-minded physical therapist will benefit young athletes and take them through a gradual, step-by-step method of building strength. Once the athlete returns to play, the key to prevent injury recurrence is to maintain a strength program for the maintenance of healthy activity.

Case 4
Shoulder pain (Little League shoulder) in 12-year-old baseball pitcher

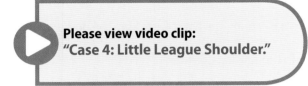

▶ **Please view video clip: "Case 4: Little League Shoulder."**

Description

In this case, a 12-year-old baseball pitcher reports pain in the shoulder with throwing. He comes into the office reporting pain in the proximal humerus.

Little League shoulder, also called pitcher's shoulder or proximal humeral epiphysitis, is a condition in which repetitive throwing activity leads to chronic changes in the cartilaginous physis of the proximal humerus. There is some debate whether the condition represents merely inflammation or a stress fracture of the physis, but some combination of both is likely, stemming from persistent and repetitive microtrauma. Closure of the physis occurs between ages 14 and 17 years, causing it to be a weak point in the shoulder during strenuous activity in adolescence, as the condition commonly presents in patients between the ages of 11 and 16 years. High-performance pitchers are most frequently affected, although tennis players, swimmers, and gymnasts may also be affected by the condition. Incidence is higher among boys than among girls, mostly because of the type of activity that each sex is performing.

The primary concern in patients with Little League shoulder is pain in the proximal humerus during the throwing motion. Pain becomes more severe the harder and more frequently the athlete throws. It is not uncommon for adolescents to present to their physician months after the onset of symptoms. Another common concern is loss of velocity of pitches. A thorough history of the number of games played and pitches thrown each week is important in evaluating potential treatment. This should include pitches thrown at full speed at practice and at home.

Workup and Management

Physical examination is focused on assessment of bony tenderness, shoulder stability, range of motion, and provocative maneuvers (Figure 5-10). The most common physical examination finding with Little League shoulder is focal pain on palpation of the proximal humeral physis. Standard tests of the shoulder examination, such as apprehension, relocation, Neer, Hawkins, supraspinatus, infraspinatus, cross-body adduction, O'Brien, Speed, and Yerguson tests, should assist in differentiating bony pathology from rotator cuff, biceps brachii tendon, AC joint pathology, or GH instability. Examination of the cervical spine is also advised, to rule out cervical radiculopathy as a cause of pain.

Radiographs may show evidence of chronic inflammatory changes or fracture of the proximal humeral epiphysis, marked by sclerosis, widening, or displacement at the physis (see red arrow in Figure 5-11). However, symptoms may precede, by several weeks, any significant bony changes appreciable on plain radiographs, in which case repeat radiographic study and meticulous comparison with the unaffected side are warranted.

As with other bony overuse injuries, treatment consists of ceasing exacerbating activity and resting the shoulder for up to 3 months. Physical therapy may begin after 1 to 2 weeks, but immobilization anytime is discouraged. Therapy should focus on stretching, rotator cuff and scapular muscle strengthening, and range-of-motion exercises.

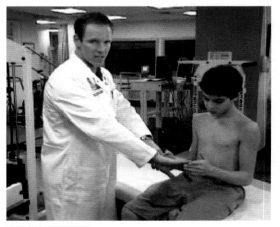

FIGURE 5-10

Internal rotation test.

Before returning to play, the athlete should demonstrate full strength, full range of motion, and no discomfort when performing the throwing motion. Patients may return to play earlier if playing positions such as first or second base, in which stresses on the arm are low. Third base is a position that should be avoided because of the long distance required to throw to first base.

Because of risk of masking pain feedback, a feedback that is important in modifying activity, the use of NSAIDs is not recommended. Patients should not resume pitching or playing positions that require hard throwing until they have been asymptomatic for a minimum of 4 weeks and have no pain both on throwing or with palpation of the proximal humeral physis, and, in cases with significant widening on the radiograph, until follow-up radiographs have been obtained.

We cannot stress enough that prevention is the best treatment. Playing in only one league at a time, beginning conditioning of the arm gradually before each season, developing proper throwing mechanics, avoiding throwing curveballs at a young

age, and limiting the number of pitches thrown each week are imperative to the prevention of serious injury. Parents, coaches, and players should all be made aware of the recommended guidelines on numbers of pitches (tables 5-1 and 5-2) and types of pitches that are safe for young baseball players.

Table 5-1. Little League Baseball 2010 Pitching Guidelines: Maximum Pitches per Game

10 y and younger	75 pitches per d
11–12 y	85 pitches per d
13–16 y	95 pitches per d
17–18 y	105 pitches per d

From Rice SG, Congeni JA; American Academy of Pediatrics Council on Sports Medicine and Fitness. Baseball and softball. *Pediatrics*. 2012;129(3):e842–e856. Reproduced with permission.

Table 5-2. Little League Baseball 2010 Pitching Guidelines: Rest Requirements for Pitchers

Pitchers 14 y and younger	
66 or more pitches in a day	Four (4) calendar days
51–65 pitches in a day	Three (3) calendar days
36–50 pitches in a day	Two (2) calendar days of rest must be observed
21–35 pitches in a day	One (1) calendar day of rest must be observed
1–20 pitches in a day	NO (0) calendar day of rest must be observed
Pitchers 15–18 y	
76 or more pitches in a day	Four (4) calendar days
61–75 pitches in a day	Three (3) calendar days
46–60 pitches in a day	Two (2) calendar days of rest must be observed
31–45 pitches in a day	One (1) calendar day of rest must be observed
1–30 pitches in a day	NO (0) calendar day of rest must be observed

From Rice SG, Congeni JA; American Academy of Pediatrics Council on Sports Medicine and Fitness. Baseball and softball. *Pediatrics*. 2012;129(3):e842–e856. Reproduced with permission.

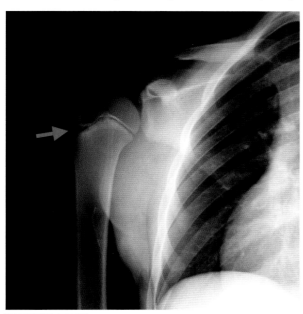

FIGURE 5-11
AP view of the shoulder showing widening of the proximal humeral physis consistent with Little League shoulder (proximal humeral epiphysitis).

Abbreviation: AP, anteroposterior.

Bibliography

Cordischi K, Li X, Busconi B. Intermediate outcomes after primary traumatic anterior shoulder dislocation in skeletally immature patients aged 10 to 13 years. *Orthopedics.* 2009;32(9)

Deitch J, Mehlman CT, Foad SL, Obbehat A, Mallory M. Traumatic anterior shoulder dislocation in adolescents. *Am J Sports Med.* 2003;31(5):758–763

Jones KJ, Wiesel B, Ganley TJ, Wells L. Functional outcomes of early arthroscopic bankart repair in adolescents aged 11 to 18 years. *J Pediatr Orthop.* 2007;27(2):209–213

Lampert C, Baumgartner G, Slongo T, Kohler G, Horst M. Traumatic shoulder dislocation in children and adolescents: a multicenter retrospective analysis. *Eur J Trauma.* 2003;29(6):375–378

Li X, Ma R, Nielsen NM, Gulotta LV, Dines JS, Owens BD. Management of shoulder instability in the skeletally immature patient. *J Am Acad Orthop Surg.* 2013;21(9):529–537

Postacchini F, Gumina S, Cinotti G. Anterior shoulder dislocation in adolescents. *J Shoulder Elbow Surg.* 2000;9(6):470–474

Rice SG, Congeni JA; American Academy of Pediatrics Council on Sports Medicine and Fitness. Baseball and softball. *Pediatrics.* 2012;129(3):e842–e856

Seybold D, Schildhauer TA, Muhr G. Rare anterior shoulder dislocation in a toddler. *Arch Orthop Trauma Surg.* 2009;129(3):295–298

Wagner KT Jr, Lyne ED. Adolescent traumatic dislocations of the shoulder with open epiphyses. *J Pediatr Orthop.* 1983;3(1):61–62

CHAPTER 6

Wrist and Elbow Injuries in the Young Athlete

Shaina A. Lipa, MD; Mark Wu, BS; and Benton E. Heyworth, MD

Anatomical Overview

1. Wrist

The wrist is exposed in most sports and therefore susceptible to injury. Basic knowledge of the anatomy of the wrist can lead to an accurate and speedy diagnosis of injury that may have potential complications if missed in the developing athlete. Football and basketball have been shown to have a high incidence of hand and wrist injuries, while swimming has the lowest.

The bony anatomy of the wrist consists of the articulation of the distal radius and ulna, with the 8 carpal bones (Figure 6-1). There are 4 bones in the proximal row of the carpus (scaphoid, lunate, triquetrum, and pisiform) and 4 bones in the distal row of the carpus (trapezium, trapezoid, capitate, and hamate). The distal radius articulates with the scaphoid and lunate carpal bones, and it accepts nearly 80% of the load on the wrist. The ulna accepts approximately 20% of the load. The distal radius also articulates with the distal ulna at the distal radioulnar joint (DRUJ), which allows supination and pronation of the wrist. The triangular fibrocartilage complex (TFCC) helps stabilize the ulna to the carpal bones and radius.

Of particular interest in pediatric and adolescent patients is the scaphoid bone, which has a tenuous blood supply. It is the most commonly injured carpal bone in these patients, particularly in adolescents. The artery to the scaphoid bone enters at the distal aspect. Any fracture to the scaphoid can cause disruption of the blood supply to the proximal portion of the bone, leading to avascular necrosis. The scaphoid can be palpated in the anatomical snuff-box on the back of the wrist, between the base of the thumb and wrist articulation.

The distal radius epiphysis usually appears between the ages of 6 months and 2 years. The epiphysis of the distal ulna appears around age 7 years. The physes generally close around the ages of 16 years in adolescent girls and 17 years in adolescent boys. The ulnar physis typically closes before the radius. Fracture involving the distal radius physis has approximately a 1% incidence of growth arrest. Growth arrest occurs up to 5% of the time with ulnar physeal fractures.

The Salter-Harris classification system, developed in 1960 for fractures of the growth plate, will be reviewed briefly (Figure 6-2). This system is helpful in determining whether a growth plate fracture requires conservative treatment or surgery. There are 5 fracture types in this classification. More severe fractures run the risk of growth arrest from disruption of the blood supply to the physis.

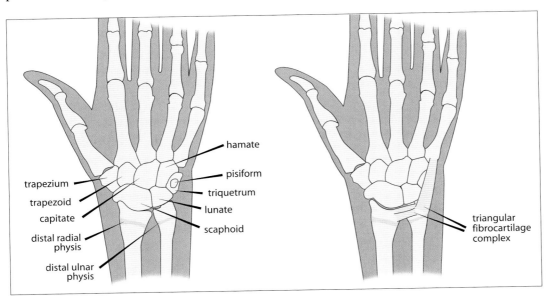

trapezium
trapezoid
capitate
distal radial physis
distal ulnar physis

hamate
pisiform
triquetrum
lunate
scaphoid

triangular fibrocartilage complex

FIGURE 6-1
Wrist anatomy.

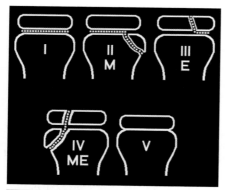

FIGURE 6-2

Salter-Harris classification system for fractures of the growth plate.

With a type I fracture, the epiphysis is completely separated from the end of the metaphysis. The likelihood is high that the bone will grow normally. A type II fracture is the most common type of growth plate fracture. The epiphysis, together with the growth plate, is partially separated from the metaphysis. Type I and II fractures almost always can be managed conservatively with cast immobilization and with low incidence of growth arrest.

Type III fractures are rare, usually occurring at the distal tibia. The fracture extends completely through the epiphysis and separates part of the epiphysis and growth plate from the metaphysis. Type IV fractures run through the epiphysis, across the growth plate, and into the metaphysis.

Surgery is needed to restore the joint surface to normal and realign the growth plate. Without surgical intervention, the risk of growth arrest and deformity is high with type III and IV fractures.

Type V fractures are also very uncommon. With this type of fracture, the growth plate has been crushed and compressed. Prognosis is poor, because premature stunting of growth is almost inevitable.

The ulnar artery and nerve, median nerve, and radial artery cross the volar portion of the wrist. The radial nerve crosses the dorsal portion of the wrist.

2. Elbow

The elbow joint, unlike the shoulder joint, is a joint with much more intrinsic stability, which is provided primarily by its bony architecture (Figure 6-3). The deep olecranon articulates with the trochlea and olecranon fossa of the distal humerus. The flexion and extension of the elbow occur at this articulation. The olecranon can be palpated as the posterior point of the elbow joint. The radial head articulates with the capitellum laterally. The coronoid process of the ulna sits anterior to the olecranon and deepens the articulating surface. It articulates with the coronoid fossa of the distal humerus anteriorly in flexion. The deep posterior olecranon fossa and shallow anterior coronoid fossa fill with fluid during elbow injuries and can be seen as the fat pad sign on lateral elbow radiographs.

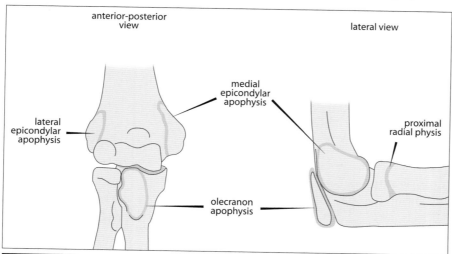

FIGURE 6-3

Bony anatomy of the elbow.

The medial and lateral epicondyles of the humerus are palpated easily on either side of the elbow, respectively. The medial epicondyle is the site of origin for the wrist flexor-pronator muscles. The lateral epicondyle is the site of origin of the wrist extensors. In full extension, the normal-functioning elbow is held at approximately 11° to 16° of valgus. This is known as the carrying angle.

In the developing elbow are 6 ossification centers that can confuse the clinician and make determination of fracture or injury difficult. These ossification centers will be reviewed briefly. Radiographs of the contralateral elbow, and knowing the progression of ossification with age, are always helpful in delineating normal anatomy from injury. The capitellum is the first ossification center to form, around the age of 2 years. The radial head follows, between the ages of 4 and 5 years, and the medial epicondyle forms between the ages of 6 and 7 years. The trochlea becomes visible between the ages of 9 and 10 years, and the olecranon forms at around age 11 years. Finally, the lateral epicondyle forms during adolescence. Ossification time can be highly variable and usually occurs in girls 6 to 12 months earlier than in boys.

Soft-tissue restraints include the joint capsule, triceps brachii posteriorly, and brachialis and biceps brachii anteriorly (Figure 6-4). Medially, the ulnar collateral ligament (UCL; also known as the medial collateral ligament, or MCL) complex provides stability to valgus stress, with the anterior bundle being the most robust. The UCL is the main medial support of the elbow during dynamic activity and if injured can greatly inhibit throwing. In athletes who are skeletally mature, rupture of the UCL in the elbow is a significant injury that requires major reconstructive surgery. Laterally, the lateral collateral ligament provides stability to varus stress.

Supination and pronation of the elbow and wrist are provided by the articulation of the radial head with the proximal ulna. The bow of the radius allows it to rotate over the top of the ulna without impinging on it.

Three nerves cross the elbow joint at different locations and are susceptible to injury. The radial nerve crosses the elbow laterally and supplies the dorsum of the hand with sensation and wrist extension. The median nerve crosses directly anterior and provides sensation to the palm, lateral 3½ fingers, and finger and wrist flexors. The ulnar nerve crosses the elbow medially in the cubital tunnel and provides sensation to the medial 1½ fingers and contributes to hand motion. This is the nerve that is irritated when the funny bone is bumped. The brachial artery accompanies the median nerve across the elbow and branches into the radial and ulnar artery.

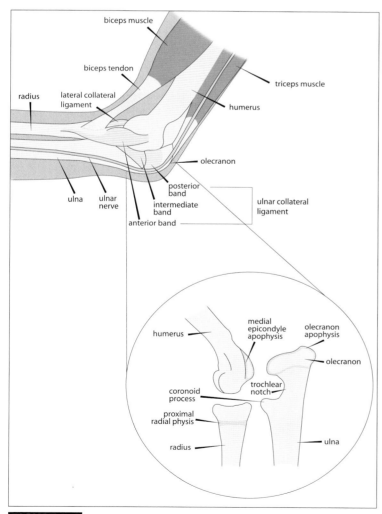

FIGURE 6-4
Soft-tissue anatomy of the elbow.

Physical Examination

1. Wrist

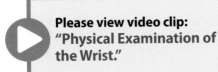

Please view video clip:
"Physical Examination of the Wrist."

- **Inspection:** To look for swelling or deformity in the wrist.

- **Range of motion (active):** Pain and limitation of motion with dorsal and volar flexion under own strength.

- **Range of motion (passive):** Pain and limitation of motion with examiner.

- **Palpation of important landmarks:** Pain with palpation of specific bony landmarks in the wrist. This is especially important in the wrist because there is little subcutaneous fat over the bony anatomy in the wrist and bone injury is palpated easily. The following 3 areas will be covered in our cases:
    - **Anatomical snuff-box (scaphoid fracture):** anatomical snuff-box (scaphoid injury)
    - **Distal radius:** site of distal radius and distal radial physeal fracture
    - **Distal ulna:** site of distal ulna and distal ulnar physeal fracture and of TFCC injury (area palmar to ulnar styloid process)

2. Elbow

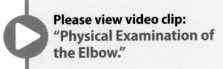

Please view video clip:
"Physical Examination of the Elbow."

- **Inspection:** Visible swelling and deformity.

- **Range of motion (active):** Active flexion, extension, pronation, and supination of the elbow. Limitation of motion in any direction suggests injury.

- **Flexion and extension:** Limitation of motion suggests injury to the humeroulnar articulation and associated soft-tissue structures.
    - **Pronation and supination:** Limitation of motion suggests injury to the radiocapitellar joint in the elbow.

- **Range of motion (passive):** Limitation of passive motion suggests structural injury in the elbow joint.

- **Palpation of important landmarks**
    - **Medial epicondyle and apophysis:** Site of Little League elbow. Pain in athlete who is skeletally mature is consistent with traction apophyseal injury or avulsion fracture at the medial epicondylar apophysis. In athletes who are skeletally mature, pain can be medial epicondylitis (golfer's elbow) or injury to the UCL.
    - **Radiocapitellar joint:** Pain in the radio-capitellar joint, with pronation and supina-tion, suggests bone overload and possible osteochondritis dissecans (OCD) in the capitellum.

- **Special testing**
    - **Ulnar collateral ligament stress test:** To stress the UCL and assess for pain or laxity, or both, that is suggestive of injury.

Radiographs

1. Wrist

Please view video clip:
"Radiographic Evaluation of the Wrist."

Wrist radiographs are generally straightforward. The standard views are anteroposterior (AP) and lateral views of the wrist (figures 6-5 and 6-6), with an ulnar deviation (scaphoid) view used for specific cases of possible scaphoid fractures (Figure 6-7).

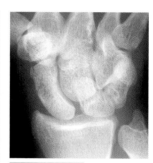
FIGURE 6-7
Scaphoid view of the wrist.

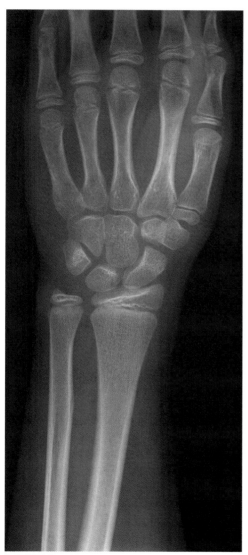

FIGURE 6-5
AP view of the wrist.

Abbreviation: AP, anteroposterior.

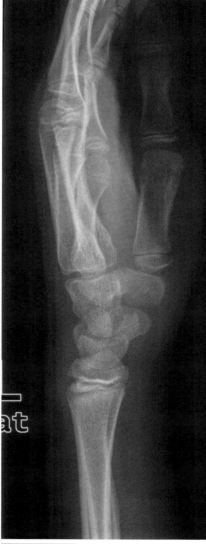

FIGURE 6-6
Lateral view of the wrist.

2. Elbow

Please view video clip: "Radiographic Evaluation of the Elbow."

Most often, the elbow is evaluated with standard AP and lateral views (figures 6-8 and 6-9), which are generally sufficient for most cases of elbow pain and injury.

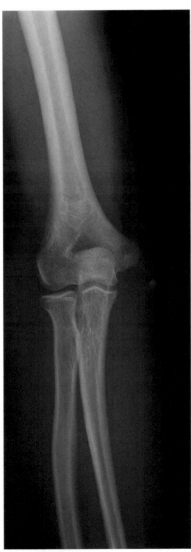

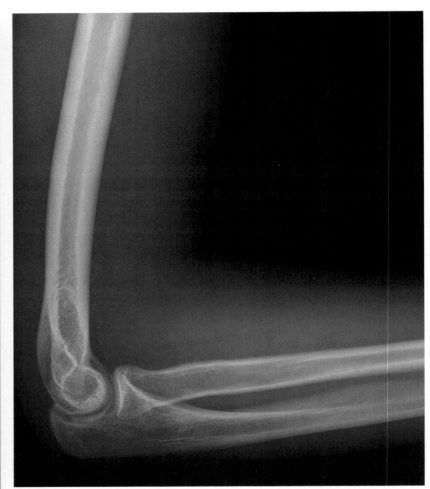

FIGURE 6-9
Lateral view of the elbow.

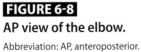

FIGURE 6-8
AP view of the elbow.

Abbreviation: AP, anteroposterior.

Case Files: Wrist and Elbow Injuries

1. Acute Trauma

Case 1

Fall onto outstretched wrist (distal radius and scaphoid bone fractures) in 13-year-old ice skater

Description

A 13-year-old ice skater comes into the office having fallen on her outstretched wrist. This case examines the fall on the outstretched hand mechanism that is the cause of many significant wrist injuries in the young athlete.

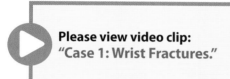

**Please view video clip:
"Case 1: Wrist Fractures."**

Fractures of the distal radius or ulna, or both, account for approximately three-fourths of bony injuries of the wrist. The carpal bones themselves are injured less frequently, but carpal bone injuries account for up to 10% of injuries to the structures of the hand. Because these injuries are frequently encountered in the primary care setting, accurate diagnosis and treatment are crucial to avoiding long-term loss of function and disability (Figure 6-10).

Workup and Management

When diagnosing and managing wrist fractures, it is important to determine whether the patient sustained an extension or flexion injury. Extension fractures result from a fall on an outstretched and pronated hand, otherwise known as a FOOSH injury. The lunate bone acts as a wedge against the articular surface of the radius and causes different injuries, depending on the age of the patient. The Colles fracture is the most common extension fracture pattern, which classically describes a fracture through the distal metaphysis approximately 4 cm proximal to the articular surface of the radius. Now the term is used loosely to describe any distal radius fracture. In children, Colles fractures require a high-energy force to cause the fracture and tend to have more complex intra-articular involvement. In adolescents, the lower epiphysis separates, with dorsal displacement or crushing. In both age groups, the fracture can be complicated by injury to the median nerve, by injury to the sensory branch of the radial nerve, by fracture of the scaphoid or dislocation of the lunate, or by a combination of those. More often, children younger than 10 years of age usually sustain a greenstick fracture of the distal radius, with or without an associated fracture of the distal ulna. Greenstick fractures are incomplete fractures with an intact cortex and periosteum on the concave side.

Flexion fractures of the distal radius are termed Smith or reverse Colles fractures. These terms are used loosely to describe fractures of the distal radius with volar displacement of the fracture fragments. Most often, they are caused by a fall onto a supinated forearm or hand. On striking the ground, the hand locks in supination, while the body's momentum forces the hand into hyper-pronation.

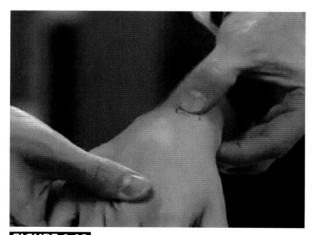

FIGURE 6-10
Palpation of the distal radius.

The scaphoid bone is based in the proximal row of carpal bones but extends into the distal row, making it more vulnerable to injury than the other carpal bones. It is the most frequently injured carpal bone, accounting for 60% to 70% of all carpal fractures.

Because 10% to 15% of scaphoid fractures are not apparent on radiograph, it is, unfortunately, a frequently missed injury. More than 75% of all scaphoid injuries occur at the narrow midportion of the scaphoid (called the waist). Because blood is supplied to the scaphoid on its dorsal surface, near the waist, fractures in this area can compromise blood flow to the bone. As a result, avascular necrosis is a serious complication of this injury (Figure 6-11).

Hyperextension of the wrist is the most common mechanism of scaphoid fracture, either by a direct blow to the palm or a fall on an outstretched hand. Often, scaphoid fractures are associated with other injuries of the wrist, including dislocation of the radiocarpal joint, dislocation between the 2 rows of carpal bones, fracture dislocation of the distal end of the radius, fracture at the base of the thumb metacarpal, and dislocation of the lunate bone.

Routine radiographic evaluations of the wrist, including AP, lateral, and oblique views, are adequate to identify most wrist fractures. When evaluating a fracture of the distal radius or ulna, it is important to check the normal anatomical alignments. The radiocarpal joint viewed on the lateral view radiograph normally has 11° of palmar angulation, with a range of 1° to 23°. Ulnar angulation on the AP view radiograph is normally 15° to 30°. Scaphoid fractures are difficult to see on routine radiographs. Scaphoid view radiographs, taken with the wrist deviated toward the ulna and slightly supinated, can help show the presence of a fracture. For a suspected scaphoid fracture without visualization on radiograph, magnetic resonance imaging (MRI) may be appropriate (Figure 6-12).

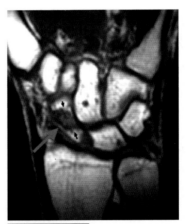

FIGURE 6-12

MRI of wrist demonstrating scaphoid bone fracture (red arrow). It is important to note that most cases of scaphoid fracture will not show on initial radiographic series. Diagnosis is made by history and physical examination. An MRI can be used to confirm presence of a scaphoid fracture.

Abbreviation: MRI, magnetic resonance image.

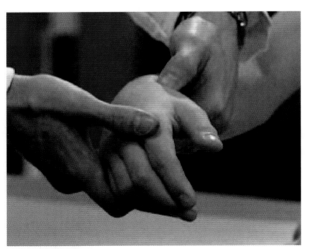

FIGURE 6-11

Palpation of the anatomical snuff-box.

To prevent inadvertent manipulation, any injury to the wrist should be immobilized, with a full forearm splint, before arrival in the emergency department. Once a full history and physical examination have been done, it is important to assess and document neurovascular status before starting reduction. To obtain good functional results, accurate reduction of the fracture is essential.

Historically, the results of nonoperative management of forearm fractures in adults have been poor. In pediatric and adolescent patients, however, treatment is primarily nonoperative because of rapid bone healing and the potential for remodeling residual deformity. Most distal radius fractures in children will heal with 3 to 6 weeks of casting. For scaphoid fractures, place the injured extremity in a short or long arm thumb spica bandage, with the distal interphalangeal joint of the thumb included. The length of the cast remains controversial; however, the long arm thumb spica bandage has been demonstrated to improve rotational stability. Proper orthopedic follow-up is required. Because of the risk of growth arrest, any fracture through the growth plate requires referral to an orthopedic surgeon.

The following video clip will explain splinting techniques for the acutely injured wrist:

Please view video clip:
"Case 1: Splinting of the Acute Wrist Injury."

TAKE-HOME POINTS

Acute Wrist Injury

▶ Acute injury to the wrist generally results from a fall onto the extended hand and wrist. Many types of significant injury can result from this mechanism. The athlete will often come into the office reporting pain and difficulty moving the wrist, and sometimes swelling is present. Physical examination is essential, particularly with the often difficult-to-diagnose scaphoid bone fracture, which is suspected in any patient presenting with pain on palpation in the anatomical snuff-box.

▶ Splinting of the acute wrist injury in the initial stage is appropriate management. This includes a short arm splint, used to immobilize the wrist in most cases, and thumb spica bandage splinting, used to immobilize the wrist and thumb in cases of suspected scaphoid fracture.

Case 2

Ulnar-sided wrist pain in a 15-year-old tennis player

Description

A 15-year-old tennis player with a history of a prior wrist fracture that healed uneventfully with routine casting 1 year ago presents with ulnar-sided wrist pain. This case examines an increasingly diagnosed cause of ulnar-sided wrist pain in adolescent athletes.

The TFCC refers to a convergence of soft-tissue structures between the distal ulna and ulnar-sided carpal bones. This structure functions as the major stabilizer of the DRUJ and cushions loads imparted to the ulnar wrist. Injury to the TFCC in the pediatric and adolescent population most often affects adolescents, rather than school-aged children, and results from trauma, such as a fall on an outstretched hand or a hyper-rotation injury. Many patients will have a history of a distal radius or ulna fracture, or both. Patients with prior distal radius fractures involving the physis can have radial growth arrest. In this scenario, the distal ulna outgrows the distal radius, which is referred to as *positive ulnar variance* (Figure 6-13) and may lead to chronic impaction of the distal ulna on the carpal bones and TFCC (ulnocarpal

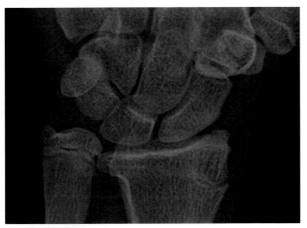

FIGURE 6-13

Plain AP radiographic view demonstrating positive ulnar variance.

Abbreviation: AP, anteroposterior.

impaction syndrome). In the pediatric population, most TFCC injuries result from acute injury, and they can be categorized into 4 types, first described by Palmer and Werner (Table 6-1). Wrist overuse can also lead to TFCC injury, particularly in sports such as gymnastics (ie, repetitive, compressive forces to the ulnar side of the wrist can lead to inflammation of the TFCC, predisposing it to subsequent tears).

Table 6-1. Palmer Classification of Acute Injuries of the Triangular Fibrocartilage Complex

Class	Description
1A	Central perforation or tear
1B	Peripheral ulnar-sided tear
1C	Distal tear (of the ulnocarpal ligaments)
1D	Radial sided tear

Patients with injury to the TFCC may present with concerns of ulnar-sided wrist pain, which is made worse with forceful grip or twisting of the wrist. Some experience popping and clicking with wrist movement. Historical findings may be subtle, as many patients will report pain during sport or more athletic activities but not with activities of daily living.[1] On physical examination, classic findings include a positive "ulnar fovea sign," which is defined as tenderness in the soft spot between the ulnar styloid process, flexor carpi ulnaris tendon, palmar surface of the ulnar head, and pisiform bone. This test has been reported to have 95% sensitivity and 87% sensitivity for foveal disruptions and ulnar-triquetral ligament injuries.[2] Patients may also report pain with ulnar or radial deviation of the wrist. The "press test," during which the patient lifts himself or herself out of a chair while bearing weight on extended wrists, is another useful maneuver. It is also important to assess for DRUJ instability, by looking for the "piano key sign," or a prominent and ballottable distal ulna with full forearm pronation.

Workup and Management

Patients should be evaluated with plain radiographs of the wrist, including neutral forearm rotation AP, lateral, and oblique views, to rule out other abnormalities (eg, physeal stress fractures, scaphoid injury, hook of hamate bone injury) and to assess for potential concomitant TFCC wrist injuries. For patients whose conservative treatment has failed or who have persistent wrist pain, advanced imaging, using MRI or magnetic resonance arthrography (MRA), may assist in diagnosing TFCC injuries, along with extensor carpi ulnaris tendon, DRUJ tendon, and chondral injuries[3] (Figure 6-14). It should be noted that MRI and MRA can be difficult to interpret and should be viewed alongside clinical history and physical. Wrist arthroscopy is currently the criterion standard for diagnosing injuries to the TFCC.

Most symptomatic, acute TFCC tears can be managed conservatively for at least 4 to 6 weeks, depending on the severity of symptoms. Nonoperative management includes immobilization with splinting, icing, restriction of exacerbating activity, and physical and occupational therapy. Therapy should focus on generalized range of motion and strengthening exercises of the wrist.[4] If pain is persistent, conservative treatment has failed, significant DRUJ instability was present on physical examination, or a tear was seen on advanced imaging, referral to an orthopedic surgeon, to discuss surgical intervention with arthroscopy and TFCC repair, should be considered.[4,5] For central TFCC tears, arthroscopic debridement has been reported as the preferred treatment, and for peripheral tears, open or arthroscopic repair is performed. Other procedures may be done at the same time to address coexisting injury, such as DRUJ instability or ulnocarpal impaction.

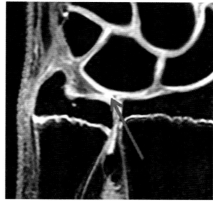

FIGURE 6-14

MRI demonstrating TFCC tear at its radial attachment (type 1D TFCC tear) (see red arrow).

Abbreviations: MRI, magnetic resonance image; TFCC, triangular fibrocartilage complex.

TAKE-HOME POINT

Triangular Fibrocartilage Complex Injury

▶ Patients with triangular fibrocartilage complex injuries often present with ulnar-sided wrist pain after acute trauma, such as a fall onto an extended wrist, or a hyper-pronation or hyper-supination event. It can also present as chronic pain in a patient with a remote history of a wrist fracture. The history may be significant only for pain during sport or strenuous activities. Physical examination findings include a positive "ulnar fovea sign," positive "press test" result, and pain with terminal wrist motions. Plain radiographs of the wrist are important in ruling out bony abnormalities. Advanced imaging, with magnetic resonance imaging or magnetic resonance arthrography, may be helpful in identifying triangular fibrocartilage complex tears and coexisting injuries, but findings can be difficult to interpret. Initial conservative treatment with immobilization, activity modification, and physical and occupational therapy is appropriate in most cases. Failed nonoperative treatment, persistent pain, and gross distal radioulnar joint instability warrant surgical consultation by an orthopedic surgeon.

2. Overuse Injury

Case 3
Wrist pain ("gymnast's wrist") in a 12-year-old gymnast

Description

A 12-year-old gymnast presents to the office with 3 months of achy right wrist pain that occurs during and after gymnastics activities.

"Gymnast's wrist" is a colloquial term used to describe repetitive stress injury to the distal radius physis. A unique aspect of gymnastics is the regular use of upper extremities to support the body weight with impact-loading activities. Events such as the pommel horse, floor exercise, and balance beam subject the wrist joint to recurrent loading. The wrist is subject to forces in gymnastics that can exceed twice the gymnast's body weight, and rates of loading up to 16 times the body weight have been reported.[6,7] Under these conditions, wrist pain is extremely common in gymnasts of both sexes, affecting approximately 45% to 80% of participants.[8-12] Risk factors include older age at initiation of gymnastics training, higher gymnastic skill levels, and higher-intensity training.[9]

The precise pathophysiology of gymnast's wrist remains incompletely understood, but it is hypothesized that repetitive compressive loads across the physis lead to vascular insufficiency and mechanical failure. Although most experts have described this as a compression injury, some have also suggested that the radiographic findings support more of a traction than compression injury at the physis, related to weight bearing on the palms and using the wrist almost as an ankle joint.[13]

Gymnasts who are skeletally immature with chronic wrist pain typically describe a vague achy pain on the dorsal and central portion of the wrist that may occur during and after gymnastics activities. In advanced cases, the wrist pain is present even at rest. It most commonly occurs in gymnasts 10 to 14 years of age. It is thought that the increased incidence in this age-group is likely related to their growth spurt in this period, during which the distal radial growth plate is undergoing its slow process of ossification, or physeal closure. Wrist pain that is limited to the ulnar side of the joint is more common in gymnasts who are skeletally mature (whose radial and ulnar physes are closed), in whom injury to the TFCC has been well described. Triangular fibrocartilage complex injuries are discussed in case 2 of this chapter.

In addition to tenderness to palpation over the dorso-central wrist, physical examination may demonstrate subtle loss of wrist extension. In advanced cases, with ulnocarpal impaction secondary to distal radius growth retardation and normal distal ulnar growth, ulnar deviation may be restricted. Tenderness to palpation over the ulnar side of the wrist may be indicative of ulnar overgrowth and possible TFCC injury.

Workup and Management

Radiographs may show characteristic features consistent with distal radial physeal stress injury, including physeal widening, cystic or sclerotic changes of the metaphysis, beaking of the epiphysis near the radial styloid process, premature physeal closure, and positive ulnar variance (Figure 6-15). The different grades of gymnast wrist based on radiographic findings are depicted in Table 6-2. As for ulnar variance, it is known that ulnar positive variance is more common in young gymnasts than in age-matched non-gymnasts, but the origin and clinical significance remain unknown.[9] It is

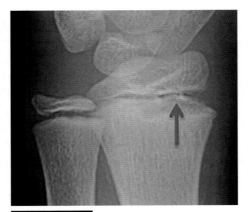

FIGURE 6-15

Radiograph demonstrating widening and irregularity (see red arrow) of the physeal borders of the distal radius.

unclear whether ulnar positive variance is an independent cause of wrist pain or result of abnormal radial growth.

Table 6-2. Radiographic Grades of "Gymnast's Wrist"

Radiographic Grade	Findings
0	Normal (on plain radiographs)
1	Physeal haziness, irregularity of physeal borders
2	Cystic changes, metaphyseal sclerosis, metaphyseal beaking
3	Physeal widening

On MRI, the findings are edema on the metaphyseal and epiphyseal sides of the physis. Cartilaginous ingrowth into the metaphysis can also be seen. This is thought to result from failure of ossification of the physeal cartilage in the metaphysis, which has been attributed to metaphyseal injury and bony bridging from epiphyseal trauma.[14,15]

As with most overuse injuries, the best treatment is prevention of the inciting event. Prevention measures such as gradual advances in training intensity during periods of rapid skeletal growth and alternating loading activities during training can be taken.[4] It remains controversial whether wrist braces have any protective effect in the prevention of gymnast's wrist. The thought is that limiting extension may limit excessive loading of the radial physis. Once the diagnosis has been made, rest of up to 2 to 3 months must be initiated, or at least until the patient is pain-free with absent signs (no tenderness or pain with extremes of range of motion). A very gradual return to play is recommended. Even with resolution of symptoms, serial radiographic evaluations are recommended every 6 to 12 months until skeletal maturity, to confirm resolution of radiographic changes and absence of radial physeal arrest.[4] Patients with radial physeal arrest and symptomatic ulnar positive variance would likely benefit from surgical intervention. The options include wrist arthroscopy, TFCC repair, DRUJ stabilization, ulnar shortening osteotomy, and distal ulnar epiphysiodesis.

TAKE-HOME POINT

"Gymnast's Wrist"

▶ Patients are most commonly 10 to 14 years of age with months of dorso-centrally located, vague, achy wrist pain. Symptoms may occur during and after gymnastics activities. Radiographs may show characteristic features consistent with distal radial physeal stress injury, including physeal widening, cystic or sclerotic changes of the metaphysis, beaking of the epiphysis near the radial styloid process, premature physeal closure, and positive ulnar variance. If the diagnosis is suspected but radiographic findings are equivocal or negative, a magnetic resonance image can be obtained and may show edema, physeal widening, or physeal cartilage extension into the metaphysis. Once the diagnosis has been made, rest must be initiated until the patient is no longer symptomatic. Patients with radial physeal arrest and symptomatic ulnar positive variance would likely benefit from surgical intervention. Prevention measures can be taken, such as gradual advances in training intensity during periods of rapid skeletal growth and alternating loading activities during training.

Case 4
Elbow pain (Little League elbow) in 13-year-old baseball pitcher

Description

A 13-year-old baseball pitcher comes into the office reporting medial elbow pain with throwing. This case examines the patient with elbow pain with throwing.

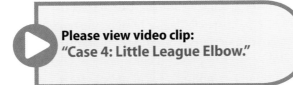

> ▶ **Please view video clip:**
> **"Case 4: Little League Elbow."**

Little League elbow describes a group of elbow problems related to the stress of repetitive throwing in young athletes. During the throwing motion, a great deal of stress is placed on the medial structures of the elbow, including the medial epicondyle, medial epicondylar apophysis, and UCL complex. As a result, the lateral structures (ie, radial head and capitellum) are compressed. When tissue breakdown exceeds tissue repair, overuse injuries ensue. Patients with Little League elbow come into the office reporting pain with throwing.

As is true with all types of overuse injury, the key issue that the practitioner is looking for is pain that limits ability to throw. If that is the case, it is important to "hold the athlete out" from throwing activities, find the proper diagnosis, and devise a treatment plan that fixes the injury and provides a framework to prevent it from recurring.

Little League elbow encompasses several conditions in the young thrower, including

- Medial epicondylar apophysitis or avulsion fractures
- Ulnar collateral ligament sprain
- Osteochondrosis and osteochondritis of the capitellum
- Deformation and osteochondrosis of the radial head

- Olecranon apophysitis, with or without delayed closure
- Hypertrophy of the ulna

It is tremendously important to emphasize that young athletes who report elbow pain should be taken seriously. As is the case with most injuries in young athletes, early detection makes treatment easier. A delay in diagnosis can lead to more substantial problems.

The most common location for elbow pain in the young thrower is the medial elbow. This is termed *medial elbow overload,* and it encompasses a range of severity, from medial apophysitis in the athlete who is skeletally immature to rupture of the UCL in the throwing athlete who is skeletally mature.

Athletes with medial epicondylar apophysitis report medial elbow pain, initially after throwing, that progresses to persistent pain. Because the medial epicondyle is the last ossification center in the elbow to close, it has the longest exposure to medial distraction forces in the elbow. Thus, medial epicondyle apophysitis is the most common elbow injury during childhood (before the appearance of all the secondary ossification centers). These patients typically present with pain directly over the medial epicondyle. The pain can be exacerbated by asking the patient to flex a closed wrist against light resistance (Figure 6-16). Other

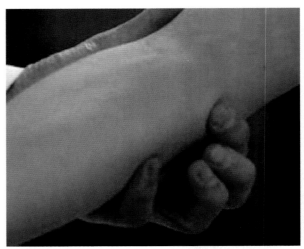

FIGURE 6-16

Palpation of the medial epicondyle.

physical examination findings include tenderness to palpation over the medial epicondyle and worsening pain with valgus stress.

Workup and Management

Radiographic findings of medial epicondylar apophysitis (irritation of the medial epicondyle) can range from normal to widening at the medial epicondyle (Figure 6-17). In general, the more the widening at the epicondyle is present, the more significant the injury.

Treatment first includes rest from throwing until symptoms subside. Typically, 2 to 4 weeks of rest is necessary for complete resolution. Ice packs to the elbow for 30 minutes every 4 hours for 48 hours can help eliminate the acute pain. Because of the possibility of masking pain symptoms, nonsteroidal anti-inflammatory drugs should be avoided.

Patients recover at different rates, so return to play should be determined individually and only when pain has fully subsided. Full strength and range of motion should be present before full return to play. Throwing should be reintroduced gradually, and it should be stopped immediately if pain recurs. Proper throwing techniques should be reinforced and practiced before each season and before return to play after injury. Physical therapists or pitching coaches, or both, can help ensure proper throwing mechanics and implement a preventive strengthening program.

The best treatment is prevention. At the beginning of each season, players should increase the number and intensity of pitches gradually. During the season, the number of pitches thrown each week should be monitored carefully. Parents, coaches, and players should be made aware of the recommended guidelines for numbers of pitches (see tables 5-1 and 5-2 in Chapter 5, Shoulder Injuries in the Young Athlete) and types of pitches that are safe for young baseball players.

Medial epicondylar avulsion fractures should be considered if the patient describes a sudden "pop" in the elbow, followed by the acute onset of pain. Physical examination findings are usually similar to the findings for the patient with medial epicondylar apophysitis. Plain radiographs will show avulsion of the medial epicondylar apophysis (Figure 6-18). Surgical consultation should be sought with more than 2 mm of displacement of the apophysis or with any ulnar nerve findings, including radicular pain into the ring and little fingers.

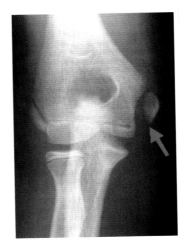

FIGURE 6-18

AP radiographic view of elbow showing medial epicondylar avulsion fracture (see red arrow). This injury can require surgery in some cases and requires referral.

Abbreviation: AP, anteroposterior.

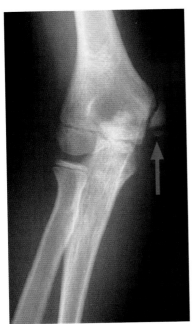

FIGURE 6-17

AP radiographic view of the elbow showing widening at the medial epicondylar apophysis (red arrow). In this case, radiographic findings indicate that the problem is more advanced Little League elbow. If patients report medial pain with throwing, radiographic findings may be normal in appearance and show no evidence of widening.

Abbreviation: AP, anteroposterior.

Ulnar collateral ligament sprains and full-thickness tears occur in throwers who are skeletally mature, as well as in other athletes who sustain valgus impact injuries to an outstretched arm. On physical examination, valgus stress at 30° of elbow flexion reproduces medial pain and instability. This test is best performed with the forearm in pronation (Figure 6-19).

Treatment for UCL strains is rest, for at least 2 to 3 months, with no throwing activities. Ice can be used to control symptoms, but nonsteroidal anti-inflammatory drugs generally are not recommended, because they can mask pain, which is an important feedback symptom of the throwing athlete with UCL pain.

Athletes with persistent UCL pain with throwing need to undergo MRI so injury to the ligament can be evaluated (Figure 6-20). Rupture of the UCL is treated surgically, with UCL reconstruction (often referred to as Tommy John surgery, named after one of the first high-profile professional baseball pitchers to undergo this procedure). This is a highly specialized surgical procedure and should be performed only by an orthopedic surgeon who is well-trained in this specific technique.

In cases of chronic medial elbow overload, it is essential to treat not only the ligament but also

the underlying reason for the injury. In general, overload to the medial elbow results from a poor throwing mechanic and insufficient shoulder girdle strength. Treatment for any case of medial elbow overload should include not only a correction of the throwing mechanic (often through the use of a pitching coach) but also referral to a physical therapist who is knowledgeable in the rehabilitation of throwing athletes.

On the lateral aspect of the elbow, the radiocapitellar joint is a common site for Little League elbow. In this compression side of the elbow, pitchers and throwers commonly report pain after releasing the ball. Injuries in this area, termed *compression injuries*, include a range from pain in the capitellum, the distal area of the humerus, to OCD, a more serious injury involving permanent bone injury in the capitellum.

Depending on the stage of the lesions, treatment for OCD lesions in the capitellum ranges from conservative to surgical. Increasingly, MRI is being used as a useful study to pick up edema (swelling) in the capitellum before a lesion progresses to full-blown OCD (Figure 6-21). For that reason, care and attention should be given to the athlete who reports lateral elbow pain, including physical examination, radiographic studies, and, if the capitellum has focal pain on pronation and supination of the elbow, an MRI study.

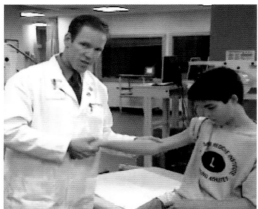

FIGURE 6-19

Valgus stress test for UCL strength.

Abbreviation: UCL, ulnar collateral ligament.

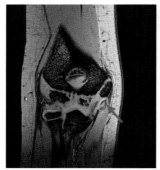

FIGURE 6-20

MRI of elbow showing rupture of the UCL (see red arrow).

Abbreviations: MRI, magnetic resonance image; UCL, ulnar collateral ligament.

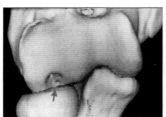

FIGURE 6-21

MRI of the elbow showing edema in the capitellum with an OCD lesion.

Abbreviations: MRI, magnetic resonance image; OCD, osteochondritis dissecans.

Finally, posterior elbow pain (pain in the olecranon) can be problematic for pediatric and adolescent throwing athletes. These athletes present to the office with pain in the posterior aspect of the elbow, usually with ball release (Figure 6-22). In this case, obtaining a radiograph is helpful to evaluate for avulsed or delayed closure in the apophysis of the olecranon (Figure 6-23). Olecranon apophysitis generally is more self-limiting than medial or lateral elbow pain, and it is treated with a combination of 6 to 8 weeks of rest and shoulder strengthening. Athletes can usually return to play when they are pain-free.

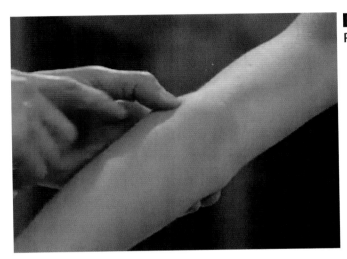

FIGURE 6-22
Palpation of the radiocapitellar joint.

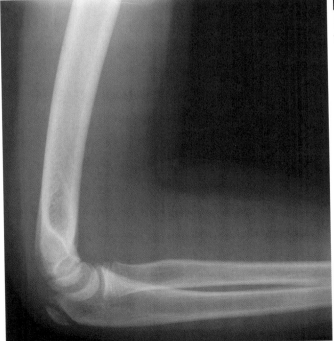

FIGURE 6-23
Lateral radiographic view of elbow showing widening at the olecranon apophysis.

Rehabilitation and Prevention Exercises

Prevention exercises for throwers are tremendously important. Any athlete who has had a previous elbow injury should be evaluated by a physician and a physical therapist before doing these exercises. This is because, in the circumstance of a previous injury, there are specific issues for each athlete, such as a specific injury, a specific area of vulnerability, or a specific area of muscular weakness, that are best addressed in a one-on-one environment.

In the overhead athlete, great demands are placed on the shoulder, elbow, and wrist. If the athlete presents with postural or scapular weakness, or both, even greater demands are placed throughout the distal kinetic chain of the upper extremity. Any overhead athlete should incorporate core stabilization and scapular and shoulder strengthening into his or her program, in addition to the wrist exercises. The following exercises are helpful for the prevention of throwing injury in the healthy adolescent athlete:

Wrist Extension (targets wrist extensors)

1. Begin with the forearm supported and with the hand hanging off the supporting surface (palm down) holding a 1- to 2-lb weight.
2. Bend the wrist up and hold this position for 2 to 5 seconds.
3. Slowly return to the starting position.
4. Perform 10 repetitions; do 2 to 3 sets.

To advance: **Increase the amount of weight by 0.5 lb.**

Wrist Pronation and Supination (targets pronators and supinators)

1. Begin with the forearm supported and with the hand holding a 1- to 2-lb weight in a palm-up position.
2. Turn palm down and turn palm up, maintaining forearm contact with the supporting surface.
3. Perform 10 repetitions; do 2 to 3 sets.

To advance: **Increase the amount of weight by 0.5 lb.**

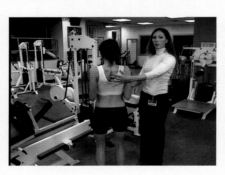

Scapular Retraction (targets middle trapezius and rhomboid muscles)

Please view video clip: **"Middle Trapezius and Rhomboid Muscle Exercises."**

1. Stand erect, holding therapeutic band lax in each hand with arms outstretched.
2. Squeeze the scapula together while bringing elbows next to the trunk.
3. Hold the position for 2 to 5 seconds, and slowly bring arms back to the starting position.

To advance: **Increase the band resistance.**

Prone Shoulder Elevation (targets lower trapezius and shoulder musculature)

1. Lie on the stomach on a raised surface, with one arm hanging over it.
2. Raise the arm with a straight elbow and thumbs up, toward the sky, until arm is parallel with the ear. Focus on squeezing the scapula closer to your spine and downward.
3. Hold the position for 2 to 5 seconds, and slowly bring the arm back to the starting position.

To advance: **Do exercise with both arms simultaneously.**

continued

Rehabilitation and Prevention Exercises, *continued*

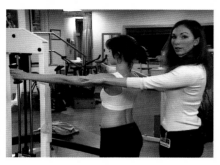

Scaption (targets synchronization of the scapular stabilizers with shoulder muscles)

Please view video clip: **"Scapular Stabilizer Exercises."**

1. Stand erect with shoulders back.
2. Elevate the arms in a V formation (as depicted) to shoulder height, with thumbs up, toward the ceiling.
3. Hold the position for 2 to 5 seconds, and slowly bring the arms back to the starting position.

***To advance:* Add 0.5 to 1 lb at a time. Do not exceed 4 lb unless you are under medical supervision.**

Wall Push-ups With a Plus (targets serratus anterior and provides proprioception while engaging scapular and rotator cuff muscles)

1. Place both hands on the wall at least shoulder width apart, and gradually walk both feet away from the wall.
2. Maintain the trunk and body in a straight line, with tight abdominal muscles.
3. Bend your elbows for the push-up.

For the "plus," straighten the elbows, and push away from the wall.

TAKE-HOME POINTS

Little League Elbow

▶ Elbow pain in throwing athletes is a common problem. It is important to try and distinguish the type of pain an athlete is describing (ie, medial, lateral, or posterior pain). Medial elbow pain is the most common and generally is a traction apophyseal injury in the athlete who is skeletally immature and an injury to the ulnar collateral ligament in the throwing athlete who is skeletally mature. Prompt diagnosis and intervention can fix this problem and prevent a more serious injury. Lateral pain in the thrower is most likely an overload of the radiocapitellar joint. If allowed to progress, this can develop into osteochondritis dissecans. Again, prompt diagnosis is essential. Magnetic resonance imaging can be useful in showing edema in the capitellum before the full osteochondritis dissecans lesion develops.

▶ Posterior pain is olecranon apophysitis in the athlete who is skeletally immature and triceps tendinitis in the athlete whose elbow is skeletally mature.

▶ In all cases of overuse injury from throwing, the keys are an evaluation of the injury and an assessment of the factors that led to the injury. These factors can include the number of pitches being thrown, the throwing mechanic, and the underlying strength of the athlete. These are all issues that can be effectively modified.

References

1. Bae DS, Waters PM. Pediatric distal radius fractures and triangular fibrocartilage complex injuries. *Hand Clin.* 2006;22(1):43–53

2. Tay SC, Tomita K, Berger RA. The "ulnar fovea sign" for defining ulnar wrist pain: an analysis of sensitivity and specificity. *J Hand Surg Am.* 2007;32(4):438–444

3. Smith TO, Drew B, Toms AP, Jerosch-Herold C, Chojnowski AJ. Diagnostic accuracy of magnetic resonance imaging and magnetic resonance arthrography for triangular fibrocartilaginous complex injury: a systematic review and meta-analysis. *J Bone Joint Surg Am.* 2012;94(9):824–832

4. Waters PM, Bae DS. *Pediatric Hand and Upper Limb Surgery: A Practical Guide.* Philadelphia, PA: Lippincott Williams & Wilkins; 2012

5. Rettig AC. Athletic injuries of the wrist and hand. Part I: traumatic injuries of the wrist. *Am J Sports Med.* 2003;31(6):1038–1048

6. Koh TJ, Grabiner MD, Weiker GG. Technique and ground reaction forces in the back handspring. *Am J Sports Med.* 1992;20(1):61–66

7. Markolf KL, Shapiro MS, Mandelbaum BR, Teurlings L. Wrist loading patterns during pommel horse exercises. *J Biomech.* 1990;23(10):1001–1011

8. DiFiori JP, Puffer JC, Aish B, Dorey F. Wrist pain in young gymnasts: frequency and effects upon training over 1 year. *Clin J Sport Med.* 2002;12(6):348–353

9. DiFiori JP, Puffer JC, Aish B, Dorey F. Wrist pain, distal radial physeal injury, and ulnar variance in young gymnasts: does a relationship exist? *Am J Sports Med.* 2002;30(6):879–885

10. DiFiori JP, Puffer JC, Mandelbaum BR, Mar S. Factors associated with wrist pain in the young gymnast. *Am J Sports Med.* 1996;24(1):9–14

11. Caine D, Roy S, Singer KM, Broekhoff J. Stress changes of the distal radial growth plate. A radiographic survey and review of the literature. *Am J Sports Med.* 1992;20(3):290–298

12. Mandelbaum BR, Bartolozzi AR, Davis CA, Teurlings L, Bragonier B. Wrist pain syndrome in the gymnast. Pathogenetic, diagnostic, and therapeutic considerations. *Am J Sports Med.* 1989;17(3):305–317

13. Rang M. Syndromology. In: Wenger DR, Rang M, eds. *The Art and Practice of Children's Orthopaedics.* New York, NY: Raven Press; 1993:627–655

14. Ecklund K, Jaramillo D. Patterns of premature physeal arrest: MR imaging of 111 children. *AJR Am J Roentgenol.* 2002;178(4):967–972

15. Jaramillo D, Laor T, Zaleske DJ. Indirect trauma to the growth plate: results of MR imaging after epiphyseal and metaphyseal injury in rabbits. *Radiology.* 1993;187(1):171–178

CHAPTER 7

Hip and Spine Injuries in the Young Athlete

Greg Canty, MD, FAAP

Anatomical Overview

1. Hip and Pelvis
2. Spine

Physical Examination

1. Hip
2. Spine

Radiographs

1. Hip
2. Spine

Case Files: Hip and Spine Injuries

1. Acute Trauma
   - Case 1: Acute hip injury (apophyseal avulsion fracture of the pelvis) in 16-year-old soccer player
   - Case 2: Acute neck injury ("burners" and "stingers") in 17-year-old football player

2. Overuse Injury
   - Case 3: Hip pain (femoral neck stress fracture) in 17-year-old runner
   - Case 4: Lumbar spine pain (spondylolysis) in 15-year-old volleyball player

Anatomical Overview

1. Hip and Pelvis

Hip injuries are quite common in the adolescent athlete. The hip is a ball-and-socket joint formed by the articulation of the proximal end of the femur, or femoral head (the ball), and the cuplike acetabulum of the pelvis (the socket). The cartilage-covered femoral head is the spherical endpoint of the femoral neck, which diverges proximally and medially from the vertically oriented shaft of the femur at an angle of approximately 135°. The epiphysis of the femoral head is the region of bone proximal to the cartilaginous growth plate, or physis, of the proximal femur. The epiphysis sits within the acetabular socket and is a relatively common site of pathology in conditions such as slipped capital

femoral epiphysis (SCFE) and Legg-Calvé-Perthes disease. At the medial, posterior base of the femoral neck is the lesser trochanter, which is the insertion point for the tendon of the iliopsoas, the major flexor of the hip. Figure 7-1 reviews the bony anatomy of the adolescent hip and pelvis.

The acetabulum represents the triangular junction of the 3 major segments of the pelvis (specifically, the ilium, ischium, and pubis). A surrounding ringlike fibrocartilaginous labrum deepens the acetabular socket to enhance hip joint stability. The hip joint is surrounded by a soft-tissue capsule, several ligaments, and several muscles and tendons, which have origination or insertion sites along the bony prominences of the pelvis. These prominences, or apophyses, are cartilaginous secondary growth centers in adolescents, which generally close around

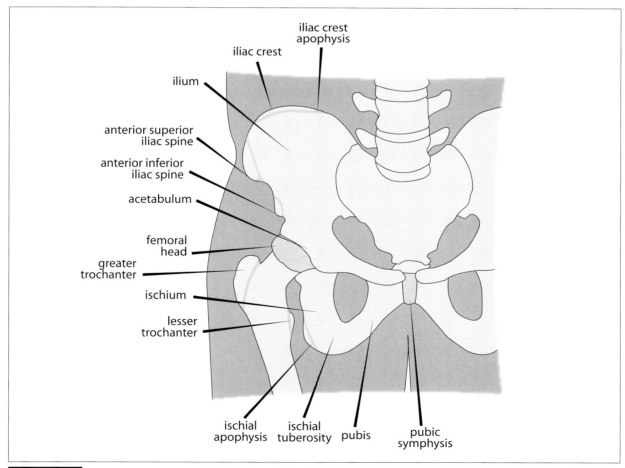

FIGURE 7-1

Anterior view of pelvis with labeled apophyses.

age 16 years in girls and age 18 in boys. Remember, growth centers close according to stages of pubertal development rather than age, so closure for each patient is independent of any one-size-fits-all formula.

The apophyses of the adolescent hip are a common site of unique avulsion injuries. These happen when the muscle-tendon attachment aggressively contracts against the immature apophysis. Examples include

- **Anterior-superior iliac spine (ASIS):** origin of the sartorius

- **Anterior-inferior iliac spine (AIIS):** origin of one belly, or head, of the rectus femoris (the central, superficial muscle of the quadriceps femoris)

- **Iliac crest:** insertion of the external and internal oblique muscles

- **Ischial tuberosity (posterior aspect):** origin of the hamstring muscles (the semimembranosus, semitendinosus, and biceps femoris)

2. Spine

The spine consists of 33 vertically aligned embryological segments, or vertebrae, in continuity with each other. The spine has 5 major divisions, running from superior to inferior: cervical (7 vertebrae, C1–C7), thoracic (12 vertebrae, T1–T12), lumbar (5 vertebrae, L1–L5), sacral (5 fused vertebrae), and coccyx (4 fused vertebrae).

Except for C1 and C2, the cervical, thoracic, and lumbar vertebrae are separated by collagenous intervertebral disks, which provide cushioning and mobility. Each individual vertebra may be divided into several parts, from anterior to posterior. Anteriorly, the vertebral body, along with the adjacent intervertebral disk, is the major weight-bearing portion of the spine. The vertebral canal sits posterior to the body and houses the spinal cord and its surrounding dura mater. The pedicles are the cylindrical bridges that connect the vertebral bodies to the posterior aspect of the spine and serve as sidewalls for the canal. The neural foramina are openings between the pedicles, through which nerve roots from the spinal cord exit the canal before becoming peripheral nerves. The laminae are thin plates of bone that sit posterior to the canal and offer protection posteriorly. Diverging horizontally on each side of the laminae are the transverse processes, and then, posteriorly, a single, central, bony extension becomes the long spine. These processes serve as attachment sites for the surrounding paraspinal muscles.

Each vertebra also has 4 facets that extend off the superior and inferior aspects of the laminae to form facet joints, which are cartilaginous articulations between adjacent vertebra. In the cervical spine, the various nerve roots exiting the neural foramina form reattachments to each other in the brachial plexus. This complex neural network lies deep in the interval between the neck and the arm to innervate the entire upper extremity. Also, lumbar and sacral plexuses provide innervation to the lower extremities and pelvis. Injury to the spine can involve any of these structures, including bone, nerve, disk, ligament, or muscle. Figure 7-2 reviews the basic anatomy of the spine.

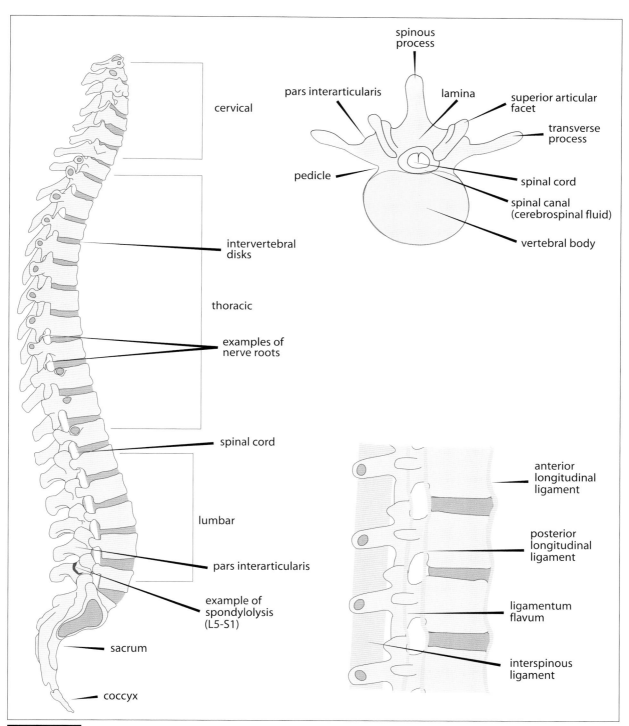

FIGURE 7-2

AP and lateral views of the spine.

Abbreviation: AP, anteroposterior.

Physical Examination

1. Hip

 Please view video clip: "Physical Examination of the Hip."

- **Gait:** patient walking and presence of antalgic gait (limp)
- **Seated hip examination (passive motion):** used to assess passive rotation of the hip joint
  - **Internal rotation:** in the seated or prone position, outward rotation of the ankle and lower leg producing an internal rotation at the femoral head
  - **External rotation:** in the seated or prone position, inward rotation of the ankle and lower leg producing external rotation of the femoral head
- **Standing hip examination**
  - **Palpation of apophyses**
    1. **Anterior-superior iliac spine:** origin of the sartorius
    2. **Anterior-inferior iliac spine:** origin of the rectus femoris
- **Prone hip examination**
  - **Palpation of ischial apophysis and tuberosity:** origin of the hamstring muscles

2. Spine

 Please view video clip: "Physical Examination of the Spine."

- **Cervical spine**
  - **Range of motion:** flexion, extension, and rotation
  - **Palpation:** long spine, looking for bone-related injury
- **Spurling test:** 45° of rotation and ipsilateral extension to assess for cervical root impingement
  - **Upper-extremity strength and reflexes:** major muscle groups of upper extremities (biceps brachii, triceps brachii, brachioradialis, hand muscles, and wrist muscles) to assess for weakness and biceps brachii, triceps brachii, and brachioradialis reflexes
- **Thoracic spine**
  - **Adams forward flexion test:** best screening test for thoracic curves, such as scoliosis and kyphosis (Patients place both palms together, extend arms, and bend forward.)
- **Lumbar spine**
  - **Visual inspection:** to assess for a hyperlordosis or scoliotic deformity in the spine, along with comparison of scapular and pelvic height
  - **Forward flexion test:** to assess for diskogenic back pain, which is often exacerbated with forward flexion
  - **Extension:** to assess for posterior element bone and facet joint pain, such as spondylolysis (Also, consider side-specific, provocative hyperextension maneuvers [eg, the Stork test].)
  - **Rotation:** to assess for the presence of pain along the paraspinal muscles
- **Neurologic assessment and strength testing**
  - **Patellar reflex**
  - **Achilles reflex**
  - **Heel walk**
  - **Toe walk**

Radiographs

1. Hip

Please view video clip: "Radiographic Evaluation of the Hip."

Because of the many ossification centers that can be injured, obtaining radiographs of the hip and pelvis is extremely important after acute injuries in the adolescent athlete. Most apophyseal avulsion injuries are visible with an anteroposterior (AP) pelvis radiographic view (Figure 7-3), which shows the major apophyses, including the ASIS, AIIS, iliac crest, and ischial tuberosity.

Anteroposterior and frog-leg lateral radiographic views of the hip and pelvis are recommended when looking for less common avulsions of the lesser trochanter or other hip conditions, such as SCFE (Figure 7-4). A simple, commonly used radiographic tool is Klein line, a straight line drawn along the lateral, or superior, border of the femoral neck extended toward the acetabulum. In a normally structured hip, Klein line bisects a portion of the femoral head and epiphysis. In mild SCFE, the line runs along the superior border of the epiphysis, and with more advanced SCFE the line clearly demonstrates slippage of the epiphysis, below Klein line.

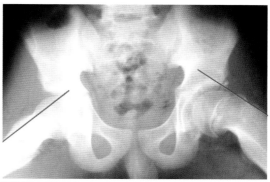

FIGURE 7-4
Frog-leg lateral view of the hip with Klein lines drawn in. The right hip shows normal structure, and the left hip shows SCFE.
Abbreviation: SCFE, slipped capital femoral epiphysis.

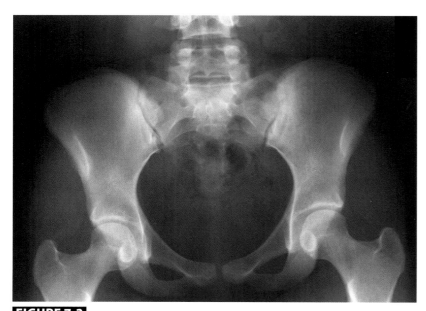

FIGURE 7-3
AP view of the pelvis.
Abbreviation: AP, anteroposterior.

2. Spine

Spine radiographs remain the best tool for initial imaging of acute and chronic spinal injuries.

- For cervical spine injuries, 3 views of the cervical spine are recommended, including AP, lateral, and odontoid views (figures 7-5–7-7). If further concerned about cervical instability or chronic injury, consider the addition of flexion and extension views (figures 7-8–7-9).

Please view video clip: "Radiographic Evaluation of the Spine."

- For thoracic spine injury, AP and lateral views are usually sufficient.
- For lumbar spine injuries, AP, lateral, and oblique views are helpful (figures 7-10–7-12). The lateral view is especially helpful for demonstrating spondylolisthesis, and the oblique views are helpful for spotting spondylolysis.

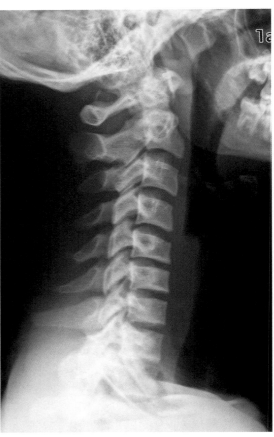
FIGURE 7-6
Lateral view of the cervical spine.

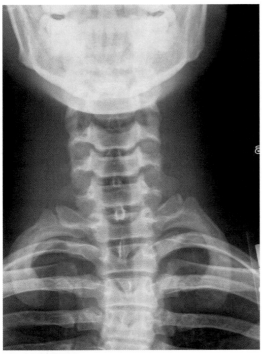
FIGURE 7-5
AP view of the cervical spine.
Abbreviation: AP, anteroposterior.

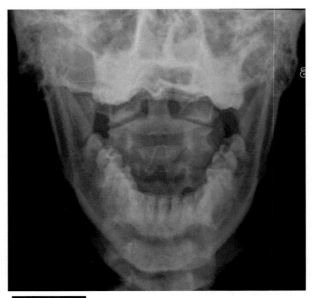
FIGURE 7-7
Odontoid view of the cervical spine.

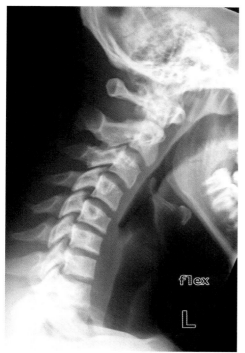

FIGURE 7-8
Flexion view of the cervical spine.

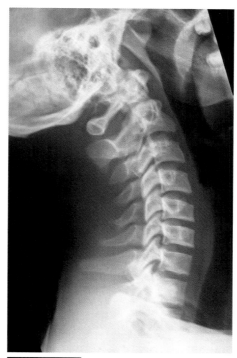

FIGURE 7-9
Extension view of the cervical spine.

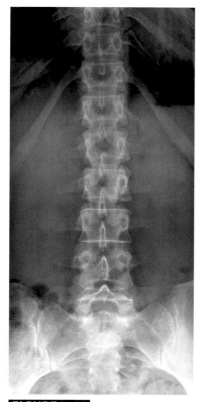

FIGURE 7-10
AP view of the lumbar spine.
Abbreviation: AP, anteroposterior.

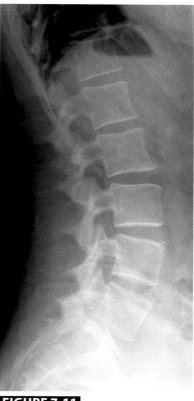

FIGURE 7-11
Lateral view of the lumbar spine.

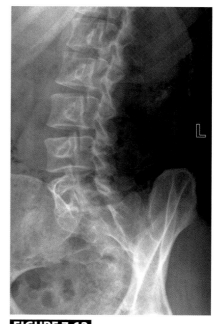

FIGURE 7-12
Oblique view of the lumbar spine.

Case Files: Hip and Spine Injuries

1. Acute Trauma

Case 1

Acute hip injury (apophyseal avulsion fractures of the pelvis) in a 16-year-old soccer player

Description

Because of the variety of possible origins and patient presentations, acute hip pain in a young athlete can represent a diagnostic challenge. In this case, a 16-year-old soccer player was running down the field, went to kick, and felt a "pop" in her hip. She comes limping into the office.

**Please view video clip:
"Case 1: Pelvis Fracture and Slipped Capital Femoral Epiphysis."**

Apophyseal avulsion fractures of the pelvis are increasingly common in athletes performing explosive maneuvers such as kicking (soccer), sprinting (track), and gymnastics. However, avulsions may occur in any sport, or even non-athletic activities. The classic history is a pop during maximal contraction of a muscle group, such as when kicking a soccer ball. The apophyses remain cartilaginous into adolescence before eventually ossifying with the larger segments of the bony pelvis. These areas are often weaker than the attached tendon, which makes them susceptible to acute avulsion and repetitive microtrauma (chronic apophysitis).

These injuries typically occur from a noncontact mechanism, and the patient "pulls up" during the course of competition. Obtaining a thorough history, with specific attention to understanding the precipitating biomechanical forces, may provide an important clue as to the affected area. For example, sudden hip flexion with accompanying knee extension (hamstring muscles) during a gymnastics

routine might signal an ischial tuberosity avulsion, whereas kicking a soccer ball aggressively downfield might lead to a differential diagnosis of ASIS (sartorius) or AIIS (rectus femoris) avulsion injury (figures 7-13 and 7-14).

Workup and Management

Once a good history of hip injury is obtained, physical examination consists of deliberate, sequential bony palpation of all potential avulsion sites, along with passive and active range of motion of the hips (Figure 7-15). Every examination should include the contralateral hip for comparison, regardless of the suspected diagnosis. The ASIS, AIIS, iliac crest, and ischial tuberosity are all easily palpated in most patients, but apophyses such as the lesser trochanter may require a higher index of suspicion during provocative testing.

When you are considering an avulsion fracture, radiographic workup always includes an AP pelvis view and occasionally a frog-leg lateral, if you suspect the lesser trochanter. On rare occasions, minimally or non-displaced avulsions can be challenging to appreciate on radiograph. When history and examination findings are highly suggestive with nondiagnostic radiography, magnetic resonance imaging (MRI) can be considered for confirmation.

In general, apophyseal avulsion injuries of the pelvis are nonsurgical problems. Initial management is ice, rest, and protected weight bearing, on crutches, until pain resolves (usually <2 weeks). Physical therapy begins after a couple weeks, with an emphasis on progressive range of motion, followed by functional hip girdle strengthening as pain resolves. Return to play requires radiographic evidence of bony healing, absence of pain with provocative maneuvers, and successful demonstration of functional testing. In rare circumstances, an avulsion will be displaced enough to warrant surgery, with the most at-risk being those of the ischial tuberosity or AIIS having significant displacement (>2 cm).

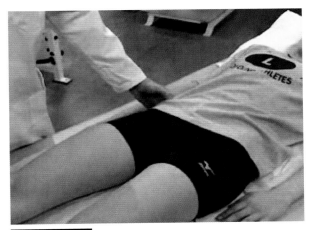

FIGURE 7-13
Palpation of the ASIS.
Abbreviation: ASIS, anterior-superior iliac spine.

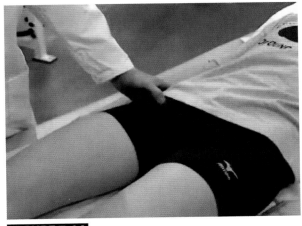

FIGURE 7-14
Palpation of the AIIS.
Abbreviation: AIIS, anterior-inferior iliac spine.

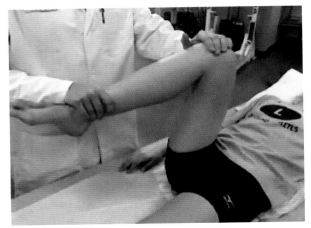

FIGURE 7-15
Internal rotation test.

Box 7-1
The Great Mimicker: Slipped Capital Femoral Epiphysis

SCFE must be considered in any adolescent with hip pain, and it may be preceded by either acute trauma or a chronic progression of symptoms. The classic patient with an increased risk has obesity, but SCFE has been described in children of all body types. The differences between SCFE and apophyseal avulsion fractures can be subtle; however, patients with SCFE are less likely to describe a distinct episode of maximum muscle loading. Furthermore, during physical examination, patients with SCFE are more likely to describe pain with passive rotation of the hip joint, while patients with avulsion injuries are more likely to describe pain with active joint motion, such as flexion and extension. When considering an SCFE, AP pelvis and frog-leg lateral radiographs are necessary. Any physeal widening, any medial displacement of the femoral head, or a superior proximal epiphysis not transected by Klein line (see Radiographs, Hip, section) is diagnostic for SCFE and warrants urgent orthopedic consultation. SCFE cases are described as stable (patient able to bear weight ± crutches) or unstable (patient cannot bear weight, even with crutches). Initial management includes making all patients with suspected cases of SCFE non–weight bearing immediately, followed by pediatric orthopedic consultation to discuss the timing for closed reduction, percutaneous pinning, or more aggressive operative treatments for the affected and contralateral hip.

Abbreviations: AP, anteroposterior; SCFE, slipped capital femoral epiphysis.

TAKE-HOME POINTS

Slipped Capital Femoral Epiphysis and Apophyseal Avulsion Fractures

► Hip pain is a common injury in the adolescent athlete. Possible causes include slipped capital femoral epiphysis (SCFE) (a slip of the growth plate at the proximal femur in the adolescent athlete). Slipped capital femoral epiphysis is characterized by pain in the hip with ambulation, an antalgic gait, and limitation of internal rotation with passive motion testing. Workup for SCFE includes anteroposterior (AP) pelvis and frog-leg lateral views, with special attention given to Klein line. Magnetic resonance imaging can aid in the diagnosis of SCFE if there is a question about the cause of pain.

► The apophyses surrounding the hip include the anterior-superior iliac spine, anterior-inferior iliac spine, iliac crest, ischial tuberosity, and lesser trochanter. Because of their strong muscular attachments, each of these apophyses is at risk for chronic traction apophysitis and acute avulsion fractures. Avulsions should be suspected with a history of an acute "pop" following a high force load of a muscle around the hip, such as a forceful kick of the soccer ball. Evaluation includes physical examination and AP pelvis radiographic view, which is usually diagnostic. If unrecognized, avulsion injuries or traction apophysitis can be made worse with continued playing.

Case 2

Acute neck injury ("burners" and "stingers") in 17-year-old football player

Description

This case is not represented in the video, but recognizing the seriousness of cervical spine injuries in young athletes is important. One of the more common neck injuries in athletes is referred to as a "burner" or "stinger." These are neurologic injuries resulting from traction or compression of the brachial plexus, or both, following an acute axial load to head, neck, or shoulder. The classic scenario is a football player who tackles headfirst, but the injury is common in players of all contact sports, including ice hockey, lacrosse, and rugby.

Patients typically present with acute onset of severe pain and paresthesias running down one arm into the hand and fingers following a direct blow to the shoulder, neck, or head. They may report that they felt like their "arm was on fire" or compare it to the sensation of striking their funny bone (ulnar nerve at the elbow). Unilateral, upper-extremity weakness and numbness may also occur, but typically symptoms last only minutes to hours before resolving spontaneously.

Workup and Management

The physical examination is extremely important because similar symptoms may be described following blows to the head, neck, or shoulder. Start with a thorough neurologic assessment of the bilateral upper extremities, testing for strength, sensation, and reflexes. The cervical spine needs to be examined closely, assessing for bony tenderness and range of motion while noting any position that replicates neurologic symptoms. Percussion over the supraclavicular fossa for tenderness and performing Spurling test (described previously) are helpful for assessing the brachial plexus and cervical roots. Concluding with an examination of the shoulder is also important, as glenohumeral instability events may produce similar symptoms caused by traction on the brachial plexus.

Be cautious if symptoms are described bilaterally, examination shows bony cervical tenderness, or neurologic findings are bilateral. Any of these findings are alarming for a cervical spine fracture or spinal cord injury. By definition, burners and stingers will produce only unilateral findings.

With suspected cervical spine injury, radiographic imaging should include 3 views of the cervical spine, including AP, odontoid, and lateral views

(Figure 7-16). With persistent symptoms or recurrent stinger injuries, consideration should be given to more advanced studies, such as MRI of the cervical spine and possibly electromyography or electroneurography, or both.

Initial management of a stinger injury depends on whether (1) symptoms have resolved, because many will recover spontaneously within a few days, and (2) the injury originates from the cervical spine or shoulder region. If symptoms persist and no fracture is present, most patients will benefit from rehabilitation with a physical therapist. Initial focus is on range of motion, with a gradual progression to strengthening of the neck and shoulder depending on the origin of symptoms. Massage, heat and cold therapy, ultrasound, and electrical stimulation may also be beneficial modalities. Strongly consider referral to a sports medicine center in cases of stinger injuries, and athletes should never return to play until symptoms have completely resolved.

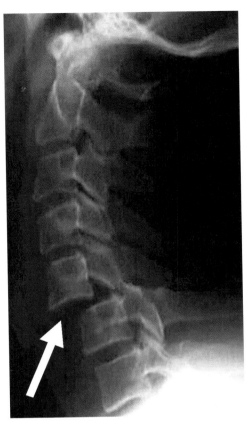

FIGURE 7-16
Lateral radiographic view of cervical spine with arrow indicating spondylolisthesis.

2. Overuse Injury

Case 3
Hip pain (femoral neck stress fracture) in 17-year-old runner

Description

Overuse injuries of the hip are generally the result of chronic, repetitive loading of the hip joint. Common overuse injuries of the hip include iliopsoas tendinitis, pelvic apophysitis, and stress fractures of the femoral neck. One has to be particularly concerned when symptoms are progressing and limiting a patient's ability to participate in sports. This overuse case involves a 17-year-old female runner coming into the office reporting vague groin pain exacerbated by running and now limiting her ability to participate.

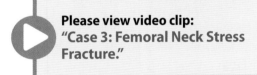

Please view video clip:
"Case 3: Femoral Neck Stress Fracture."

Femoral neck stress fractures often occur in female athletes having the female athlete triad, a classic constellation of symptoms including amenorrhea, disordered eating, and premature osteoporosis. These stress fractures are one of the more worrisome overuse syndromes seen in adolescent athletes, and they most often occur in runners. Chronic bone stress from vigorous exercise, along with abnormal bone mineralization caused by alterations in eating habits, can lead to weakness in the femoral neck and subsequent fracture. Amenorrhea or irregular menses may be one of the earliest signs of female athlete triad and should be an essential part of the examination and history for all female athletes.

Patients with femoral neck stress fracture often present with groin or anterior thigh pain that is most severe when the foot strikes the ground during running. Pain may also occur during any exercise with high strain in the hip, such as kicking or jumping. Femoral neck stress fractures may occur on either the tension or compression side of the femoral neck. Failure to recognize a femoral neck stress fracture of the hip may result in displacement of the fracture and avascular necrosis of the hip, so early detection is essential. Other causes of pain and overuse injury of the hip include pelvic apophysitis, tendinitis, femoroacetabular impingement, and labral tears of the acetabulum.

Workup and Management

On initial examination, palpation of the hip may not be diagnostic. Passive range of motion in the hip or active abduction may reveal groin pain (Figure 7-17). The Trendelenburg test result is often positive, with the patient leaning away from the affected hip when asked to stand on the affected extremity. An abductor lurch may be present when observing ambulation. The "hop" test (during which patients hop on the affected leg) result is positive with femoral neck stress fractures, but be cautious performing this test until after radiographic evaluation if highly suspicious of a stress fracture.

When evaluating a possible femoral neck stress fracture, initial radiographs should include AP and frog-leg lateral views of the hip and pelvis. Radiographs may be nondiagnostic early in the disease process, with visible changes not occurring until 2 to 3 weeks after presentation. If a femoral neck stress fracture is strongly suspected, urgent MRI is the criterion standard for diagnosing it (Figure 7-18).

As soon as a femoral neck stress fracture is suspected, weight bearing of the affected extremity should be protected with crutches. It is imperative to reinforce patient adherence to weight-bearing precautions. Both the teen and parent should be warned about the possible risk of further fracture displacement and subsequent avascular necrosis if non-adherent.

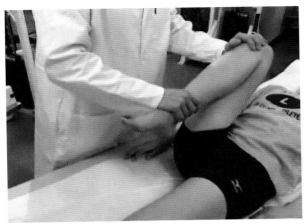

FIGURE 7-17
Passive flexion and impingement test.

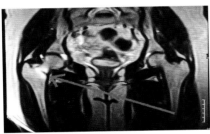

FIGURE 7-18
MRI of the hip showing femoral neck stress fracture in a 17-year-old runner.
Abbreviation: MRI, magnetic resonance image.

As mentioned, femoral neck stress fractures exist in 2 forms: tension and compression. Tension fractures occur on the lateral (superior) side of the neck and are the most serious. Because of the high risk of progression to a complete transverse fracture without management, tension fractures require surgical fixation by an orthopedic surgeon. Compression fractures occur on the medial (inferior) side of the neck, and they are typically treated without surgery. Close observation, frequent radiographic evaluation, non–weight bearing with crutches, and an adherent patient are the keys to successful conservative treatment for this injury. Protected weight bearing is usually prescribed for 1 to 2 months, with no weight bearing until the patient is able to walk without pain or an abductor lurch. Complete healing may take up to 3 months. Physical therapy and other activity modifications, such as water jogging, may be considered during later stages of recovery.

Before an athlete returns to play, a thorough assessment of strength and biomechanical factors, such as running gait analysis, should be performed. Also, consider laboratory testing for vitamin D or calcium deficiency, or both, along with a bone density dual-energy x-ray absorptiometry study looking for other contributing factors.

Rehabilitation and Prevention Exercises

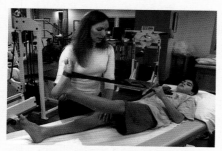

Hamstring Muscle Stretch (targets hamstring muscles)

Please view video clip: "Hamstring Muscle Exercises."

1. Begin lying on your back with a towel or strap wrapped around one foot.
2. Raise the leg (with knee straight) with the towel or strap until a stretch is felt in the back of the thigh.
3. Hold this position for 30 seconds, and repeat 5 times on each leg.

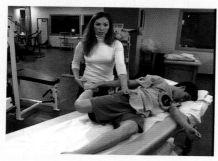

Thomas Test (targets hip flexors, rectus femoris, and iliotibial band)

Please view video clip: "Hip Flexor, Rectus Femoris, and Iliotibial Band Exercises."

1. Begin lying with both knees pulled into the chest.
2. Release one leg so it extends off the supporting surface.
3. Maintain the extended leg in neutral rotation, in line with your body.
4. A stretch should be felt across the hip and thigh.
5. Hold this position for 30 seconds.
6. Return to the starting position.
7. Repeat 5 times on each leg.

Abdominal Set With Alternating Legs (targets core stabilization while moving legs)

1. Begin lying with both knees bent and with feet supported on surface.
2. Tighten abdominal muscles, flattening the lumbar spine into the surface.
3. Maintain the abdominal activation (without holding breath) while lifting one knee to chest.
4. Return leg to starting position without movement in the lumbar spine.
5. Repeat with opposite leg.
6. Perform 10 times on each leg; do 2 sets.

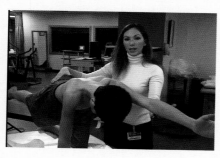

Quadruped Alternating Arms (targets core stabilization while moving arms)

Please view video clip: "Core Stabilization Exercises."

1. Begin on hands and knees with the spine in neutral.
2. Raise one arm (with thumb pointing up) next to your ear.
3. Hold this position for 2 to 5 seconds.
4. Return your arm to starting position.
5. The key to this exercise is maintaining a stable, neutral spine.
6. Perform 10 times each arm; do 2 to 3 sets.

continued

Rehabilitation and Prevention Exercises, *continued*

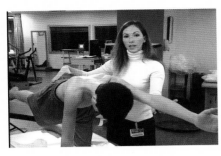

Quadruped Alternating Legs (targets core stabilization while moving legs)

Please view video clip: **"Core Stabilization Exercises."**

1. Begin on hands and knees with the spine in neutral.
2. Lift one leg so it is in line with your body.
3. Hold this position for 2 to 5 seconds.
4. Return your leg to starting position.
5. The key to this exercise is maintaining a stable, neutral spine.
6. Perform 10 times on each leg; do 2 to 3 sets.

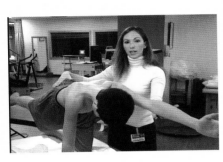

Quadruped Alternating Arms and Legs (targets core stabilization while moving arms and legs)

Please view video clip: **"Core Stabilization Exercises."**

1. Begin on hands and knees with the spine in neutral.
2. Lift one leg while simultaneously lifting the opposite arm.
3. Hold this position for 2 to 5 seconds.
4. Return your arm and leg to starting position.
5. The key to this exercise is maintaining a stable, neutral spine.
6. Perform 10 times, alternating opposite arms and legs; do 2 to 3 sets.

TAKE-HOME POINTS

Femoral Neck Stress Fracture

▶ Like all the cases of stress fracture discussed in this workbook, a stress fracture of the femoral neck is a serious condition that can be made worse if insufficient attention is paid to the initial symptoms. Because of the high risk of complication from delay in diagnosis, these injuries are best diagnosed early, through a combination of patient history, physical examination, radiographic evaluation, and magnetic resonance imaging if necessary.

▶ The causative factors for a femoral neck stress fracture include increased training, biomechanical problems such as hip and core muscle weakness, poor recovery, insufficient nutrition, and low bone density in the form of adolescent osteopenia or osteoporosis. These factors should all be considered when evaluating an athlete with this type of injury.

▶ Return to play should be considered only when the athlete is completely asymptomatic and able to run, jump, and do dynamic sporting activities without difficulty.

Case 4

Lumbar spine pain (spondylolysis) in 15-year-old volleyball player

Description

Overuse injuries of the lumbar spine are common in young athletes. A classic example is spondylolysis, a stress fracture in the pars interarticularis region of the lumbar spine. This chronic injury to the posterior elements of the lumbar spine can occur in any athlete, but athletes who do repeated lumbar hyperextension maneuvers are most at risk. Athletes such as gymnasts, ballet dancers, tennis players, and football lineman may present describing discomfort whenever they "bend backward." In our case, a volleyball player comes to the office reporting pain whenever serving or "arching her back."

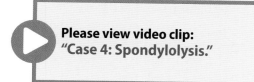

Please view video clip: "Case 4: Spondylolysis."

Spondylolysis is found in up to 6% of the general population, but incidence increases dramatically in adolescents who participate in sports requiring repetitive hyperextension of the lumbar spine, such as gymnastics, diving, volleyball, and dance. Over time, increased stress on the posterior elements of the lumbar spine can cause bony edema, stress fracture, and, occasionally, progression to spondylolisthesis, a condition in which one lumbar vertebra slips forward on another. Spondylolysis and spondylolisthesis are most commonly seen at the level of the L5 vertebra.

Studies have shown that up to 30% of adolescents experience lower back pain. Many of these concerns may seem benign and self-limited, but pay close attention to differentiate pathology such as muscle strain, stress fracture, herniated disks, and tumors. If patients report intermittent lower back pain starting to limit activity, investigate whether it is worse during sport-specific maneuvers such as serving and back bends, during which lumbar

extension is present. These features are rather specific for spondylolysis.

Workup and Management

As discussed in the video, lumbar spine examintion generally can be divided into 3 motions (pain with flexion, pain with extension, and pain with rotation) (figures 7-19 and 7-20). Patients who describe radicular pain, particularly with forward flexion, should be suspected of having a disk-related cause of back pain. While this is less common in adolescent athletes than adult athletes, it does occur. Patients having pain with extension are concerning for injury to the posterior elements, pedicles, and pars interarticularis. The most common example of posterior element injury is spondylolysis. Finally, patients having pain with rotation, but no radicular symptoms, are likely to have an injury with muscular origin. These patients often describe pain along the paraspinal region with rotation.

Physical examination for spondylolysis may also reveal lumbar spine tenderness, tight hamstring muscles, and a bent-knee, flexed-hip gait. A "step off" in the lumbar spine may even be palpable if spondylolisthesis has occurred. A thorough neurologic assessment is essential, but findings are typically normal with this condition.

Radiographic workup includes AP, lateral, and oblique views of the lumbosacral spine (figures 7-21 and 7-22). The lateral view may show a fracture or spondylolisthesis, the slipping of one vertebra on another. The oblique view, taken at 45° from midline, looks for a pars interarticularis fracture, classically described as the collar on a "Scottie dog" profile. Frequently, radiographic findings are negative for stress fractures associated with spondylolysis, but when suspicion remains high, consider more advanced studies, such as single-photon emission computed tomography, bone scintigraphy, computed tomography (Figure 7-23), or MRI. Magnetic resonance imaging is clearly the choice if any suggestion of diskogenic pain or neurologic findings on examination. Otherwise, each of these advanced techniques has advantages and drawbacks that should be discussed with your radiologist to ensure the best, advanced study is performed.

Conservative, nonoperative treatment for spondylolysis is usually successful, with few patients ever requiring surgical intervention. In most cases of spondylolysis, because of repetitive hyperextension, the goal of management is resolution of clinical symptoms with a successful return to play without pain. These injuries rarely have complete bony healing but demonstrate a more fibrous healing pattern.

The mainstay of treatment for spondylolysis is activity modification, relative rest, and avoidance of any activity causing lumbar hyperextension. Once pain-free, patients are prescribed physical

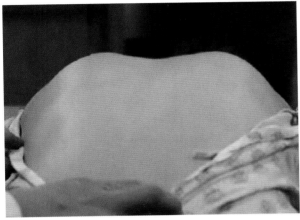

FIGURE 7-19
Forward flexion test.

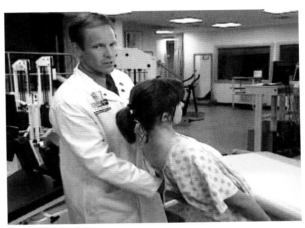

FIGURE 7-20
Extension test.

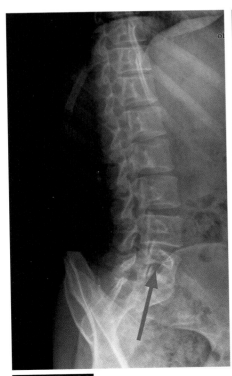

FIGURE 7-21
Oblique view of lumbar spine with arrow demonstrating spondylolysis.

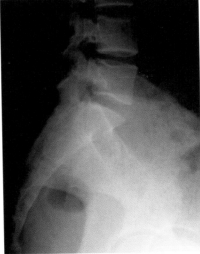

FIGURE 7-22
Lateral view of lumbar spine showing grade 1 spondylolisthesis.

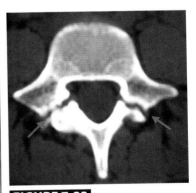

FIGURE 7-23
CT scan of lumbar spine with arrows showing spondylolysis.
Abbreviation: CT, computed tomography.

therapy to guide stabilization of the core muscles supporting the spine and to address the many biomechanical factors contributing to lower back stress. Slow and deliberate guidance back to play based on performance in therapy is essential. Patients such as the one discussed in our vignette may find bracing helpful to reduce pain and prevent lumbar extension. The long-term benefit or need for bracing continues to be an area of debate within spondylolysis management.

Most patients with spondylolisthesis can be treated similarly to those with spondylolysis. The degree of slippage forward on the adjacent vertebrae guides management. Most patients have a slip of less than 25% and have the same treatment goals and strategies as discussed above for spondylolysis, mainly activity restrictions, physical therapy, and progressive guidance back to activity. When the degree of slippage is 50% or greater, and anytime the degree of slippage appears to be progressing, referral to an orthopedic surgeon for surgical stabilization is indicated.

Conservative, nonoperative treatment for spondylolysis is usually successful, with few patients ever requiring surgical intervention. In most cases of spondylolysis, because of repetitive hyperextension, the goal of management is resolution of clinical symptoms with a successful return to play

Rehabilitation and Prevention Exercises

Physical therapy for spondylolysis and spondylolisthesis emphasizes lumbar flexion through abdominal strengthening and improving flexibility around the hip. These treatment principles decrease the stress on the pars fracture sites and, when used in conjunction with bracing, may prevent slips from increasing. The abdominal strengthening and core stabilization decreases the bias toward lumbar hyperextension that initially puts patients at risk for injury. When a patient has tightness in hip muscles, he or she may compensate with increased movement in the lumbar spine. Thus, patient education in avoiding lumbar extension and in altering body mechanics, as well as improving core stability and muscle flexibility, will assist in returning to play without pain. All patients participating in higher-risk hyperextension activities (eg, gymnastics, dancing, volleyball, tennis) should consider preventive exercise programs to decrease stress on the lumbar spine.

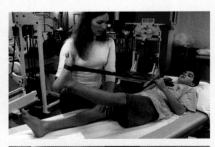

Hamstring Muscle Stretch (targets hamstring muscles)

Please view video clip: "Hamstring Muscle Exercises."

1. Begin lying on your back with a towel or strap wrapped around one foot.
2. Raise the leg (with knee straight) with the towel or strap until a stretch is felt in the back of the thigh.
3. Hold this position for 30 seconds, and repeat 5 times on each leg.

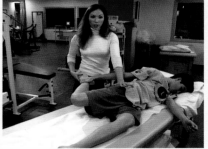

Thomas Test (targets hip flexors, rectus femoris, and iliotibial band)

Please view video clip: "Hip Flexor, Rectus Femoris, and Iliotibial Band Exercises."

1. Begin lying with both knees pulled into the chest.
2. Release one leg so it extends off the supporting surface.
3. Maintain the extended leg in neutral rotation, in line with your body.
4. A stretch should be felt across the hip and thigh.
5. Hold this position for 30 seconds.
6. Return to the starting position.
7. Repeat 5 times on each leg.

continued

Rehabilitation and Prevention Exercises, *continued*

Abdominal Set With Alternating Legs (targets core stabilization while moving legs)

1. Begin lying with both knees bent and with feet supported on surface.
2. Tighten abdominal muscles, flattening the lumbar spine into the surface.
3. Maintain the abdominal activation (without holding breath) while lifting one knee to chest.
4. Return leg to starting position without movement in the lumbar spine.
5. Repeat with opposite leg.
6. Perform 10 times on each leg; do 2 sets.

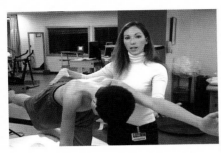

Quadruped Alternating Arms (targets core stabilization while moving arms)

Please view video clip: "Core Stabilization Exercises."

1. Begin on hands and knees with the spine in neutral.
2. Raise one arm (with thumb pointing up) next to your ear.
3. Hold this position for 2 to 5 seconds.
4. Return your arm to starting position.
5. The key to this exercise is maintaining a stable, neutral spine.
6. Perform 10 times on each arm; do 2 to 3 sets.

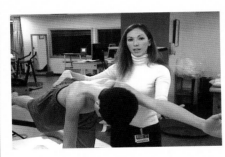

Quadruped Alternating Legs (targets core stabilization while moving legs)

Please view video clip: "Core Stabilization Exercises."

1. Begin on hands and knees with the spine in neutral.
2. Lift one leg so it is in line with your body.
3. Hold this position for 2 to 5 seconds.
4. Return your leg to starting position.
5. The key to this exercise is maintaining a stable, neutral spine.
6. Perform 10 times on each leg; do 2 to 3 sets.

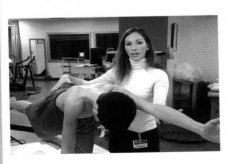

Quadruped Alternating Arms and Legs (targets core stabilization while moving arms and legs)

Please view video clip: "Core Stabilization Exercises."

1. Begin on hands and knees with the spine in neutral.
2. Lift one leg while simultaneously lifting the opposite arm.
3. Hold this position for 2 to 5 seconds.
4. Return your arm and leg to starting position.
5. The key to this exercise is maintaining a stable, neutral spine.
6. Perform 10 times, alternating opposite arms and legs; do 2 to 3 sets.

without pain. These injuries rarely have complete bony healing but demonstrate a more fibrous healing pattern.

The mainstay of treatment for spondylolysis is activity modification, relative rest, and avoidance of any activity causing lumbar hyperextension. Once pain-free, patients are prescribed physical therapy to guide stabilization of the core muscles supporting the spine and to address the many biomechanical factors contributing to lower back stress. Slow and deliberate guidance back to play based on performance in therapy is essential. Patients such as the one discussed in our vignette may find bracing helpful to reduce pain and prevent lumbar extension. The long-term benefit or need for bracing continues to be an area of debate within spondylolysis management.

Most patients with spondylolisthesis can be treated similarly to those with spondylolysis. The degree of slippage forward on the adjacent vertebrae guides management. Most patients have a slip of less than 25% and have the same treatment goals and strategies as discussed above for spondylolysis, mainly activity restrictions, physical therapy, and progressive guidance back to activity. When the degree of slippage is 50% or greater, and anytime the degree of slippage appears to be progressing, referral to an orthopedic surgeon for surgical stabilization is indicated.

Treatment

- Relative rest (Encourage fitness while avoiding hyperextension activity.)
- Full assessment of degree of bone injury (stress fracture versus stress reaction or injury)
- Referral to physical therapist for lumbar and hamstring muscle stretching and abdominal and core muscle strengthening
- Gradual return to play
- Possible use of brace for return to play during ongoing strengthening

For patients with spondylolysis, return to play is based on resolution of pain, and for patients with spondylolisthesis, it is based on the degree of slip of one vertebra on another. Patients with less than a 25% slip may return to full play when symptoms have subsided and physical therapy has been completed. Patients with greater than a 25% slip should avoid hyperextension activities, and patients with greater than a 50% slip should be referred to an orthopedic surgeon to evaluate for surgical stabilization if they are skeletally mature and bracing and physical therapy has failed. Patients may return to full play after surgical stabilization, although decreased range of motion of the lumbar spine may exist.

TAKE-HOME POINTS

Spondylolysis

▶ Spondylolysis is an overuse injury of the lumbar spine that results from increased forces on the lumbar spine with repetitive extension maneuvers. As with all bony overuse injuries, there is a spectrum, from stress injury to stress fracture. As such, pain with extension can be as simple as a stress injury, which is managed with relative rest, core strengthening, and guided return to play. A more serious variety is the full-blown stress fracture, which tends to cause significant pain as a bony crack forms in the region of the pars interarticularis and significantly limits activity. For preadolescents, treatment can be focused on trying to obtain a bony union of the lesion. With adolescents and adults, the chances of bony healing in the lesion are minimal, so symptomatic relief becomes the goal. The mainstays of treatment include activity modification, rest, physical therapy, and gradual progression back to activity. Some patients may also find the use of a supportive brace helpful to alleviate pain.

▶ The workup for suspected spondylolysis includes patient history, physical examination, lumbar radiographs (anteroposterior, lateral, and oblique views), and, often, advanced studies such as magnetic resonance imaging or single-photon emission computed tomography scan.

CHAPTER 8

Concussions in the Young Athlete

Thomas L. Devries, MD, and David T. Bernhardt, MD, FAAP

Case File: Concussion in a 17-Year-Old Hockey Player

A senior high school hockey player presents to your office for follow-up of a concussion that was sustained 3 days ago. The patient describes a helmet-to-ice collision in a game when he fell after colliding with another player. He had no loss of consciousness, but he does not remember a few seconds to minutes from the time of impact or the time the coaches hovered over him on the ice. He reports feeling woozy and nauseated (no vomiting), and he had an immediate headache. He reports significant improvement occurring during the trip to the emergency department (ED). No diagnostic studies were performed in the ED because his clinical picture appeared to be normal.

In your office today, he still has a headache, across the back of his skull, but no neck pain, nausea, or other symptoms. No significant abnormalities are found in the complete neurologic assessment. The patient has 2 games left in the season, and he is anxious to return to play (practice and competition).

Background

Concussion is a subtype of mild traumatic brain injury that commonly occurs in players of contact sports. Historically, it has been defined as a low-velocity injury that causes the brain to "shake" within the skull, resulting in clinical symptoms. In reality, the mechanism of injury is variable, including high velocity, rotational velocity, and low velocity.

The science of concussion has been a rapidly evolving field. The definition of concussion has changed over the years and usually includes verbiage related to trauma to the head causing neurologic symptoms. A recent expert consensus from the 2012 International Conference on Concussion in Sport in Zurich, Switzerland, defines it as a "complex pathophysiological process affecting the brain, induced by biomechanical forces." Other features that characterize a concussion include rapid onset of short-lived neurologic impairment, lack of abnormal findings from standard structural neuroimaging studies, and resultant clinical symptoms that may involve a loss of consciousness and, in some cases, may be prolonged.[1]

This chapter will highlight the important aspects of concussion related to sport, including sideline evaluation, clinical symptoms and signs, imaging and scanning studies, complications, return to play, and injury prevention, while following the clinical case example from your office back to school and the playing field.

Epidemiological Studies

Concussions are inherently underreported because of the nature of their often mild and nonspecific symptoms. Athletes' fear of losing playing time and their lack of knowledge about signs and symptoms may also contribute to underreporting. The Centers for Disease Control and Prevention reports that of the estimated 1.7 million annual concussions, 20% are sports related.

A recent systematic review of concussion incidence rate in youth athletes reported an overall incidence of 0.23 injuries per 1,000 athlete exposures per year.[2] This same review found that incidence of concussion varied widely among different sports. Of the 12 sports examined in the various studies, incidence ranged from 0.03 associated with volleyball to 4.18 associated with rugby. The sports with the highest incidence in addition to rugby included American (tackle) football and hockey (1.20 and 0.53, respectively).

Overall, higher contact sports are associated with higher incidence of concussion. Ongoing research suggests higher incidence among older age-groups in pediatric patients and among girls compared with boys playing like sports.

As you approach this adolescent boy in your office, what are your concerns? He seems to have been treated appropriately on the ice and in the ED. His memory is intact, but his brief period of fogginess is clearly indicative of a concussion. His clinical improvement is common among athletes with concussion.

Sideline Evaluation

Evaluation of concussion on the sideline can be difficult. The practitioner is often under time constraints, athletes may not be forthcoming in reporting their symptoms, and findings from neurologic assessment can be completely normal. In diagnosing a concussion, no single test is perfect, and it is important to have a standardized method to assess potential concussions on the sideline. Additionally, knowledge of the injured athlete's baseline mental status is paramount to assessing mild cognitive deficits.

Prior to administering any assessment tool on the sideline, standard emergency management protocols, with a focus on ruling out spinal cord injury, should be pursued. Urgent transport to the nearest hospital should be considered in athletes with deteriorating mental status, potential spinal cord injury, progressively worsening symptoms, or new neurologic signs. Acute concussion should be viewed as an evolving injury; players with an injury should undergo serial monitoring and should not be left alone for the first 48 hours. Any player diagnosed as having a concussion should not return to play on the day of injury.

The 2012 Zurich consensus statement advocates for the use of the SCAT3 (Sport Concussion Assessment Tool, third iteration) or another assessment tool. The SCAT3 assesses mental status and cognitive function with the Glasgow Coma Scale, Standardized Assessment of Concussion, and Maddocks score (Figure 8-1). It also includes a comprehensive symptom evaluation and examination of the neck, balance, and coordination. While this tool is a useful guide in establishing a

diagnosis during a sideline assessment, it can also be used in return-to-play decisions when baseline testing is available.

Consider actually being at the game or in the ED when this athlete first presented. While you are evaluating the adolescent boy on the sideline, he starts to report a more severe headache and becomes more stuporous before your eyes. Are there other, more severe, forms of head injuries that must be considered when evaluating the athlete with a concussion? On-site preparation, of spine board, cardiopulmonary resuscitation equipment, and an emergency plan, is the key to early management.

Symptoms, Signs, and Studies

The classic symptoms of concussion are headache, confusion, and amnesia. While loss of consciousness can occur, most concussions occur without loss of consciousness. Additional symptoms can follow the injury immediately or can have a more gradual onset. Headache, dizziness, mental fogginess, nausea, and vomiting tend to occur earlier (minutes to hours). Sensitivity to light and noise, emotional lability, and sleep disturbances may develop over hours to days.

Concussions can commonly occur without any observed findings and relatively normal findings from neurologic assessment. Signs can include a vacant stare, delayed verbal expression, inattentiveness, disorientation, slurred speech, gross incoordination, and any loss of consciousness. Subtle findings may include postural sway (Romberg sign), nystagmus, and difficulty with tandem gait.

Findings from conventional structural imaging and scanning are typically normal with concussion and are therefore not of routine use. However, in situations of deteriorating mental status, progressively worsening symptoms, or focal neurologic signs, it is important to obtain a head computed tomography scan to evaluate for intracranial bleeding or skull fracture, or both. These findings would be supportive of a more significant traumatic brain injury rather than concussion.

Research relating to more advanced studies and concussion are ongoing. Functional magnetic resonance imaging has been shown to demonstrate activation patterns that correlate with concussion symptom severity.[3] Other studies, including positron emission tomography, magnetic resonance spectroscopy, and diffusion tensor imaging, are currently being used in the research setting.

One week later, the patient is reporting headaches, dizziness, loss of appetite, and fatigue. On obtaining further history, you find that he had a concussion a year ago with similar symptoms that lasted for approximately 4 days. Is it "normal" for an athlete with a concussion to continue to be symptomatic for days to weeks?

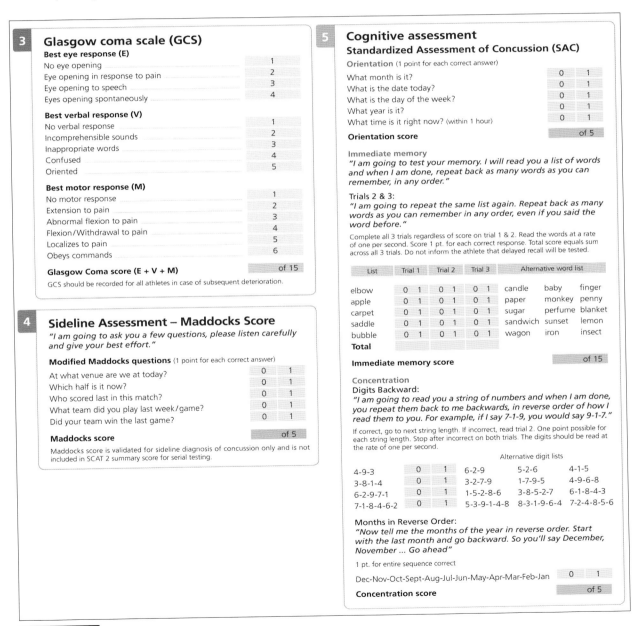

FIGURE 8-1

Selected elements of the Sport Concussion Assessment Tool, third iteration.

From the Concussion in Sport Group, originally published in the *British Journal of Sports Medicine* Injury Prevention and Health Protection, 2013, volume 47, issue 5. Reproduced with permission.

Complications

Most concussions resolve over a period of 7 to 14 days, although children and adolescents tend to have longer recovery times. The literature suggests that athletes with previous concussions, greater number of reported symptoms, or more severe symptoms will be at risk for having a prolonged recovery. Other risk factors for a prolonged recovery include preexisting depression, anxiety, and migraine headaches. The term *post-concussion syndrome* is reserved for cases with persistent symptoms. These lingering symptoms can last as long as a few weeks to months. In these cases, it is important to consider alternative diagnoses, as the symptoms are not specific to concussion.

Second impact syndrome is a potentially fatal complication that can occur when an athlete experiences a concussion while the athlete is still recovering from a prior concussion. It is theorized to be caused by disordered cerebral autoregulation, resulting in cerebral vascular congestion, subsequent diffuse cerebral edema, and, ultimately, brain herniation. Second impact syndrome is rare in the literature, and its existence is somewhat controversial.[4]

Much attention has been paid to the idea that repeated concussions may lead to chronic pathological changes. Personality change, depression, suicidal ideation, and parkinsonism have been described in what is labeled as chronic traumatic encephalopathy (CTE). A 2016 review article elaborates that CTE is a distinctive neurodegenerative disease that, at present, can be diagnosed only with postmortem brain tissue.[5] There is significant concern over increasing evidence that CTE may affect both amateur and professional athletes involved in contact sports. Given the large number of those participating in sports (estimated 7 million adolescents, in high school sports, in the United States), CTE has become a major public health concern. There is still a significant knowledge gap as to the exact origin of CTE and whether subclinical blows to the head, genetics, preexisting conditions, or other unexplained factors may contribute to this condition.

When should you allow an athlete to return to play? How will you explain your medical decision-making to the athlete and his family?

Return to Learning and Return to Play

The main aspects of concussion management are physical and cognitive rest. Physical rest initially involves avoiding any activity that increases the heart rate or worsens symptoms. Cognitive rest is similar: any activity that worsens symptoms should be avoided, including TV, computers, video games, cell phones, and loud music. It is sometimes necessary to keep an athlete out of school to achieve appropriate cognitive rest. The degree and duration of rest has not been determined in the literature, but it is generally accepted that relative rest in the initial 24 to 48 hours after injury is of benefit. The 2012 Zurich consensus statement adds that it is not recommended for the athlete to rest until symptom-free, as prolonged rest can have negative consequences, including fatigue, depression, and deconditioning. In addition, there is more evidence that graded exercise can improve cerebrovascular blood flow and can be beneficial in recovery.

Typically, the school-aged athlete will fully recover within 3 weeks of the head injury. During the recovery process, the athlete with a concussion may have attention and processing problems. This is similar to many patients who have been previously diagnosed as having a learning disorder and receive academic accommodations. As pointed out in a 2013 clinical report by Halstead, a student returning to a learning environment may benefit from a multidisciplinary team, to support the physical, psychological, social, and exercise needs of the student as the student recovers.[6] Students may require quiet environments, extra time to complete assignments and tests, notetakers, or physical education class modification.

A stepwise approach is taken toward returning to play. Generally, the sequence involves progressing from light aerobic activity; to noncontact, sport-specific exercise; to full-contact practice, with eventual return to play. If the athlete experiences any significant worsening of symptoms during the stepwise progress, the athlete should return to the previous step, during which she or he was asymptomatic (Box 8-1). No evidence-based timeline has been established for returning to play; rather, it is based on avoidance of significantly aggravating symptoms.

Box 8-1
Stepwise[a] Return to Play Guideline

Step 1
Relative Rest

Minimal physical and cognitive activity based on symptoms

Step 2
Light Aerobics

Avoid resistance training, and keep heart rate at <70% of maximum.

Step 3
Sport-Specific, Noncontact Training

Avoid head impact, and athlete can begin resistance training.

Step 4
Full-Contact Practice

Resume normal training.

Step 5
Return to Game Play

[a] The athlete should spend ≥24 h in each step prior to advancing. If the athlete develops any symptom recurrence, the athlete should stop and resume the previous asymptomatic step.

Adapted from Halstead ME, Walter KD; American Academy of Pediatrics Council on Sports Medicine and Fitness. Sport-related concussion in children and adolescents. *Pediatrics*. 2010;126(3):597–615, with permission.

Overall, it is never appropriate for an athlete to return to play on the same day of injury. When dealing with children and adolescents, it is recommended to take a conservative approach, given their propensity to take longer to recover. The emphasis should be placed on return to learning rather than return to play.

Injury Prevention

Any athlete participating in a contact sport should have a thorough concussion history reviewed as part of anticipatory guidance during pre-participation examination. The athlete with a history of multiple concussions presents a management dilemma for the specialist and primary care physician. Those who become increasingly symptomatic with less severe trauma and take longer to recover with each successive concussive injury should be counseled to pursue athletic endeavors that involve less contact.

There is no evidence to support that currently used protective equipment reduces the risk of concussion. Although helmets and mouth guards have not been shown to reduce incidence of concussion, they play an important role in protection against other types of head, facial, and dental injury.[7] The concept of risk compensation is important to consider when discussing protective equipment. Essentially, the use of protective equipment may lead to the adoption of more dangerous play style, paradoxically increasing injury rates.

Rule changes in sport may pick up where protective equipment falls short. Rule changes that support fair play and limit violence have been implemented in the National Football League. A study looking at the effects of a "zero tolerance for head contact" policy change in youth hockey found that the rule change did not reduce in-game concussion incidence. However, the authors noted that the increased concussion awareness and education after the policy change may have obscured the results.

There is growing evidence that athletes at the collegiate level are at increased risk for sustaining a musculoskeletal, lower-extremity injury when they return to play after recovering from concussion.[8] Slowed reaction time or impaired proprioception may increase risk of injury.

TAKE-HOME POINTS

Concussion

▶ All contact sports carry a risk of concussion. Evidence-based research relating to concussions is limited but growing. The final determination on diagnosis, management, and return to play is ultimately based on clinical judgement. Important points to consider when taking care of any athlete with a head injury include

1. Be prepared when responsible for game coverage (ie, know how and when to initiate emergency protocols).

2. Return-to-play decisions should be conservative. There is no reason to risk further brain injury, especially in children and adolescents.

3. Recognition of post-concussion syndrome is essential. Students may need additional support in the classroom and a stepwise return-to-learning and return-to-play plan.

▶ Of note, the 2016 Berlin consensus statement on concussion in sport, published in April 2017, represents the most current expert consensus guidelines on sport-related concussion.[9] This chapter was based on the 2012 Zurich consensus guidelines and all salient points remain consistent with the current guidelines.

References

1. McCrory P, Meeuwisse WH, Aubry M, et al. Consensus statement on concussion in sport: the 4th International Conference on Concussion in Sport held in Zurich, November 2012. *Br J Sports Med.* 2013;47(5):250–258

2. Pfister T, Pfister K, Hagel B, Ghali WA, Ronksley PE. The incidence of concussion in youth sports: a systematic review and meta-analysis. *Br J Sports Med.* 2016;50(5):292–297

3. Chen J, Johnston KM, Collie A, McCrory P, Ptito A. A validation of the post concussion symptom scale in the assessment of complex concussion using cognitive testing and functional MRI. *J Neurol Neurosurg Psych.* 2007;78(11):1231–1238

4. McCrory PR, Berkovic SF. Second impact syndrome. *Neurology.* 1998;50(3):677–683

5. McKee AC, Stein TD, Kiernan PT, Alvarez VE. The neuropathology of chronic traumatic encephalopathy. *Brain Pathol.* 2015;25(3):350–364

6. Halstead ME, McAvoy K, Devore CD, Carl R, Lee M, Logan K; American Academy of Pediatrics Council on Sports Medicine and Fitness, Council on School Health. Returning to learning following a concussion. *Pediatrics.* 2013;132(5):948–957

7. Schneider DK, Grandhi RK, Bansal P. Current state of concussion prevention strategies: a systematic review and meta-analysis of prospective, controlled studies. *Br J Sports Med.* 2016; doi: 10.1136/bjsports-2015-095645

8. Brooks MA, Peterson K, Biese K, Sanfilippo J, Heiderscheit BC, Bell DR. Concussion increases odds of sustaining a lower extremity musculoskeletal injury after return to play among collegiate athletes. *Am J Sports Med.* 2016;44(3):742–747

9. McCrory P, Meeuwisse W, Dvorak J, et al. Consensus statement on concussion in sport—the 5th International Conference on Concussion in Sport held in Berlin, October 2016 [published online April 26, 2017]. *Br J Sports Med.* doi: 10.1136/bjsports-2017-097699

Part ❸
Sports

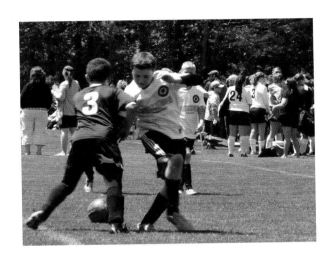

CHAPTER 9
Soccer and the Young Athlete

Hamish Kerr, MD, MSc, FAAP, FACSM, and Jeffrey M. Mjaanes, MD, FAAP, FACSM

Overview

History of Child and Youth Soccer

Soccer is the most popular team sport in the world. According to the Fédération Internationale de Football Association, more than 270 million adult athletes participated in soccer worldwide in 2006. The relative simplicity of soccer's rules, along with the lack of need for expensive equipment, permits a high level of participation in countries across the globe.

In the United States, soccer is also one of the most popular child and youth team sports, with more than 3 million participants younger than 19 years each year (Figure 9-1). Its popularity continues to grow; from 1990 to 2014, the number of children and youths officially registered with U.S. Soccer programs increased by almost 90%.

Several reasons exist for this increasing popularity. Since the National Collegiate Athletic Association enacted Title IX in 1972, the number of girls and women engaged in sports has increased dramatically. The success of the U.S. Soccer Women's National Team in recent years has also heightened interest in the sport, as has the acquisition of high-level international players and increased competitiveness in the nation's men's professional league, Major League Soccer.

Because of growing popularity among both girls and boys, soccer injuries and preventive strategies are increasingly of concern to pediatricians who are eager to keep their young athletes healthy and on the field. As the science of prevention continues to evolve, much work is to be done in preventive health strategies for pediatricians and pediatric health care professionals.

Physiologic Demands of Child and Youth Soccer

Soccer is described as a high-dynamic, low-static sport, typically with a vigorous intensity (7–10 metabolic equivalents). It is played most often over a 90-minute duration; however, child and youth soccer games may be scheduled for 60 minutes or less. Play is continuous, and players will spend the duration of the match alternating between walking, jogging, sprinting, and resting (while the ball is out of play). As such, it is a hybrid sport with intermittent bouts of short intense activity alternating with low-level, moderate intensity. Aerobic conditioning is the most advantageous preparation for soccer participation.

At the elite level, soccer players can cover greater than 10 km (6 mi) a match at intensity close to the anaerobic threshold (80%–90% of maximum heart rate). For an elite team to play more than twice a

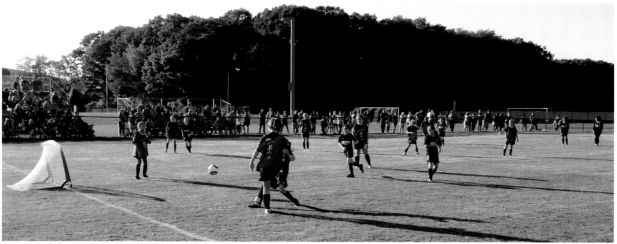

FIGURE 9-1
Youth soccer.

week is uncommon, as it takes 72 hours to recover from such high intensity and the contact inherent in a soccer match.

Differences in aerobic conditioning tend to become evident after puberty, with maximum oxygen consumption of elite, male players measured at 63.7 ± 8.5 mL/min and a higher heart rate response than that of nonelite, indicating elite players are more aerobically fit and spend less time walking and standing during a game. Elite, female players have similarly high aerobic capacity (eg, 57.6 mL/min in English national team players).

Players' fitness profile will also include measurements for calf muscle, hamstring muscle, and quadriceps femoris strength, as well as conditioning needed to be able to run, jump, and kick for 60 to 90 minutes. Foot skills are essential for the sport, and most practice for child and youth players involves the coaching of passing, dribbling, and controlling the soccer ball. Balance and coordination are also important, and evidence is evolving that losing one's balance and falling is a leading cause of injury from child and youth soccer. Males and females have similar fitness requirements.

Epidemiology of Child and Youth Soccer Injuries

Recent studies indicate that injury rates associated with child and youth soccer are increasing. While increased participation may certainly contribute to this rise, the overall incidence of injuries seems to be increasing as well. Determining the exact incidence of injuries in the medical literature is challenging, as incidence and injury rates vary depending on study design, methodology, populations studied, and the definition of injury. Although there is a general perception that soccer has a lower injury rate than that associated with other contact sports, evidence indicates that soccer actually has a higher rate of injury than that associated with many other sports, including field hockey, rugby, basketball, and even American football. Players younger than 15 years have a higher relative injury risk and greater prevalence

of injury than older players do. Female children and youths may be at higher risk for injuries than male children and youths of the same age, although rates vary by study. In general, though, girls have a higher relative risk of anterior cruciate ligament injuries and concussion. Lower-extremity injuries tend to occur more frequently than upper-extremity or head and neck injuries. In general, injury rates seem to be similar regardless of location (indoor vs outdoor) or field type (artificial turf vs grass), although, during child and youth soccer, injury risk is greater with competition than with practice.

General Injury Patterns

Sprains, Strains, and Fractures

Lower-extremity trauma is inherent in soccer, whether caused by contact mechanisms, twisting, or falls. In a recent investigation of soccer injuries presenting to the emergency department in the United States, sprains or strains accounted for 34.6% of injuries, and fractures, 23.2%, with patients 7 to 11 years of age more likely to sustain a fracture (relative risk = 1.34; 95% CI, 1.29–1.39).

Given the relative weakness of the physes compared with the ligaments and tendons, youth soccer players may be more susceptible to growth plate issues than to soft-tissue injuries, especially in the lower extremities (Figure 9-2). These are particularly common in the growing athlete because of a combination of increased strength gain and diminished flexibility during puberty. These 2 factors, increased strength and decreased flexibility, combine to create a window of vulnerability for the developing soccer athlete. Pediatricians are encouraged to promote preventive strategies during this growth stage.

Ankle sprains are one of the most common injuries caused by soccer, similar to injuries caused by other team sports played on grass or turf. The susceptible position of the ankle to inversion injury, in plantar flexion, means that many of the actions associated with soccer have this risk. Players sprinting and kicking the soccer ball with the laces are particularly at risk for inversion.

Challenging an opponent for the ball with one's feet is termed a *tackle,* and it adds the risk of direct trauma to the ankle, both for the player tackling and the player tackled. When opponents attempt to win the ball, but they enter a tackle over the ball (high tackle), they place the tackled player at risk for distal tibial or fibular fracture, or both. The laws of the game prohibit such dangerous play, and players must wear shin guards to help protect against such injuries.

Knee ligament injuries are another common occurrence, principally because of contact. A valgus stress to the knee from trauma to the distal extremity (eg, challenging for a ball with an opponent) can result in a medial collateral ligament sprain. Anterior cruciate ligament injuries can have contact or noncontact mechanisms. Prevalence of anterior cruciate ligament injuries is particularly high among female soccer players. This risk can be mitigated to some extent by neuromuscular coordination programs for prevention. Such programs minimize the risk of injury occurring with non-contact mechanisms such as cutting, twisting, and landing awkwardly by decreasing quadriceps femoris dominance during these activities and increasing hamstring muscle activation.

Muscle strains are very common in soccer players because of the high-intensity activity involving sprinting, changing direction quickly, and kicking. Lower-extremity strains predominate, with strains of the calf muscles (ie, gastrocnemius, soleus), hamstring muscles, and quadriceps femoris being the most common. The distal muscle-tendon junction is the most frequent site of injury; however intrasubstance muscle partial or complete tears can occur. Hematoma formation may be palpable as a "cord," or ecchymosis may develop overlying the injury. Musculoskeletal ultrasound, and in rare circumstances magnetic resonance imaging (MRI), can be helpful in diagnosing the extent of the injury.

Groin Injuries

Groin injuries are common in soccer. The "sports hernia," a chronic groin strain, has been described with frequency among adolescent and young adult soccer players. Studies indicate that groin injuries account for 2% to 13% of all injuries. The nature of the game predisposes the soccer player to hip and groin pathology. Movements in soccer such as rapid acceleration, frequent and sudden changes in direction, kicking, and quick side-to-side motions increase shear stresses across the pelvis and axial loads to the hip joint and pubis.

As discussed, one of the most common injury patterns associated with soccer, especially in older adolescents, involves lower-extremity muscle-tendon strains. Hip adductor muscle strains occur from overuse as well as from sudden, rapid, lateral movements, especially when the hip is in an abducted and externally rotated position. Injury may occur within the substance of the muscle, at the myotendinous junction, or at the tendon attachment. Clinical grading of the injury depends on presence and degree of functional loss. First-degree strains, in which a small number of fibers are torn, but no function or strength is lost, tend to heal in 1 to 3 weeks. Second- and third-degree strains involve tears to all or a significant amount of muscle fibers and can result in significant morbidity. These often require rest and physical therapy; recovery can take up to 6 weeks, or longer.

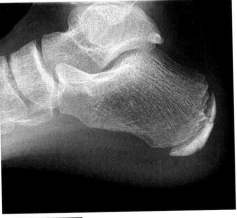

FIGURE 9-2
Calcaneal apophysitis.

In athletes who are skeletally immature, the cartilaginous growth plates, or physes, tend to be more susceptible to injury than the adjacent muscles, tendons, or mature bone. Physes are primary growth plates that contribute to the length of the bone. An example of a physis in the hip is the growth plate in the proximal femur. Apophyses are accessory growth plates that serve as an attachment point for muscle-tendon units. There are several apophyses about the hip and pelvis, including the anterior-superior iliac spine (ASIS) (attachment of the sartorius muscle), anterior-inferior iliac spine (AIIS) (rectus femoris), ischial tuberosity (biceps femoris), lesser trochanter (iliopsoas), greater trochanter (gluteus medius, piriformis, and obturator muscle) iliac crest (abdominal oblique muscles, gluteus medius, and tensor muscle of fascia lata), and pubic symphysis (rectus abdominis and gracilis) (Figure 9-3). Apophysitis can occur at any of these sites and is typically the result of overuse and repetitive traction, leading to inflammation and micro-injury. Radiographic findings are typically normal, and diagnosis is often clinical. An MRI is typically unnecessary for diagnosis but, if obtained, will often reveal an increase in fluid (high signal intensity) at the apophysis. Treatment for apophysitis includes rest, rehabilitation, and gradual return to play.

A sudden, forceful concentric or eccentric contraction of one of the hip muscles can result in an acute injury to the apophysis, known as an apophyseal avulsion fracture. These injuries tend to occur from older adolescence into young adulthood and often result in significant disability, especially if not diagnosed and managed promptly. Radiographic findings usually confirm the diagnosis. Treatment involves protected weight bearing as well as rehabilitation focusing initially on pain-free range of motion and then on strengthening. Progression back to sport should be gradual and may take several months. Surgical treatment may be indicated if the avulsed fragment is displaced greater than 2 to 4 cm.

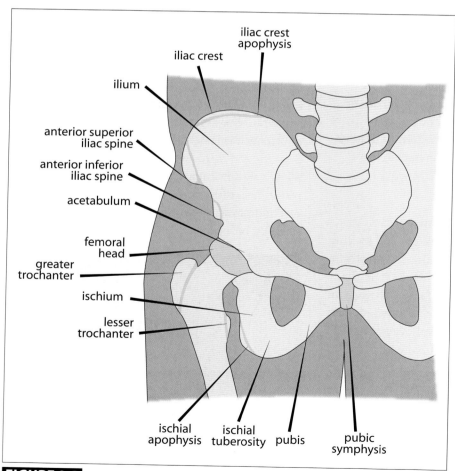

FIGURE 9-3

Diagram indicating apophyses of the hip and pelvis.

Courtesy of Lurie Children's Hospital.

Osteitis pubis is a common cause of pain in adult soccer players, although it is less prevalent in child and adolescent athletes. The term describes inflammation at the pubic symphysis and is thought to represent chronic degenerative changes at the symphysis caused by repetitive shear forces across the pubis. Radiographs and MRIs can aid diagnosis. Treatment is often conservative and consists of relative rest, nonsteroidal anti-inflammatory drugs, rehabilitation, and, occasionally, corticosteroid injections.

The intense forces and shear stress across the pelvis in soccer players also contribute to development of a sports-related condition, known as athletic pubalgia. Also referred to (somewhat controversially) as a sports hernia, *athletic pubalgia* is actually a generic term used to describe an injury to one of the core abdominal or adductor muscles, or both, or their attachments to the pubis. The injury spectrum includes tearing of the external abdominal oblique muscle or rectus abdominis aponeurosis, or both; disruption in the conjoint tendon or tearing of the tendon from the pubic tubercle or dehiscence between conjoint tendon and inguinal ligament; or tearing of the adductor muscle near its proximal attachment. Athletes will often report vague lower abdominal or groin pain, which worsens with activities. The affected player may have tenderness at the pubic tubercle and pain with resisted abdominal contraction or hip adduction, or both. Diagnosis of athletic pubalgia can be difficult. Magnetic resonance imaging and dynamic ultrasound may reveal the anatomical disruption at the level of the muscle or tendon, although are helpful at ruling out other potential causes of groin pain, such as osteitis pubis, stress fractures, masses, or intra-articular hip pathology. Conservative treatment, focusing on rest, rehabilitation, and physical therapy, is often attempted initially, although most experts agree that surgical repair is the definitive treatment for a core muscle injury in a high-level athlete.

Concussion

Several epidemiological studies indicate that concussions may account for 1.2% to 8.0% of all soccer injuries, although significant concern exists for underreporting of symptoms. Rates of concussion seem to be higher in female soccer players than in males at the same level of play. In one study by Kiani et al, female soccer players sustained more concussions than male players by a ratio of 1.8:1.0 in practice and 5.8:1.0 in games. Studies indicate that the most common mechanism of head injuries from soccer seems to be contact with another player's head, elbow, or foot, followed by contact with the ball or with ground or goalpost. Purposeful heading does not seem to contribute to acute concussive injury or the development of cumulative brain damage, although further studies are needed to elucidate the potential neuropsychological effects, both short- and long-term.

Any athlete with a suspected concussion should be removed from play and evaluated by a health care professional. Sideline evaluation includes an assessment of symptoms; a neurologic assessment, with emphasis on ocular function and balance; and a cognitive assessment. Several sideline evaluation tools are available for general use, including ones developed specifically for use with elementary school–aged children. Management of concussion centers on relative cognitive and physical rest and avoidance of activities that exacerbate symptoms. Once the athlete has been free of new symptoms at rest, he or she begins a graduated exercise program, commonly known as a return-to-play protocol, to ensure no symptoms develop with increasing physical load. To return to play, the athlete should be back to baseline symptoms at rest and with exertion, be on no medications that might mask symptoms, and have neuropsychological testing results consistent with results from baseline testing, if performed prior to the start of the season. Most concussions resolve clinically within 7 to 10 days; however, some athletes may take weeks or months to recover.

Case Files: Soccer Injuries

Case 1

18-year-old with mid-substance biceps femoris grade 2 strain

A college freshman from Germany presents after the first week of preseason soccer. He had a clean bill of health on his pre-participation physical examination over the summer. He says he has a "tight" right leg muscle since the conditioning session last night, when the team did a lot of running on the turf field and then practiced long ball passes, from touchline to touchline. He says he has never had any injury problems when playing soccer in Germany for a second-tier club side, whose practices and games were all on grass fields. He plays center back, and he was offered a scholarship on the basis of scouting reports that he was a fast, dominant defender and had a very hard shot when given the chance to take free kicks.

He is 193 cm (6 ft 4 in) and weighs 86 kg (190 lb). He has a full range of motion of his lumbar spine in flexion and extension, non-tenderness to palpation of the spine, and 120° of hip flexion, with 30° of internal rotation and 45° of external rotation of the hip flexed to 90°. Once his compression shorts are removed, there is no visible hematoma or ecchymosis. His popliteal angle of the right hip is tight, with approximately 50° from full knee extension with the hip flexed to 90°. His left leg popliteal angle is 40°. He has tenderness to palpation over the biceps femoris belly in the posterolateral leg. The ischial tuberosity and hamstring muscle origin is nontender, and the distal attachments at the knee are nontender.

He wants to know whether he will be able to play in the season opener in 3 weeks, whether the turf field is responsible for his injury, and if he might undergo MRI of his leg.

In the acute care setting, a musculoskeletal ultrasound of the thigh, with the player prone, identifying an 8- to 10-cm (3- to 4-in) heterogeneous signal intensity in the posterolateral thigh over the area of maximal tenderness is just as good a study as MRI. The ultrasound in this case shows no significant fluid collection, just fiber disruption and echogenicity (Figure 9-4). This indicates that he will need to take his rehabilitation week by week but that the natural history of muscle strains makes a return to play possible in a 3- to 4-week period. He can initiate eccentric strengthening almost immediately under his athletic trainer's guidance, and he must not attempt to try kicking the ball until he is told to do so.

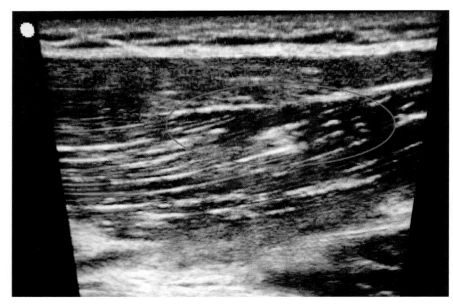

FIGURE 9-4
Ultrasound sound image showing discontinuity of fibers consistent with partial tearing of biceps femoris muscle.

Case 2
13-year-old with fifth metatarsal apophyseal avulsion fracture

A 13-year-old soccer player presents with lateral foot and ankle pain. He first noticed discomfort during his spring travel season. It improved over the summer, while he was on vacation, but has recurred with his participation on the middle school "modified" team this fall. He says his coach has been making the team do a lot of running for conditioning, and he has been getting a lot of playing time on the field during games. He is a center midfielder and is expected to get from "box to box," to help his team on offense and defense, throughout the game. At the game a couple of nights ago, he was "cleated" when an opponent attempted to tackle him; he missed the ball, striking his foot instead. He was able to get up and walk off the field after this incident, but it has hurt to weight bear.

On examination, his ankle has a full range of motion in dorsiflexion, plantar flexion, inversion, and eversion; however, a fully inverted foot reproduces pain. There is no swelling or ecchymosis and no deformity. He has a well-developed arch and good muscle tone in his calves. He has tenderness over the fifth metatarsal and non-tenderness over the lateral malleolus, midfoot, and heel. Resisted eversion is painful and 4/5 strength.

Imaging reveals open growth plates, some calcaneal sclerosis, and widening without frank displacement of the apophysis at the base of the fifth metatarsal–peroneal attachment. An oblique foot comparison view of the unaffected side is obtained, which also shows the apophysis but has less of a gap.

Although the father expresses concern that this was an overuse injury, the examinations indicate there was likely some inflammation of the growth plate (apophysitis) that was preexisting, since the spring, particularly since he has grown 2 foot sizes over the last 6 months. However, the susceptibility of the growth plate to trauma has resulted in a widening of the apophysis, which can completely avulse the tendon from the bone. The patient is recommended a period of relative rest, an ankle brace, and some rehabilitation for the peroneal muscle group.

Case 3
14-year-old with chronic hip pain

A 14-year-old left wing who plays on an elite travel team presents to the office with 4 weeks of insidious-onset left hip pain. She does not recall experiencing any trauma. The pain occurs primarily with sprinting and long kicks and has been gradually worsening over the last few weeks. She has only minimal pain at rest and with ambulation. She indicates that the site of her discomfort is centered over the anterior aspect of the hip, near the proximal aspect of her quadriceps femoris. She has not had any swelling or discoloration. She has no prior history of hip pain.

On physical examination, no swelling or deformity of the hip is appreciated nor is any erythema or ecchymosis seen. Her active hip range of motion is intact in all directions, but she reports pain with active hip flexion on the left. Passive internal rotation and flexion does not cause discomfort, but she has mild anterior pain with passive hyperextension of the left hip. Manual muscle testing reveals pain and minimal weakness with resisted straight-leg raise but normal, pain-free strength with adduction and abduction. On palpation, she has focal tenderness on the left AIIS but nowhere else.

Radiographs are obtained, including an anteroposterior view of the pelvis and a frog-leg lateral view of the left hip. Apophyses are open but appear symmetric. No evidence is appreciated of avulsion fractures or slipped capital femoral epiphysis.

On the basis of her examination, a diagnosis of apophysitis of the AIIS is determined. She needs to rest from activities that cause pain, such as sprinting and long kicks, but should stay active with pain-free activities, such as jogging. It is recommended that she start physical therapy or a home exercise program focused first on stretching, then on eccentric strengthening of the rectus femoris. Requirements for return to full play include full pain-free range of motion, full strength, and ability to perform functional movements, such as sprinting and kicking, without pain.

Case 4
17-year-old with acute anterolateral hip pain and limp

A 17-year-old high school senior presents with acute-onset right hip pain. He plays center back and made a breakaway sprint but felt a sudden pop in the anterior aspect of his right hip and fell to the ground. He came off the field limping and was told by the athletic trainer that he has a muscle strain. Despite applying ice, he has increased pain this morning.

On examination, he appears uncomfortable with ambulation and has an antalgic gait. No deformity of the hip is appreciated, although he has subtle swelling over the anterior iliac crest on the right. He has pain with active hip flexion and abduction but not with passive motion. He has significant tenderness to palpation over the anterior aspect of the iliac crest at the origin of the sartorius. He has weakness and difficulty performing an active straight-leg raise.

Radiographs are obtained, including with an anteroposterior view of the pelvis, and show widening of the right ASIS compared with the left. The displacement is measured at 1.5 cm. The remainder of the radiographic findings appear to be normal.

This young man has an avulsion fracture of his right ASIS growth plate. Recommendations include 1 to 2 weeks of protected weight bearing, with crutches, and early range of motion exercises and pain-free stretching. Given the relative severity of the injury, his rehabilitation plan should be directed by a physical therapist. Eventually, he will advance to strengthening and then functional exercises, but this injury often requires 4 to 8 weeks to heal completely.

Injury Prevention

An inherent risk of injury exists during all contact sports. Nevertheless, many injuries from soccer could be prevented with consistent use of recommended protective equipment and adherence to the rules of fair play.

Protective Equipment

The shin guard is standard equipment for soccer at all levels. It helps protect against contusions in the anterior ankle. Referee inspection of shin guards prior to competition occurs at the high school level and in most child and young adult leagues. The shin guard must be the appropriate size for the height of the athlete and must be worn under the stockings.

Ocular injuries can occur in soccer players from direct impact from the ball or contact with another player's body, typically the elbow or finger. The American Academy of Pediatrics recommends protective eyewear for all soccer players, given the potential for injury to the eye in this contact sport. The American Academy of Pediatrics and the American Academy of Ophthalmology believe eye protection should be mandatory for athletes with only one functional eye or those with a history of major eye surgery or trauma. The protection should consist of properly fitted polycarbonate lenses.

The use of soccer headgear, such as headbands or padded head covers, to prevent concussion is controversial. Several companies promote the headgear as a means to dissipate the forces on the head from collisions and thereby reduce the risk of concussion. However, quality studies on the effectiveness of headgear in preventing concussion are lacking. In addition, many question whether the use of headgear could give players a false sense of security and actually increase the risk of head injuries. At this time, a critical review of the medical literature does not support the use of headgear during soccer to reduce the risk of concussion.

Laws, Fair Play, and Coaching

Soccer originated in England and Scotland, and the laws of the game became globalized in the 20th century by Fédération Internationale de Football Association. The laws of the game are almost universal; however, there can be local interpretation of rules, such as the number of players on each team, the size of the playing field, the number of substitutions allowed, and the consequences of a game tied at the end of regulation time. Child and youth soccer rules vary by age in the United States. Coaches, players, and referees must familiarize themselves with local nuances, such as the implementation of the "offside law," the size of ball to be used, and weather-related decisions, for heat, lightning, and water on the field.

Soccer is a contact sport; as such, not every player-to-player contact is illegal (Figure 9-5). The need for some contact leaves enormous room for interpretation of what constitutes illegal contact. The guiding principal should be whether a player attempted to play the ball and, if the ball was played, whether contact was incidental or purposeful, with intent to harm. Even during kindergarten soccer, there can be disagreement of what is a fair attempt to get the ball, as opposed to an intentional shove of an opponent. Player welfare must be the principal consideration, and a tackle that is deemed too aggressive because of excessive force or the lack of an attempt to play the ball may

be disciplined. Whistling for a foul, issuing a yellow card as a warning, or issuing a red card and dismissing the player responsible for the remainder of the game are options for a referee. Referees are encouraged to take a tough stance on dangerous play, such as a player's use of an elbow in a contest for a loose ball. Consistent refereeing can help educate child and youth players on what constitutes fair play and what is illegal.

Coaching soccer is an enjoyable and immensely rewarding activity, and it must be undertaken with a responsibility to educate players about playing within the rules and spirit of the game (Figure 9-6). The professional sport of soccer is unfortunately littered with incidents of intentional foul play and attempts to con the referee; thus, the child or youth coach's job is to counteract what can be watched on TV with encouragement of conscious decisions to play fair and never attempt to harm an opponent. U.S. Soccer provides guidance, with online modules and a certification process, that can be of benefit to coaches who did not play the game themselves.

The age for introduction of heading the ball into the game of soccer has come under scrutiny. Currently, the United States Soccer Federation recommends that players 10 years and younger not engage in heading in games or practices. Concern is that these players may not possess enough coordination or core and cervical strength to avoid injury, given their larger head to body ratio and relatively weaker muscle strength. Nevertheless,

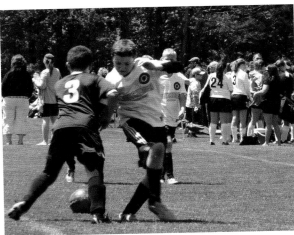

FIGURE 9-5
Youth soccer is a contact sport.

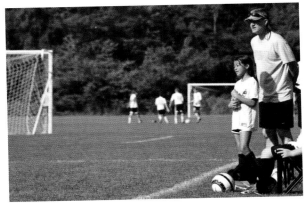

FIGURE 9-6
Coaching youth soccer.

the skill must be introduced at some stage, as it is a fundamental component of the game. If introduced by certified coaches in a manner that follows guidance from governing bodies, heading can be executed safely and effectively in the 10- to 12-year-old age-groups. To reiterate, intentional heading the ball per se does not typically cause concussion.

Summary

Soccer is a popular sport among young athletes in the United States, and rates of participation among boys and girls are on the rise. Unfortunately, the incidence and rates of injury in young soccer players are increasing as well. Clinicians who care for young athletes need to be aware of the typical injury patterns seen in soccer players.

Bibliography

Connell DA, Schneider-Kolsky ME, Hoving JL, et al. Longitudinal study comparing sonographic and MRI assessments of acute and healing hamstring injuries. *AJR Am J Roentgenol.* 2004;183(4):975–984

Cross KM, Saliba SA, Conaway M, Gurka KK, Hertel J. Days to return to participation after a hamstrings strain among American collegiate soccer players. *J Athl Train.* 2015;50(7):733–741

Davis JA, Brewer J. Applied physiology of female soccer players. *Sports Med.* 1993;16(3):180–189

Ekstrand J, Tropp H. The incidence of ankle sprains in soccer. *Foot Ankle.* 1990;11(1):41–44

Emery CA, Meeuwisse WH, Hartmann SE. Evaluation of risk factors for injury in adolescent soccer: implementation and validation of an injury surveillance system. *Am J Sports Med.* 2005;33(12):1882–1891

Francisco AC, Nightingale RW, Guilak F, Glisson RR, Garrett WE Jr. Comparison of soccer shin guards in preventing tibia fracture. *Am J Sports Med.* 2000;28(2):227–233

Fuller CW, Dick RW, Corlette J, Schmalz R. Comparison of the incidence, nature and cause of injuries sustained on grass and new generation artificial turf by male and female football players. Part 2: training injuries. *Br J Sports Med.* 2007;41(suppl 1):i27–i32

Fuller CW, Ekstrand J, Junge A, et al. Consensus statement on injury definitions and data collection procedures in studies of football (soccer) injuries. *Br J Sports Med.* 2006;40(3):193–201

Junge A, Rösch D, Peterson L, Graf-Baumann T, Dvorak J. Prevention of soccer injuries: a prospective intervention study in youth amateur players. *Am J Sports Med.* 2002;30(5):652–659

Kerr H. Concussion risk factors and strategies for prevention. *Pediatr Ann.* 2014;43(12):e309–e315

Kiani A, Hellquist E, Ahlqvist K, Gedeborg R, Michaëlsson K, Byberg L. Prevention of soccer-related knee injuries in teenaged girls. *Arch Intern Med.* 2010;170(1):43–49

Koutures CG, Gregory AJ; American Academy of Pediatrics Council on Sports and Fitness. Injuries in youth soccer. *Pediatrics.* 2010;125(2):410–414

Little T, Williams AG. Specificity of acceleration, maximum speed, and agility in professional soccer players. *J Strength Cond Res.* 2005;19(1):76–78

Mohr M, Krustrup P, Bangsbo J. Match performance of high-standard soccer players with special reference to development of fatigue. *J Sports Sci.* 2003;21(7):519–528

Nichols AW. Does eccentric training of hamstring muscles reduce acute injuries in soccer? *Clin J Sport Med.* 2013;23(1):85–86

Polman R, Walsh D, Bloomfield J, Nesti M. Effective conditioning of female soccer players. *J Sports Sci.* 2004;22(2):191–203

Reilly T. Energetics of high-intensity exercise (soccer) with particular reference to fatigue. *J Sports Sci.* 1997;15(3):257–263

Silvers HJ, Mandelbaum BR. Preseason conditioning to prevent soccer injuries in young women. *Clin J Sport Med.* 2001;11(3):206

Smith NA, Chounthirath T, Xiang H. Soccer-related injuries treated in emergency departments: 1990–2014. *Pediatrics.* 2016;138(4):1–9

Stølen T, Chamari K, Castagna C, Wisløff U. Physiology of soccer: an update. *Sports Med.* 2005;35(6):501–536

Strayer SM, Reece SG, Petrizzi MJ. Fractures of the proximal fifth metatarsal. *Am Fam Physician.* 1999;59(9):2516–2522

Strøyer J, Hansen L, Klausen K. Physiological profile and activity pattern of young soccer players during match play. *Med Sci Sports Exerc.* 2004;36(1):168–174

U.S. Soccer. Coaching education: digital coaching center. U.S. Soccer Web site. http://www.ussoccer.com/coaching-education. Accessed July 1, 2017

Wisløff U, Helgerud J, Hoff J. Strength and endurance of elite soccer players. *Med Sci Sports Exerc.* 1998;30(3):462–467

CHAPTER 10

Baseball and Softball and the Young Athlete

Kristina Wilson, MD, MPH, CAQSM, FAAP, and Peter K. Kriz, MD, FACSM, FAAP

Overview

Baseball and softball remain popular sports among child and adolescent athletes. According to The Aspen Institute's *State of Play 2016* data, baseball remains the second most popular sport among children aged 6 to 12 years; 13.2% of children who play sports regularly in this age-group participate in baseball (Table 10-1).[1]

With year-round participation and travel and club team involvement becoming more of the norm, the injury risk potential has increased. Overuse injuries are prevalent in both baseball and softball, with upper extremity injuries dominating the spectrum. Research conducted at the American Sports Medicine Institute in Birmingham, AL, has shown a

staggering rise in ulnar collateral ligament (UCL) reconstructive surgeries in child and high school throwers over the past 2 decades. Of the UCL surgeries performed at the American Sports Medicine Institute involving child, high school, college, and pro baseball players, child and high school players now consistently comprise approximately 30% of patients undergoing these surgeries annually.[2]

While the explanation for this rise in injuries is multifactorial and includes better detection and better diagnostic testing such as magnetic resonance imaging (MRI), undeniably, there has been an increase in volume and intensity of throwing among child and high school pitchers. A disturbing injury trend that sports medicine physicians have witnessed is an increase in shoulder and elbow

Table 10-1. Core Participation in Team Sports. Percent of Children Ages 6-12 Years Who Played These Sports on a Regular Basis

	2008	2009	2010	2011	2012	2013	2014	2015	2008-15	2014-15
Basketball	16.6	14.4	15.3	15.5	14.1	16.0	14.7	14.7	⬇	➡
Baseball	16.5	14.5	14.1	14.9	12.5	14.2	12.9	13.2	⬇	⬆
Outdoor soccer	10.4	10.4	10.9	11.2	9.2	9.3	9.1	8.9	⬇	⬇
Tackle football	3.7	4.0	3.8	3.2	3.6	3.5	3.3	3.3	⬇	➡
Gymnastics	2.3	2.9	2.8	4.1	3.5	2.9	3.0	2.7	⬆	⬇
Flag football	4.5	3.3	3.0	3.0	2.8	2.8	2.4	2.6	⬇	⬆
Volleyball (court)	2.9	2.2	2.6	1.8	2.4	2.7	2.8	2.5	⬇	⬇
Ice hockey	0.5	0.7	0.7	0.9	0.8	1.1	1.1	1.1	⬆	➡
Track and field	1.0	0.8	1.2	1.5	1.7	1.1	1.2	1.0	➡	⬇
Lacrosse	0.4	0.7	0.6	0.9	0.7	0.8	0.9	0.7	⬆	⬇
Wrestling	1.1	1.1	1.1	1.0	0.8	0.7	0.6	0.7	⬇	⬆
Field hockey	0.4	0.7	0.6	0.3	0.5	0.6	0.4	0.5	⬆	⬆

From Aspen Institute Sports & Society Program. *State of Play 2016: Trends and Developments.* Washington, DC: Aspen Institute; 2016. https://www.aspeninstitute.org/publications/state-play-2016-trends-developments. Accessed July 1, 2017. Reproduced with permission.

injuries among pitchers in the off-season, occurring during showcases for coaches at "the next level," when they are relatively deconditioned or have had inadequate rest from intensive seasons of play. Pediatricians, with an eye toward prevention and keeping players on the field, are encouraged to consider preventive strategies for young baseball players in their offices.

More times than not, a shoulder or elbow injury results from a weak link further up the kinetic chain. Poor hip flexibility, weak core (eg, lower abdominal muscles, gluteus medius) strength, and poorly coordinated motions between the lower extremities, trunk, and upper extremities result in altered mechanics of the shoulder and elbow throughout the phases of throwing. Recent research has shown that child and high school athletes that have better throwing mechanics subject their shoulders and elbows to lower forces during the phases of throwing.[3] Learning proper throwing mechanics at an early age seems to be essential to both reduce injury risk and enhance performance. Two-dimensional video analysis is an emerging tool for the kinematic assessment and observational measurement of throwing mechanics. Sports medicine programs that use screening of pitching biomechanics as a component of injury risk assessment are becoming more readily available to communities in the United States.[4]

This chapter will highlight, through case examples, some of the more common injuries seen in baseball and softball players, with brief explanations of the injury, diagnosis, and treatment. The chapter will conclude with strategies to help children and adolescents participate safely in baseball and softball by taking steps to reduce their risk of overuse injuries.

Baseball-Specific Injuries

Elbow

The skeletally immature pediatric and adolescent elbow is particularly vulnerable to injury because of the presence of open physes, growth areas located at the ends of adolescent bones. Because the closure of these physeal areas depends on sexual maturity, not chronological age, it is not uncommon for baseball players of the same chronological age to have vastly different sexual and skeletal maturity. This is particularly important in baseball because increased muscle strength leads to increased force while throwing, which can lead to overload of physeal anatomy. For that reason, it is essential to consider every adolescent athlete as unique; no one size fits all when considering the young thrower.

Physes are relatively weak links in the kinetic chain when compared with surrounding tendons, ligaments, and bone. They are prone to inflammation from repetitive muscular contraction and overuse. The repetitive stress of throwing can result in muscle fatigue, which can lead to muscle, tendon, ligament, and physeal injury.[5] Most elbow injuries occur because of stresses incurred during the acceleration phase, when valgus torque can reach 64 N · m, shear forces experienced by the medial elbow approach 300 N, and compressive forces at the radiocapitellar joint near 500 N.[6]

Medial Elbow Injuries

Injuries to the medial elbow are caused by traction forces produced during the late cocking and early acceleration phases of throwing. In the child and adolescent thrower, medial traction forces can cause inflammation, separation, or avulsion of the humeral medial epicondylar apophysis and overuse injury in the common flexor tendon,[5] as well as overuse injuries involving the flexor-pronator mass (FPM), the UCL, and the ulnar nerve. The following injuries scenarios are common in the developing thrower:

Case 1
Medial elbow pain in a 12-year-old Little Leaguer

Sammy is a 12-year-old baseball player who started playing baseball 6 years ago. He is an excellent pitcher and catcher, and he has not been able to decide which position he prefers. For the past 2 years, he has been following Pitch Smart/USA Baseball guidelines[7] for pitch counts and days of rest. Typically, he throws 50 to 60 pitches per game once or twice per week between his recreational league, travel team, and school teams. He generally catches only for his travel team, but he has been utilized as a catcher by his school team coach as well. He has been experiencing medial elbow pain intermittently for the past year, which progressively worsened once he started practicing daily with his school team 1 month ago. He has not noticed any swelling and does not recall a specific injury. Initially, he experienced pain after pitching, which would improve over his 2 to 3 days of rest with icing, but now he has constant pain while pitching that occurs during the early acceleration phase.

Little League Elbow

Little League elbow (LLE) is a general term encompassing a group of injuries that occur in athletes who are skeletally immature. It results from repetitive valgus stress to the medial aspect of the elbow, as well as inadequate periods of rest. In early phases, irritation to the medial epicondylar physeal plate or apophysis (apophysitis) occurs, which may progress to accelerated apophyseal growth with delayed closure of the epicondylar growth plate or an avulsion fracture of the medial epicondyle. It frequently presents in young throwers (usually 9–14 years of age) with gradual onset of progressively worsening medial elbow pain during throwing activities. Throwers typically present with a combination of elbow pain, loss of throwing velocity and distance, and reduced effectiveness (eg, accuracy, location). Often encountered in pitchers, LLE can lead to fracture. Many athletes with LLE typically pitch in addition to playing shortstop or other infield positions, such as catcher or third base. Ultimately, the weak link, the physis, fails, resulting in a medial epicondylar apophyseal stress fracture. On examination, athletes commonly have tenderness over the medial epicondyle and pain with resisted wrist flexion.

While LLE is a clinical diagnosis, radiographs may demonstrate subtle widening of the medial epicondylar apophysis with anteroposterior (AP) view (Figure 10-1), but often findings can be normal, especially when obtained early in the disease process. A comparison view of the opposite elbow is often helpful.

Treatment typically involves restriction of all throwing activities for a minimum of 6 weeks. Initial treatments are ice, nonsteroidal anti-inflammatory drugs (NSAIDs), and a short course of elbow immobilization (severe cases) in conjunction with a thrower's rehabilitation program focusing on correcting the defects in the kinetic chain that led to the development of LLE. Prevention efforts are directed at adhering to Pitch Smart/USA Baseball guidelines[7] and learning proper throwing mechanics.

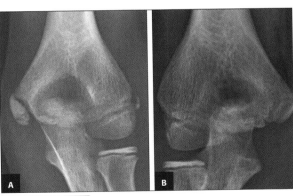

FIGURE 10-1

(A) Medial epicondyle apophysitis: asymmetric hypertrophy, widening, and mild fragmentation of the apophysis in the throwing arm. (B) Normal contralateral view.

Medial Epicondylar Avulsion Injuries

Medial epicondylar avulsion fractures are experienced by school-aged and adolescent throwers. These injuries occur acutely, characterized by immediate pain over the medial elbow after an especially hard throw, and are usually accompanied by an audible pop or crack. Athletes have limited elbow extension and focal tenderness over the medial epicondyle on examination; radiographs reveal minimally displaced avulsion fractures with variable physeal (growth plate) widening (Figure 10-2). Obtaining specialized images or scans (eg, flexed-elbow AP view in 40° flexion, stress radiographs, 3-dimensional computed tomography scan) may be helpful to assess displacement, but carry the risk of increased radiation exposure (particularly computed tomography scan). While optimal treatment for medial epicondylar avulsions remains a highly debated topic, most authors recommend a brief (eg, 5–7 days) course of immobilization in a sling or splint for stable, minimally (<5 mm) displaced fractures, followed by activity restriction and physical therapy emphasizing early range of motion. For athletes who have sustained more substantial trauma, demonstrate elbow laxity or instability,

or have significant (≥4 mm) fragment displacement, surgical consultation is advised, with reduction and internal fixation recommended for fragments displaced by 5 mm or greater.[6,8–9] A hinged elbow brace is often used during the rehabilitative phase to protect and provide some restraint to traction forces generated on the elbow. Return to play in less than 1 year is the norm for both nonoperative and operative options. Attention is also given to review the importance of pitch counts and proper throwing mechanics.

Case 2

Medial elbow pain in a 16-year-old high school pitcher

Aaron is a 16-year-old varsity baseball pitcher who reports medial right elbow pain following a return to his high school team's fall conditioning program. Aaron, who hopes to sign a letter of intent with a Division I collegiate program imminently, worked intensely over the summer to increase velocity and accuracy of his fastball, and he participated in 6 showcase tournaments. Unfortunately, during the last 2 showcases, he started to develop elbow pain and swelling with pitching. He has been resting since and had resolution of the pain with daily activities but continues to have limited extension in the elbow. He recently resumed an interval throwing program and immediately had return of the pain, which he describes as a constant, dull ache on the medial aspect of the elbow. His pain can be sharp when pitching, especially in late cocking and early acceleration phases. He reports having had a similar pain last year, but it was less severe and it improved throughout the year, until its recurrence this summer. He has recently experienced intermittent numbness and tingling of his ring and little fingers. He has not had any imaging to date.

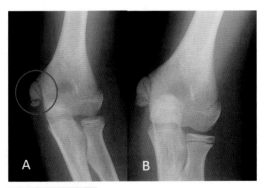

FIGURE 10-2

A, Medial epicondylar avulsion fracture (circled region). B, Repeat radiograph 6 months into conservative treatment demonstrates interval healing.

On examination, Aaron has tenderness to palpation approximately 2 cm distal to the medial epicondyle with the elbow in 60° of flexion. A moving valgus stress test elicits pain from 70° to 120° of flexion. He demonstrates scapular dyskinesis and limited glenohumeral internal rotation (loss of 25° of his arc of motion) in comparison with his nondominant arm. He also has tight hip flexors and a positive Trendelenburg test result of bilateral hips and corkscrewing with single-leg squat, highlighting his poor core stability with weak hip abductor muscles and gluteal musculature.

Overuse Injury of the Ulnar Collateral Ligament

Aaron's story and examination findings are concerning for an overuse injury of the UCL. The UCL complex is the primary restraint to valgus forces on the elbow. It typically fails from repetitive valgus stress causing chronic microtrauma, resulting in an acute (rupture) or chronic (instability) presentation. Of the 3 bundles of the UCL complex, the anterior oblique ligament is the only significant restraint to valgus stress.[10] Although the curveball has been implicated as a cause of elbow injury, and recommendations have been made on limitations on numbers of curveballs thrown and the appropriate age to begin throwing breaking pitches,[7,11] recent literature has refuted this concern, suggesting that the biomechanics of throwing indicate that the fastball puts the greatest valgus load on the elbow.[12–14] The fastball as the culprit is further supported by maximum pitch velocity being significantly associated with risk of elbow injury, particularly in those whose injury requires surgery.[15] In addition, pitch count during games and cumulative counts over a season were significantly associated with elbow injuries in child and youth pitchers.[11,15–17]

Physical examination of the child or adolescent thrower with a suspected UCL injury begins with inspection, which may show ecchymosis in the setting of ligament or (concurrent) tendon rupture. An elbow effusion may also be present with loss of terminal elbow extension.[10] Elbow range of motion, forearm rotation, glenohumeral internal rotation, and assessment for scapular dyskinesis should be performed when assessing any elbow injury. Isolated loss of elbow extension is not necessarily pathological, as up to 50% of professional throwers possess this adaptive change.[10] Palpation of the UCL should be performed in 50° to 70° of flexion, to expose the ligament by moving the medial muscle mass anterior. Provocative and special tests for UCL injury include valgus stress testing at 20° to 30° of elbow flexion, modified milking maneuver, and moving valgus stress tests. Valgus stress tests will elicit pain between 120° and 70° of flexion in the setting of UCL insufficiency, and they have a reported 100% sensitivity and 75% specificity, using arthroscopic valgus stress testing and surgical exploration as the criterion standard.[10,18]

Imaging evaluation of UCL injuries generally starts with plain radiographs, which may demonstrate an avulsion fragment in acute injuries. In chronic UCL injuries, ossification of the UCL, osteophytic changes of the radiocapitellar joint or posteromedial compartment, loose bodies, or olecranon stress injury may be demonstrated.[10,18] While dynamic musculoskeletal ultrasound examination with an applied valgus stress is an emerging study that can be performed in the office setting to assess UCL injuries, examination is operator dependent, limiting the reliability of this study. The image of choice to evaluate for injuries to the UCL is a magnetic resonance arthrogram of the elbow, which increases the sensitivity of diagnosing partial tears over an unenhanced MRI,[10–18] although non-contrast MRI remains the preferred study at many institutions (Figure 10-3).

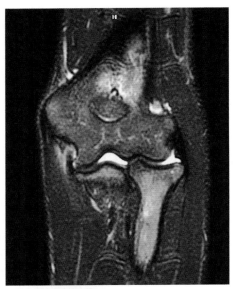

FIGURE 10-3

MRI of the elbow demonstrating UCL tear in an adolescent pitcher. Treatment for UCL overuse injuries depends on the severity of the injury. Nonoperative treatment is indicated for low-grade partial tears confirmed by magnetic resonance arthrography, whereas UCL reconstruction surgery is typically recommended in the following settings:

- High-grade or complete tears of the anterior oblique ligament in athletes desiring to return to throwing sports.
- Throwing athletes with partial UCL tears whose comprehensive rehabilitation program has failed.
- Non-throwing athletes who remain symptomatic despite conservative treatment.[10]

Abbreviations: MRI, magnetic resonance image; UCL, ulnar collateral ligament.

Flexor-Pronator Mass Strains

Repetitive contraction of the flexor-pronator muscles during the acceleration phase, and with wrist flexion during ball release, leads to overuse injuries of the FPM, which can include acute partial tears or chronic tendinopathy. Complete rupture of the common flexor-pronator origin is rare. Differentiating FPM injuries from UCL injuries can be difficult. Tenderness anterior to the medial epicondyle midline is typically consistent with FPM injury, while tenderness posterior to the medial epicondyle midline is usually related to a UCL injury. However, concurrent FPM and UCL injuries are not uncommon, and MRI is often used to clarify the diagnosis.

Conservative treatment for FPM injuries (tendinopathy and partial tears) includes throwing restrictions, NSAIDs, physical therapy, and, eventually, an interval throwing program prior to return to play. Complete ruptures of the flexor-pronator origin are treated with prolonged rest and rehabilitation. Operative treatment may be required if pain or weakness recurs with resumption of throwing.

Ulnar Neuropathy

Throwing athletes are susceptible to ulnar neuropathy, which is rarely an isolated injury but rather occurs in the setting of multiple medial elbow problems. Compression, traction, and irritation of the ulnar nerve during elbow flexion and wrist extension, as occurs during the throwing motion, renders it susceptible to mechanical factors. Medial epicondylitis, osteophytic changes in the posteromedial elbow associated with valgus extension overload, chronic valgus instability, and ulnar nerve subluxation or dislocation are all conditions that are either associated with or contribute to injury to the ulnar nerve and surrounding soft tissues.

A positive Tinel sign over the cubital tunnel, paresthesias involving the ring and little finger, and, in more severe cases, atrophy of the hypothenar muscles in the palm can be detected in patients with ulnar neuropathy. Passive elbow flexion with palpation of the cubital tunnel may elicit ulnar nerve subluxation or dislocation, which can also be visualized easily if musculoskeletal ultrasound is available (Figure 10-4). The medial head of the triceps brachii can sometimes be visualized snapping over the cubital tunnel, with or without ulnar nerve subluxation or dislocation. Anconeus epitrochlearis is also a rare cause of snapping over the cubital tunnel. While electromyographic and electroneurographic studies may be useful, electrodiagnostic changes are seldom present unless disease is advanced.

Conservative treatment for ulnar neuropathy includes throwing restrictions, NSAIDs, icing, and night splinting, with a towel wrap (elbow extended at 0° flexion). Surgical treatment typically involves ulnar nerve transposition to a more anterior location, and it is indicated in the setting of nonoperative treatment failure, persistent ulnar nerve subluxation, traction neurapraxia, and concurrent medial elbow injuries that require surgical intervention.

Lateral Elbow Injuries

Injuries to the lateral aspect of the elbow are caused by compression forces on the lateral structures, primarily the radiocapitellar joint. Osteochondritis dissecans (OCD) lesions involving injuries in child and adolescent throwers that can have an insidious onset can result in significant morbidity and require a high index of suspicion among the examining clinician.

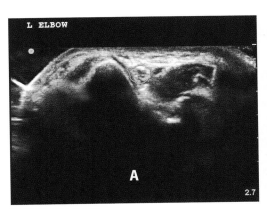
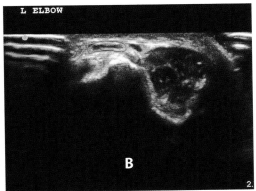

FIGURE 10-4
Dynamic musculoskeletal ultrasound image of the left elbow demonstrating dislocation of the ulnar nerve out of the cubital tunnel in an adolescent pitcher with symptoms of ulnar neuropathy. Ulnar nerve outlined by blue line. A, Elbow in extension. B, Elbow in terminal flexion.

Case 3
Lateral elbow pain in a 12-year-old baseball pitcher

Casey is a 12-year-old boy who has played organized baseball since he was 5 years of age. He started pitching 3 years ago and is currently playing for 2 teams, his middle school team and his travel team, the latter which plays doubleheaders on weekends. His middle school team plays on the "big diamond," where he pitches from a distance of 18 m (60 ft 6 in).

He presents to your office reporting elbow pain that started 6 weeks ago. The pain is localized to the lateral aspect of his elbow. Mild swelling is noted on examination. He has limited range of motion, lacking 10° of terminal elbow extension, and he is not able to flex past 130°. He has tenderness to palpation over the capitellum, and valgus stress causes pain on the lateral aspect of the elbow.

This case highlights the current culture of child and youth sports participation. There is a misconception that "more is better" and early sport specialization allows children and youths to get to the next level. Casey has multiple risk factors for developing an OCD lesion of the capitellum. Casey is pitching for 2 teams in the same season, which significantly increases his pitch counts during a given week, particularly if pitch counts and days of rest guidelines are not adhered to, which is common when pitchers play for multiple teams in multiple leagues. Year-round participation does not provide adequate time for recovery from injury. Additionally, transitioning from a Little League field (12-m [46-ft] pitching distance, 18-m [60-ft] base paths) to the big diamond (18-m [60 ft 6 in] pitching distance, 27-m [90-ft] base paths) is a big adjustment for adolescent throwers to make, as pitching and throwing requires generation of more force throughout the kinetic chain to successfully make longer throws. Casey most likely did not possess core and upper back stability necessary to throw with the same velocity at an increased distance.

Osteochondritis Dissecans of the Capitellum

Osteochondritis dissecans of the capitellum is a common cause of lateral elbow pain in throwing athletes typically 11 to 16 years of age. While the following etiology is not universally accepted, OCD likely results from compression and shear forces to the radiocapitellar joint during late cocking and early acceleration phases of throwing. Overload on the lateral structures with repetitive valgus stress, especially when the supporting musculature fatigues, contributes to microtrauma in the radiocapitellar joint. Ischemic injury to the tenuous blood supply of the developing capitellum is another potential cause.

Throwing athletes typically present with a several months' history of poorly localizable elbow pain, which is progressive and typically relieved by rest. Examination of the radiocapitellar joint (best performed in elbow flexion) is imperative, which commonly elicits tenderness. Plain radiographs may demonstrate lucency of the capitellum or flattening of the articular surface (Figure 10-5). Magnetic resonance imaging plays a vital role in detecting early OCD lesions and assisting in determining whether lesions are stable or unstable.

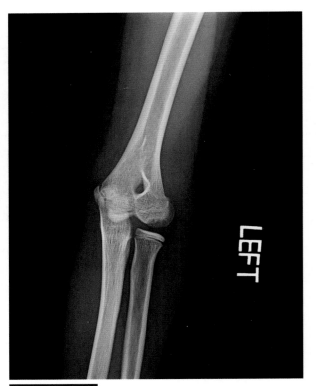

FIGURE 10-5

Radiolucency of the capitellum, indicating an OCD lesion.

Abbreviation: OCD, osteochondritis dissecans.

Nonoperative treatment is indicated for stable lesions, and it typically involves elbow rest for up to 6 months, with physical therapy for stretching and for strengthening starting once pain has resolved, generally around 2 to 3 months. Radiographs are obtained at selected intervals to assess for healing. Repeat MRI is typically performed after 6 months of conservative treatment. If an MRI demonstrates healing of the lesion and the athlete is pain-free, a dedicated throwing program under close supervision is begun.

Posteromedial Elbow Injuries

Injuries to the posteromedial compartment are caused by compression or impingement and shear forces, leading to stress fractures or spurring of the olecranon.

Valgus Extension Overload Syndrome

Valgus extension overload syndrome commonly presents with posteromedial elbow pain with extension that occurs during the late acceleration and follow-through phases of throwing. Osteophytes form in the olecranon fossa posteromedially. Contributors to valgus extension overload syndrome include repetitive valgus stress from throwing, adaptive elbow laxity, and UCL injury or insufficiency.[6] Conservative treatment includes throwing restrictions, ice, NSAIDs, and iontophoresis (consider dexamethasone). Intra-articular corticosteroid injections should be reserved for throwers who are skeletally mature and should be used judiciously. Surgical treatment, consisting of arthroscopic debridement and loose body removal, should be reserved for athletes with persistent pain with presence of loose bodies.

Olecranon Stress Injuries

Stress injuries of the olecranon include proximal olecranon stress fractures and avulsion fractures of the tip of the olecranon. These conditions should be differentiated from a persistent olecranon apophysis, which is commonly identified on radiographs of a thrower who is skeletally immature. Proximal olecranon stress fractures are the result of traction forces from the triceps tendon, olecranon impingement against the olecranon fossa, and

repetitive microtrauma, which is common in young pitchers playing competitively.[6] An MRI often shows high signal intensity in the posteromedial aspect of the olecranon, particularly on short tau inversion recovery sequences. Conservative treatment includes throwing restrictions, rest, and immobilization in certain circumstances. All activities that generate valgus stress should be avoided for a minimum of 6 weeks. Use of a splint or hinged elbow brace, which limits terminal extension, should be considered for the first 4 weeks of treatment. Physical therapy can be initiated at 4 weeks, with an interval throwing program at 8 weeks. Surgical fixation is reserved for complete olecranon stress fractures, which are fortunately rare.

Shoulder

Potential shoulder injuries in child and adolescent throwing athletes include proximal humeral epiphysiolysis (Little League shoulder), rotator cuff and biceps tendon injuries, shoulder impingement (internal and external), and glenohumeral labral tears, with superior labrum AP lesions being the most common labral tear.

Case 4
Shoulder pain in a 13-year-old pitcher

A 13-year-old, left-handed boy presents to your office with a 2-month history of left shoulder pain. He plays on multiple teams, including his middle school team, his recreational league, and an Amateur Athletic Union team, the last which typically plays 2 doubleheaders on a weekend. He is a pitcher and an outfielder. This year, he moved up to the big diamond. He is experiencing pain when throwing his fastball or when making throws to the cutoff man from the outfield. He has lost velocity when pitching and is struggling to make long throws from the outfield. On physical examination, you elicit tenderness over the lateral aspect of the proximal left humerus, with his shoulder externally rotated. You obtain radiographs with AP internal and external rotation views of the left shoulder as well as comparison views of the right shoulder.

There is diffuse widening of the proximal left humeral physis, best appreciated with AP external rotation view, consistent with proximal humeral epiphysiolysis, or Little League shoulder. You initiate a conservative treatment plan, including rest from all skilled throwing for 12 weeks. If adherence can be assured, one treatment option includes allowing the athlete to play first base but limiting all skilled throws in practice and games. Having the athlete field ground balls, or take throws from the other infielders, and drop the ball into a 19-L (5-gal) bucket is a practical method to allow the athlete to continue some skill development and participation. Additionally, limitations on hitting seldom need to be implemented. Initiating a comprehensive kinetic chain strengthening and stabilization program and identifying muscle imbalances and inflexibility issues during the 12-week throwing restriction, with a physical therapist experienced with throwing athlete injuries, is advised. Screening for improper pitching mechanics with 2-dimensional video analysis (if available) once the athlete has completed a gradual return to throwing program can be invaluable and potentially reduce the risk of reinjury. Injury prevention counseling includes discouraging year-round pitching and limiting play to 1 team per season.

Little League shoulder, also known as proximal humeral epiphysiolysis, is an injury of adolescent throwers (typically 11–16 years of age) caused by shear stress from external rotation torque in the late cocking phase of throwing. This injury is directly related to the amount and intensity of throwing, and it is more common in pitchers and year-round throwing athletes. Athletes present with progressively worsening shoulder pain with throwing. Tenderness over the lateral portion of the proximal humerus is common, and it seems to correlate with radiographic widening, most commonly seen with AP external rotation views. Obtaining radiographs with AP internal and external rotation views as well as comparison views of the unaffected shoulder should be

considered (Figure 10-6). Treatment involves rest from throwing for 12 weeks, followed by implementation of proper pitching mechanics, with a gradual return to throwing, typically following a comprehensive kinetic chain strengthening and stabilization program. Prevention involves limiting the number of skilled throws, avoiding year-round pitching, and limiting play to 1 team per season.

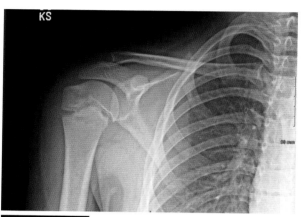

FIGURE 10-6
Widening of the proximal humeral physis, left shoulder, in an adolescent pitcher consistent with Little League shoulder.

Softball-Specific Injuries

Softball injuries most commonly involve the back, shoulder, forearm, wrist, and hand. Pitchers, catchers, and infielders have similar injury rates, although windmill pitching injuries differ from position player injuries because of the demands that the windmill motion place on the back, neck, shoulder, forearm, and wrist.[19]

Windmill pitching biomechanics associated with fast-pitch softball differ significantly from those of overhand baseball pitchers. Consequently, windmill softball pitchers are subject to different injury patterns, which tend to be overuse in nature. Similar to baseball, the shoulder and elbow joint represent most injuries, with strains and muscular injuries occurring most commonly. Shoulder, elbow, forearm, and wrist tendinitis are the most common upper-extremity pitching injuries. Back and neck pain are also common in windmill pitchers.

The deceleration phase of the windmill pitching delivery has been theorized to be the primary cause of injury to the posterior shoulder capsule and the glenoid labrum, as the compression and distraction forces about the shoulder are of high magnitude during this phase.[20] Additionally, windmill pitchers seem to be at increased risk of proximal biceps tendinitis, because of the high levels of biceps brachii activation that occur during the later phases of delivery (eg, ball release, follow-through). Forearm stress fractures, particularly of the ulna, are unique to windmill pitchers. Pitching volume and the pronation release that some windmill pitchers use to throw a drop ball have been implicated as risk factors for ulnar stress fractures.

Ulnar neuropathy is a common injury in softball position players and pitchers, as it is in baseball players, because of similar mechanical factors. However, the unique delivery of a windmill pitcher is responsible for an additional injury mechanism. Windmill pitchers tend to strike the medial aspect of their throwing elbow on their hip just prior to

ball release. This is considered to be a flaw in technique, which slows pitch velocity because of dissipation of force.[21]

Back and knee problems, as well as overhead throwing shoulder problems, predominate for catchers, while overhead shoulder and, occasionally, elbow problems are most common for positional players.[19] Please note that positional softball players that throw overhand are at risk of similar overuse and growth-related injuries seen in child and adolescent baseball players, such as Little League shoulder.

Thoracolumbar Junction of the Spine

Injuries of the thoracolumbar junction of the spine in young throwing athletes can be categorized as follows:

- Muscular
- Bone-related
- Discogenic[22]

Muscular

Acute strains of core muscles such as the internal and external abdominal oblique muscles, transversus abdominis, and rectus abdominis are common in young throwing athletes. In baseball and softball, oblique muscle strains typically present with a sharp, sudden onset of side pain after throwing, swinging, or twisting movements. Location is near or on the rib cage and is associated with localized tenderness. Reinjury rates of core muscle strains are relatively high, and predisposing factors for reinjury are thought to include lack of complete healing and failure to modify training techniques, form, or preparation. Upper segment–lower segment strength imbalances in the pediatric and adolescent throwing athlete can also contribute to injury. Young pitchers demonstrate increased trunk and leading hip rotation velocity from cocking to acceleration phases compared with adult pitchers, likely because of a decreased ability to generate lower core force. Consequently, this upper trunk–lower trunk rotational disassociation results in a tendency for young pitchers to "open up" with their throwing arm positioned behind their trunk, with increased anterior loads across the shoulder and increased valgus loads across the medial elbow.

Bone-Related

The adolescent spine has areas of growth cartilage and immature ossification centers that are susceptible to compression, distraction, and torsional injury. In the athlete who is skeletally immature, these areas are often the weakest link of energy transfer. Consequently, injuries to the anterior column (vertebral body and intervertebral disc) and the posterior column (pedicles, facet joints, pars interarticularis, spinous process) of the spine can manifest in throwing athletes, due in part to the sheer volume and intensity of repetitive pitches and throws performed.

Vertebral end-plate injuries are common among young throwing athletes. Risk factors include the vulnerable growth period of adolescence, trauma, and overload. Examples include

- Ring apophyseal abnormalities (including Schmorl nodes)
- Lumbar spine (L2–L5) vertebral osteophytes

Typically, such injuries present with localized pain in the thoracolumbar junction associated with flexion, extension, or axial loading.

Injuries to the posterior elements of the lumbar spine related to rotation, hyperextension, and flexion during repetitive activities, such as pitching and bat swinging, are relatively common injuries in baseball players, as they are in many players of overhead and throwing sports. Stress reactions and fractures of the pars interarticularis (spondylolysis) and the pedicles may present in the adolescent throwing athlete as extension-based lower back pain. Overhead and throwing sports that distribute an asymmetric load on the trunk and shoulders have been associated with an increased reported incidence of scoliosis. However, the rotational curves of these athletes seem to be small (Cobb angles <15°) and asymptomatic. It is not uncommon to encounter one-sided hypertrophy of back and shoulder muscles in overhead and throwing athletes, which may result in a falsely positive result on the Adams forward flexion test for scoliosis.

Discogenic

Disc-related disease, while less common in pediatric and adolescent throwing athletes than in adult competitors, is prevalent among young athletes, compared with their sedentary peers, particularly athletes older than 12 years. Throwing athletes are susceptible to disc injury caused by axial loading, hyperextension or hyperflexion, and rotational forces involved in training and conditioning as well as in the biomechanics of throwing and swinging. Pain worse with forward flexion is typically located in the lower back, buttock, posterior thigh, or leg, or a combination of those, because of L4-L5 and L5-S1 disc and herniated nucleus pulposus injuries in adolescents. While there are no available studies assessing the prevalence of degenerative disc disease in adolescent baseball players, a study of college athletes found baseball players to be at the highest risk of lumbar disc degeneration compared with other groups of athletes, at a rate greater than 3 times that of nonathlete controls.[23,24] Baseball players are known to develop lumbar disc herniations, comprising 13% to 35% of reported cases in studies of elite athletes.[25,26]

Treatment for Thoracolumbar Junction Injuries

Assessment of core, peripelvic, and lumbar dynamic stabilization is critical in the evaluation of a throwing athlete with a thoracolumbar junction injury, as is the development of an appropriate treatment program. Single-leg bridge and single-leg squat testing are clinical assessments of the lower abdominal and hip abductor musculature, as well as trunk neuromuscular control, that can be performed rapidly during a clinical evaluation. Additionally, postural assessment (eg, anterior pelvic tilt, lumbar lordosis) and flexibility testing (ie, Thomas testing for hip flexor tightness, popliteal angles for hamstring tightness) can provide clues to muscle imbalances, which may be predisposing a young throwing athlete to injury anywhere along the kinetic chain. Rehabilitation of thoracolumbar injuries in the young throwing athlete involves provision of therapeutic exercises to correct identifiable muscle imbalances that result from deficits in flexibility, strength, endurance, and balance.

Return to Play Issues With Thoracolumbar Junction Injuries

Pain-free range of motion, stabilization of the lumbar-pelvic-hip core complex, and progression through sport-specific phases of rehabilitation are the prerequisites for a throwing athlete to return to play following a thoracolumbar injury. To some extent, injury type and severity dictate the amount of time loss and recovery. Abdominal muscle strains take several weeks for recovery, particularly in baseball pitchers. For athletes with lumbar spondylolysis, return to full play has been accomplished within 4 to 6 weeks of treatment initiation, with a lumbar orthosis and pain-free extension. Athletes who undergo surgical treatment (eg, single-level spinal or lumbosacral fusion, micro-discectomy) and are not participating in collision sports are typically allowed to return to play 6 to 12 months' postoperatively.

Injury Prevention

Preventive measures for reducing injury risk during baseball and softball can be divided into the following categories:

- Age- and developmentally appropriate rule modifications
- Playing and protective equipment
- Environmental
- Overuse injury precautions[5,7,19,27]

The following are recommendations endorsed by the American Academy of Pediatrics[5,7]:

Age- and Developmentally Appropriate Rule Modifications

- Distance between bases set at 14 m (45 ft) for T-ball, 18 m (60 ft) for ages 10 to 12 years, 21 to 23 m (70–75 ft) for 13 to 15 years, and 27 m (90 ft) for boys and young men 16 to 18 years (although variation exists between organizations)
- Pitcher's mound distance to home plate set at 14 to 15 m (46–50 ft) for 9 to 12 years and 18.4 m (60.5 ft) for 13 to 18 years (although variation exists between organizations)
- Avoidance of headfirst sliding by child players, particularly younger than 10 years

Playing and Protective Equipment

- Use of low-impact (softer) baseballs by children younger than 10 years
- Bat standards (eg, composition, length, diameter) to reduce injuries to fielders
- Use of breakaway bases in baseball and softball to reduce foot and ankle injuries
- Use of an orange "runner's base" adjacent to the white regular base at first base to avoid collisions during child and youth softball
- Face and eye protection for batters (baseball and softball) and infielders and pitchers (softball)
- Hard plastic athletic cup for boys (Catchers, pitchers, and infielders are at greatest risk.)
- "Knee savers" for catchers and shin guards and elbow protective pads for batters
- Rapid access to automated external defibrillators in the event of commotio cordis or sudden cardiac arrest

Environmental

- Use of an emergency action plan and automated warning systems in the event of severe weather (eg, lightning)

- Use of dugouts behind a fence, elimination of the on-deck circle, and use of batting helmets by first- and third-base coaches to reduce likelihood of injuries occurring on or near the playing field

Overuse Injury Precautions

Overuse injuries, particularly involving the shoulder and elbow, are preventable. In an era of single-sport specialization and year-round training, the parent and the athlete are responsible for adhering to age-appropriate published guidelines regarding throwing and pitching, given that many players play in multiple leagues with different affiliations during different times of the year.[7] Table 10-2 provides concise guidelines derived from expert opinion resources.[5,7,19,27]

Table 10-2. Injury Prevention Guidelines for Baseball and Softball

Guideline	Baseball	Softball
Warm-up	Consistently engage in a dynamic warm-up before practices and games. This includes running, followed by stretching, followed by easy, gradual throwing. Properly warm up before pitching. Consider a resistance band warm-up for all throwers.	
Volume of play, positional restrictions, and periods of rest	• Take at least 4 mo off from throwing each year, with at least 2–3 of those months being continuous. • Avoid playing for multiple teams at the same time. • Avoid playing catcher while not pitching. • Rotate playing other positions, besides pitcher. • Play other sports throughout the year. • **Baseball:** Do not exceed 60 combined innings (≤8 y), 80 combined innings (9–12 y), or 100 combined innings in any 12-mo period (ages 13–18 y).	
Pitch counts and days of rest	Age dependent. See PitchSmart/USA Baseball Web site for details.[7] Make sure to follow guidelines across leagues, tournaments, and showcases. Monitor for signs of fatigue. Do not pitch with elbow or shoulder pain.	Age dependent. See AOSSM Web site for details.[19] Make sure to follow guidelines across leagues, tournaments, and showcases. Monitor for signs of fatigue. Do not pitch with elbow or shoulder pain.
Pitch type and biomechanics	≤8 y and 9–12 y: only fastballs and changeups 13–18 y: can begin breaking balls after developing consistent fastball and changeup Emphasize control, accuracy, and good mechanics.	Fastball, changeup, drop pitch, curveball, and rise ball are the most common pitches.[20] No consensus exists regarding introduction of pitch types. Emphasize control, accuracy, and good mechanics.
Sport-specific training	With baseball and softball injuries, the upper extremity (eg, shoulder, elbow) is typically the "victim," while the "culprit" is a weak lower segment. Off-season and preseason conditioning programs should include gluteal strengthening and peripelvic stabilization exercises in addition to core and periscapular strengthening.	
Post-practice and postgame	Icing of the shoulder and elbow following pitching and throwing activity should be encouraged to reduce soreness and inflammation. Commercially available icing sleeves and cold wraps may improve compliance.	

Abbreviation: AOSSM, American Orthopaedic Society for Sports Medicine.

References

1. Aspen Institute Sports & Society Program. *State of Play 2016: Trends and Developments.* Washington, DC: Aspen Institute; 2016. https://www.aspeninstitute.org/publications/state-play-2016-trends-developments. Accessed July 2, 2017

2. Fleisig GS, Andrews JR. Prevention of elbow injuries in youth baseball pitchers. *Sports Health.* 2012;4(5):419–424

3. Davis JT, Limpisvasti O, Fluhme D, et al. The effect of pitching biomechanics on the upper extremity in youth and adolescent baseball pitchers. *Am J Sports Med.* 2009;37(8):1484–1491

4. Defroda SF, Thigpen CA, Kriz PK. Two-dimensional video analysis of youth and adolescent pitching biomechanics: a tool for the common athlete. *Curr Sports Med Rep.* 2016;15(5):350–358

5. Rice SG, Congeni JA; American Academy of Pediatrics Council on Sports Medicine and Fitness. Baseball and softball. *Pediatrics.* 2012;129(3):e842–e856

6. Patel RM, Lynch TS, Amin NH, Gryzlo S, Schickendantz M. Elbow injuries in the throwing athlete. *JBJS Rev.* 2014;2(11):1–11

7. Pitch Smart/USA Baseball. Guidelines for youth and adolescent pitchers. Pitch Smart/USA Baseball Web site. http://m.mlb.com/pitchsmart/pitching-guidelines. Accessed July 2, 2017

8. Osbahr DC, Chalmers PN, Frank JS, Williams RJ III, Widmann RF, Green DW. Acute, avulsion fractures of the medial epicondyle while throwing in youth baseball players: a variant of Little League elbow. *J Shoulder Elbow Surg.* 2010;19(7):951–957

9. Lawrence JT, Patel NM, Macknin J, et al. Return to competitive sports after medial epicondyle fractures in adolescent athletes: results of operative and nonoperative treatment. *Am J Sports Med.* 2013;41(5):1152–1157

10. Dugas JD, Chronister J, Cain EL Jr, Andrews JR. Ulnar collateral ligament in the overhead athlete: a current review. *Sports Med Arthrosc.* 2014;22(3):169–182

11. Lyman S, Fleisig GS, Andrews JR, Osinski ED. Effect of pitch type, pitch count, and pitching mechanics on risk of elbow and shoulder pain in youth baseball pitchers. *Am J Sports Med.* 2002;30(4):463–468

12. Grantham WJ, Iyengar JJ, Bryam IR, Ahmad CS. The curveball as a risk factor for injury: a systematic review. *Sports Health.* 2015;7(1):19–26

13. Nissen CW, Westwell M, Ounpuu S, Patel M, Solomito M, Tate J. A biomechanical comparison of the fastball and curveball in adolescent baseball pitchers. *Am J Sports Med.* 2009;37(8):1492–1498

14. Dun S, Loftice J, Fleisig GS, Kingsley D, Andrews JR. A biomechanical comparison of youth baseball pitches: is the curveball potentially harmful? *Am J Sports Med.* 2008;36(4):686–692

15. Bushnell BD, Anz AW, Noonan TJ, Torry MR, Hawkins RJ. Association of maximum pitch velocity and elbow injury in professional baseball pitchers. *Am J Sports Med.* 2010;38(4):728–732

16. Petty DH, Andrews JR, Fleisig GS, Cain EL. Ulnar collateral ligament reconstruction in high school baseball players: clinical results and injury risk factors. *Am J Sports Med.* 2004;32(5):1158–1164

17. Olsen SJ II, Fleisig GS, Dun S, Loftice J, Andrews JR. Risk factors for shoulder and elbow injuries in adolescent baseball pitchers. *Am J Sports Med.* 2006;34(6):905–912

18. Hariri S, Safran MR. Ulnar collateral ligament injury in the overhead athlete. *Clin Sports Med.* 2010;29(4):619–644

19. American Orthopaedic Society for Sports Medicine. Preventing softball injuries. STOP Sports Injuries Web site. http://www.stopsportsinjuries.org/STOP/Prevent_Injuries/Softball_Injury_Prevention.aspx. Accessed July 2, 2017

20. Lear A, Patel N. Softball pitching and injury. *Curr Sports Med Rep.* 2016;15(5):336–341

21. Briskin SM. Injuries and medical issues in softball. *Curr Sports Med Rep.* 2012;11(5):265–271

22. Kriz P. Throwing sports and injuries involving the young athlete's spine. In: Micheli L, Stein C, O'Brien M, d'Hemecourt P, eds. *Spinal Injuries in Young Athletes.* New York, NY: Springer; 2014:67–74

23. Roberts DW, Roc GJ, Hsu WK. Outcomes of cervical and lumbar disk herniations in Major League Baseball pitchers. *Orthopedics.* 2011;34(8):602–609

24. Hangai M, Kaneoka K, Hinotsu S, et al. Lumbar intervertebral disk degeneration in athletes. *Am J Sports Med.* 2009;37(1):149–155

25. Mochida J, Toh E, Nomura T, Nishimura K. The risks and benefits of percutaneous nucleotomy for lumbar disc herniation. A 10-year longitudinal study. *J Bone Joint Surg Br.* 2001;83(4):501–505

26. Watkins RG. Lumbar disc injury in the athlete. *Clin Sports Med.* 2002:21(1):147–165, viii

27. American Orthopaedic Society for Sports Medicine. Preventing baseball injuries. STOP Sports Injuries. http://www.stopsportsinjuries.org/STOP/Prevent_Injuries/Baseball_Injury_Prevention.aspx. Accessed July 2, 2017

CHAPTER 11

Collision Sports and the Young Athlete: Football, Hockey, Lacrosse, and Rugby

Katherine H. Rizzone, MD, MPH, FAAP; Peter K. Kriz, MD, FACSM, FAAP; and Sarah A. Vengal, MD

Overview

Collision sports, defined as sports during which athletes generate great force and purposely hit or collide with other players or inanimate objects (eg, the ground),[1] continue to be popular activities for young athletes. American (tackle) football, ice hockey, lacrosse, and rugby compose the team collision sports, with the greatest participation numbers among children and youths in the United States, although changing trends in participation among these sports are occurring. For the pediatrician, collision sports present a dilemma between encouraging sport participation, on one hand, while simultaneously considering the greater risk for injury that these sports present, on the other. Often caught between these conflicting viewpoints, pediatricians are placed in a difficult position. This has been made even more challenging because of the increased amount of medical and media attention focused on concussion. The goal of this chapter is to educate pediatricians about becoming the most helpful resource possible for patients and families under their care who chose to participate in collision sports.

According to Sports and Fitness Industry Association data compiled between 2009 and 2014, child and adolescent tackle football experienced a 17.9% loss in participants between ages 6 and 17 years during this time period, while ice hockey, lacrosse, and rugby experienced significant increases in participation (Table 11-1).[2] While boxing is a collision sport, participation by children and youths is not recommended by the American Academy of Pediatrics. Rodeo is also considered a collision sport.[1] This chapter will highlight the sport history, epidemiology, common injuries, case-based scenarios of major issues, and injury prevention issues for the aforementioned team collision sports.

American Football

American football remains the most popular collision sport among American children and adolescents, with players between 6 and 13 years of age comprising 70% of the 5 million American football participants in the United States.[3] According to high school injury data (2005–2010), the overall injury rate associated with high school football was 4.1 injuries per 1,000 athletic exposures (AEs) per year. Player-player contact was the leading mechanism of injury, with being tackled and tackling, more specifically, resulting in the most common cause of injury.[4] For all ages, the most commonly injured body parts in football players are the knee, ankle, hand, and back. Contusions, strains, and sprains comprise most injuries. With the rule changes in 1976 rendering spear tackling (leading with the crown of the helmeted head while tackling by defensive players) illegal, cervical spine fractures, subluxations, and dislocations have declined at the high school level by 70%. Catastrophic head and neck injury risk during football has decreased substantially, with annual estimates between 0.19 and 1.78 events for every 100,000 participants. Head and neck injuries are a small percentage of overall injuries (5%–13%). Most football concussions result from tackling or being tackled. Head-to-head contact is one of the leading causes of child and youth football concussions. The incidence of concussion associated with football is higher than that associated with most other team sports and seems to increase with age.[5]

Ice Hockey

In the 2015–2016 season, nearly 365,000 child and youth players participated in ice hockey, according to USA Hockey registration statistics.[6] Historically a regional sport (eg, Northeast, Upper Midwest), ice hockey has experienced steady growth and increasing participation over the past few decades, with expansion of professional teams into southern and western states. Additionally, USA Hockey's successful American Developmental Model, which has implemented concepts such as cross-ice play and rule changes such as eliminating bodychecking from peewee (ages ≤12 years) programs, has contributed to a 44% participation increase from 2009 to 2014 among 6- to 17-year-olds.[7]

Concussion has been reported to be the most common ice hockey injury, representing greater than 15% of all injuries in 9- to 16-year-old players[8,9] and nearly 25% of injuries among boys' high school players.[10] According to high school injury data (2008–2013), concussion was the most frequent injury in boys' ice hockey players (0.6 injuries per 1,000 AEs per year). Bodychecking was the mechanism of injury responsible for greater than 46.0% of all injuries recorded. The head, face, and neck region (33.0%) and upper arm and shoulder region (20.6%) were the most commonly injured body sites, and just greater than 6.0% of injuries required surgery.[11]

While recent rule changes in child and youth hockey have been implemented in an effort to decrease contact to the head and neck, reduce risk of injury related to bodychecking, and encourage skill development at younger age levels,[12] bodychecking remains legal among male youths at bantam (ages ≤14 years), midget (≤18 and ≤16), and junior levels and in high school ice hockey. A 2010 child and youth ice hockey study showed a threefold increased risk of all game-related injuries in the categories of concussion, severe injury (time loss >7 days), and severe concussion (time loss >10 days) in leagues that permitted bodychecking compared with leagues that prohibited bodychecking at the same age level.[13]

Lacrosse

Child and adolescent lacrosse remains one of the fastest growing sports in the United States. Research involving child and adolescent lacrosse injuries remains limited. A one-season observational study involving 550 boys' lacrosse players aged 9 to 15 years from 8 leagues in 4 states was conducted in 2015. The overall injury rate was 13.0 injuries per 1,000 AEs per year. Sixty percent of injuries occurred during games, with 83.9% of injuries resulting in time loss less than 24 hours. Also, 45.2% of injuries involved the lower extremity, with contusions comprising 51.6% of these injuries. Ten of the 155 recorded injuries (6.5%) were concussions, with 35.5% and 14.2% of concussions resulting from stick and ball contact, respectively.[14] According to high school injury data (2008–2012), the overall injury rate associated with high school boys' and girls' lacrosse was 2.0 injuries per 1,000 AEs per year. Boys had higher injury rates than girls did (2.3 vs 1.5 per 1,000 AEs). Sprains and strains were the most common injuries (35.6% for boys, 43.9% for girls), followed by concussions (21.9% for boys, 22.7% for girls). The head and face were most commonly injured during competitions (32.0%), followed by the lower leg, ankle, and foot (17.8%) and knee (12.2%). For boys, contact with another player (40.9%) and no contact (21.1%) were the most common mechanisms of injury, while no contact (26.2%), contact with playing apparatus (24.0%), and overuse and chronic injuries (17.7%) were most common for girls. Finally, 6.9% of all injuries required surgery.[15]

Rugby

The first recorded American rugby game took place in Cambridge, MA, in 1874, with Harvard defeating McGill in an intercollegiate contest. Rugby grew popular in America in the early 20th century, and it was included in 4 Olympics between 1900 and 1924. However, following the International Olympic Committee's removal of rugby from the Olympics after 1924, the sport's growth in the United States collapsed, remaining essentially dormant for the next half-century. During the 1960s and 1970s, rugby experienced a renaissance, highlighted by the formation of the United States of America Rugby Football Union (now known as USA Rugby). In 2009, the International Olympic Committee voted rugby back into the 2016 Olympics. By 2011, USA Rugby reached more than 100,000 members.[16] From 2009 to 2014, rugby experienced the greatest percentage of participation increase of any team sport, doubling its participation among 6- to 17-year-olds (Table 11-1).[2]

Data regarding rugby injuries among US child and youth players are sparse. However, a systematic review published in 2016 of rugby injuries among children and youths younger than 21 years included 2 studies from the United States, and a total of 35 studies, including Australia, New Zealand, South Africa, Great Britain, Ireland, and Canada. A pooled estimate of injury incidence of 26.7 injuries per 1,000 player hours per year was calculated. For injuries requiring at least 7 days' absence from games, a pooled estimate of injury incidence of 10.3 per 1,000 player hours was determined. Twenty-eight percent of child and adolescent rugby players were likely to sustain an injury during their season, and about 12.0% were likely to sustain an injury severe enough to require at least 7 days' absence from play. Being tackled was the phase of play during which most injuries occurred. Concussion ranged from 2.2% to 24.6% of all injuries recorded, while ligament injuries, sprains, and strains comprised 15.7% to 47.2% of all injuries recorded. Fractures ranged from 3.0% to 27.0% of all reported injuries, while lacerations, contusions, and hematomas ranged from 2.7% to 46.0% of all injuries recorded. Of all injuries, 0.5% to 10.8% were dislocations and subluxations. Injuries to the head and neck ranged from 4.6% to 41.2%, while trunk injuries comprised 6.5% to 12.5% of all injuries. Upper-extremity injuries ranged from 19.3% to 38.4%, while lower-extremity injuries ranged from 3.4% to 46.8%.[17]

Table 11-1. 6-17 Year-Old Team Collision Sport Participation Data in the United States

Sport	2009	2014	% Change
Tackle Football	3,962,000	3,254,000	−17.9%
Ice Hockey	517,000	743,000	+43.7%
Lacrosse	624,000	804,000	+28.8%
Rugby	150,000	301,000	+100.7%

From Sports & Fitness Industry Association. *2015 U.S. Trends in Team Sports: The Ultimate Report on the State of Team Sports.* Silver Spring, MD: Sports & Fitness Industry Association; 2015. https://www.sfia.org/reports/409_2015-U.S.-TRENDS-IN-TEAM-SPORTS. Accessed July 2, 2017. Reproduced with permission.

Common Injuries From Collision Sports

Brachial Plexus Neurapraxia ("Burners" and "Stingers")

Cervical root and brachial plexus neurapraxias are known by several colloquialisms, including "burners" and "stingers." The terms are used to describe a transient sensation of burning, pain, numbness, or tingling in a unilateral upper extremity; motor weakness may accompany this sensation.[18] The burner-stinger syndrome is one of the most common injuries in American football players, with up to 65% of collegiate football players experiencing this injury during their 4-year collegiate careers.[19] Rugby is another common sport in which burners and stingers are prevalent. A recent study demonstrated that among high school and collegiate rugby players, 21% of players experienced at least 1 stinger during a single season of exposure, while one-third of rugby players surveyed had histories of stingers.[20] Most athletes underreport this syndrome, given its frequent occurrence.

Burners and stingers are thought to result from traction on the brachial plexus (Figure 11-1A); extension-compression of the cervical roots (C5 and C6), a mechanism more common in older players with degenerative changes of the cervical spine (Figure 11-1C), such as foraminal narrowing or degenerative disk disease; or direct compression at Erb point (Figure 11-1B), where the brachial plexus is most superficial.

Athletes typically present coming off the playing field shaking their arm or holding their arm close to their side for comfort. Burning or stinging down the arm into the hand is usual. Weakness in the biceps brachii, deltoid and rotator cuff muscles, and wrist extensors may also occur, consistent with a C5 and C6 distribution. Most athletes will have normal physical

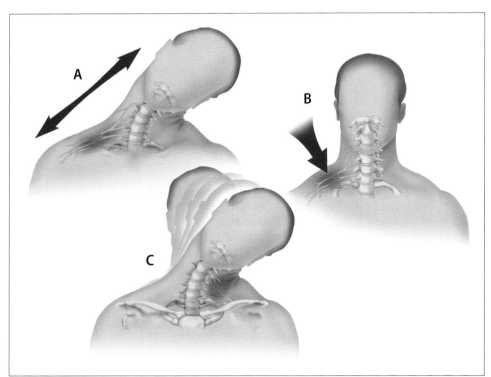

FIGURE 11-1

Mechanisms of "burners." (A) Traction to the brachial plexus from ipsilateral shoulder depression and contralateral neck flexion. (B) Direct blow to the supraclavicular fossa at Erb's point. (C) Compression of the cervical roots or brachial plexus from ipsilateral flexion and hyperextension.

Courtesy of Renee Cannon. Reproduced with permission.

examination findings by the time they reach the sideline.[19] Pain generally resolves in minutes, with full sensorimotor symptoms typically resolving within 1 to 2 days.[21]

In athletes with prolonged or recurrent symptoms, abnormal physical examination findings, or bilateral extremity involvement, the differential diagnosis must be broadened to consider a more central process. Cervical spine radiographs (anteroposterior [AP], lateral, odontoid, and lateral flexion and extension views) should be considered to assess for spinal and foraminal stenosis and instability. The Torg-Pavlov ratio compares the AP diameter of the spinal canal to the AP width of the vertebral body to evaluate for cervical canal stenosis. A spinal canal to vertebral body ratio of less than 0.8 has been associated with 3 times greater risk of incurring a stinger compared with players with ratios greater than 0.8.[22] However, the Torg-Pavlov ratio has limited value, as it was not developed to assess for foraminal narrowing,[22] and, while it has high sensitivity, it has a low positive predictive value in screening for cervical stenosis and determining future injury.[22] Many mature football players have a large vertebral body size, which decreases the ratio, even when the spinal canal diameter is within a reference range.[23] Cervical spine magnetic resonance imaging (MRI) can be used to assess for nerve root injuries, disk herniations, ligament and facet injuries, and non-displaced fractures. Electromyography should be considered if symptoms persist more than 2 weeks, to differentiate between cervical root and brachial plexus injury as well as the level of peripheral nerve injury, but an electromyogram should not be obtained until 3 weeks' post-injury, to avoid false-negative testing results.[19,21]

Regarding return to play following a stinger, an athlete is allowed to return or resume participation when he or she has complete resolution of symptoms, return-to-baseline range of motion of the cervical spine, and return-to-baseline strength in the affected upper extremity. Athletes that have a sustained stinger (ie, not transient) for the first

time should not be allowed to return to play until cervical MRI is performed to assess for structural abnormalities. While management of recurrent stingers remains controversial, the following guidelines have been established:

1. A previous history of 2 stingers within the same or multiple seasons is not a contraindication to return to play.

2. Three or more stingers in the same season is a relative contraindication to return to play.

3. Magnetic resonance imaging evidence of a cervical spinal cord abnormality is an absolute contraindication to participation.[22]

Glenohumeral Instability

Glenohumeral instability, a term that encompasses both dislocation and subluxation, is common in collision sport adolescent athletes. Young athletes in contact sports have the highest risk of initial glenohumeral instability, with nonoperative treatment leading to recurrent instability in 39% to 94% of athletes, according to numerous studies.[24] Anterior shoulder instability is most common (90%), generally occurring after a traumatic event. Typically, the arm is abducted and externally rotated when a posteriorly directed force is applied to the affected shoulder, leading to anterior displacement of the humeral head. A combination of forces that stress the anterior glenohumeral ligaments and force the humeral head out of the glenoid fossa of the scapula contribute to dislocation. For acute dislocations, the glenohumeral joint should be reduced as soon as possible, typically on the field, on the sidelines, or in the on-site training room.

Post-reduction radiographs, including with an axillary lateral view, should be obtained to confirm reduction and assess for bony injury. Posterior shoulder instability, while less common, can occur in athletes, including football linebackers, when the at-risk position of forward elevation, adduction, and internal rotation presents itself, such as falling on an outstretched arm or receiving a blow in the aforementioned position. Most posterior shoulder instability episodes are subluxation events, and many athletes present with pain alone, typically with exercises such as bench-pressing and push-ups.

It is important to distinguish glenohumeral instability from atraumatic multidirectional instability, a condition in which the glenohumeral joint demonstrates excessive translation in 2 or more directions (eg, anterior, posterior, inferior). Patients with multidirectional instability present with histories of multiple subluxations or dislocations that can often be self-reduced.

Management of glenohumeral instability is discussed in-depth in Chapter 5, Shoulder Injuries in the Young Athlete.

Acromioclavicular Joint Injuries

The acromioclavicular (AC) joint is very susceptible to injury during collision sports, and it is the second most commonly dislocated major joint, following the glenohumeral joint.[25] The AC joint has 3 main stabilizers: the AC, coracoclavicular (CC), and coracoacromial ligaments. The CC ligaments can be subcategorized into the trapezoid and conoid ligaments. Most AC joint injuries result from falling directly onto the joint while the arm is adducted or a direct blow to the area. The first ligament injured is the AC ligament, followed by the CC ligaments with more severe injury; the coracoacromial ligament remains intact. Out of 25 National Collegiate Athletic Association sports, football had the highest prevalence of AC sprains, accounting for 50% of the sprains reported, with ice hockey having the second highest prevalence.[26] Male athletes are more likely to have AC joint injuries than female athletes are.[26,27] In men's college lacrosse, 50% of shoulder injuries were related to the AC joint, according to a recent epidemiological study.[28]

Patients typically present with pain over the AC joint area. The athlete may hold the shoulder at the side of the body for comfort, and shoulder asymmetry is common. The presence of swelling may obscure obvious deformity or displacement

of the distal clavicle. Palpation of the AC joint will be painful, while overhead motion and cross-body adduction increase pain.

Plain radiographs should be obtained to assess the degree of displacement and to rule out concurrent clavicular fractures. A bilateral AP view (both AC joints on a single image) and Zanca view (AP view with 10°–15° cephalic tilt) can best assess the injured side vs the contralateral side for displacement. Stress views are of little diagnostic benefit, and they are no longer recommended.[25]

There are 6 types of AC joint injuries, with types I to III being the most commonly experienced (Figure 11-2). *Type I* injuries involve AC ligament sprain without tearing or rupture of the ligament. Examination findings are minimal, with tenderness over the AC joint but no palpable "step off" of the distal clavicle. There is no increase in radiographic CC distance. *Type II* injuries result in disruption of the AC ligament and sprain of the CC ligaments, both without tearing. Swelling and appreciable asymmetry, compared with the uninjured side, are apparent. Coracoclavicular distance is increased less than 25% of the clavicular diameter, compared with the contralateral shoulder. *Type III to VI* injuries involve complete disruption of the AC and CC ligaments. *Type III* injuries involve a distinct step off of the distal clavicle clinically and 25% to 100% increase in radiographic CC distance. *Type IV* injuries are associated with posterior distal clavicle displacement; *Type V,* with a 100% to 300% increase (superiorly) in radiographic CC distance; and *Type VI,* with inferior displacement of the distal clavicle.

Types I to II of AC joint injuries are typically managed with a sling for immobilization and for pain control in addition to rest, oral analgesics or nonsteroidal anti-inflammatory drugs, ice, and activity modification. Generally, an arm sling is used for approximately 1 week with type I and 2 to 3 weeks with type II AC joint injuries. Physical therapy should be initiated when pain subsides, with strengthening exercises begun after full active range of motion is achieved.

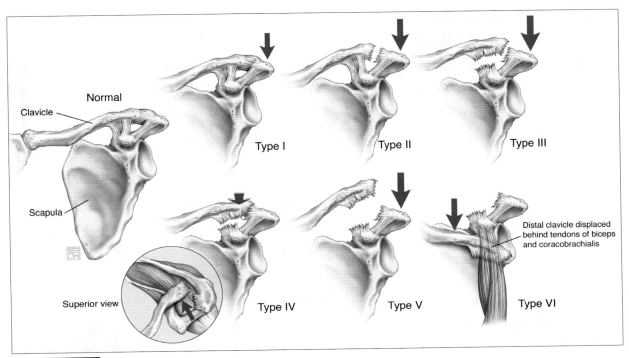

FIGURE 11-2
Types of acromioclavicular separations.
Courtesy of Steve Oh. Reproduced with permission.

Type III AC joint injury initial management remains controversial and without consensus. However, a 2007 survey of American Orthopaedic Society for Sports Medicine members reported that 86.3% preferred nonsurgical treatment for uncomplicated type III AC joint injuries.[29] Some argue that contact as well as collision sport athletes should consider delaying surgical management until their playing careers are over, given the high likelihood of injury recurrence. Sling immobilization duration for type III injuries is typically longer (2–4 weeks); otherwise, the treatment approach is similar to that for types I and II. Surgical management is indicated for types IV to VI.[25]

Type I injuries typically result in return to play 2 weeks following injury, although this can vary. Type II to III injuries typically require 2 to 3 weeks of rest before rehabilitation can be initiated, with contact and collision sports usually avoided for a total of 8 to 12 weeks.[25]

Concussion

Concussion remains a common injury among collision sport athletes at the middle school, high school, and collegiate levels. Studies from youth football have shown that youth players are capable of generating high-magnitude forces that result in concussion in other high school and collegiate football players.[3] Second impact syndrome, defined as brain injury associated with cerebral edema that occurs in the setting of a second (often minor) blow to the head before full recovery from concussion, is a devastating entity that has been described in collision sport athletes typically younger than 20 years.[5] Concussion and second impact syndrome are discussed more in-depth in Chapter 8, Concussions in the Young Athlete.

Transient Cervical Cord Neurapraxia

Transient cervical cord neurapraxia, or transient quadriplegia or paresis, is an acute neurologic episode associated with sensory changes, with or without motor weakness or complete paralysis of at least 2 extremities. At time of injury, the cervical area is usually pain-free, with painless range of motion. Generally, complete recovery occurs within 10 to 15 minutes, although symptoms may last up to 36 hours. Cervical spinal stenosis is believed to be the primary causative factor predisposing an athlete to cervical cord neurapraxia. Magnetic resonance imaging is the preferred screening study for cervical spinal stenosis, as football players can have large vertebral bodies that make the traditional Torg-Pavlov ratio on lateral cervical spine radiographs a poor screening tool for athletic participation. A previous history of a single episode of transient quadriplegia or paresis in athletes with a Torg-Pavlov ratio of 0.8 or less is a relative (not absolute) contraindication to return to play. Athletes returning to play must have full return-to-baseline strength and cervical range of motion, with imaging demonstrating mild to moderate spinal stenosis. More than 1 recurrence of transient quadriplegia or paresis, neurologic symptoms lasting more than 36 hours, ligamentous instability, and MRI evidence of cord defects or swelling are absolute contradictions to continued participation.[30]

Fractures

"Clay Shoveler's Fracture"

"Clay shoveler's fracture" is a colloquial term originated in the 1930s when posterior spinal avulsion fractures occurring in the lower cervical (C6 and C7) or upper thoracic vertebrae were identified in ditchdiggers in Australia.[31] With collision sports, a sudden or forced hyperflexion of the neck (eg, tackling during football or rugby, being checked into the boards during ice hockey) leads to large forces generated from the trapezius, rhomboid muscles, or serratus posterior muscles. It represents a stable vertebral fracture, as it involves only the posterior spinal column.

Athletes experiencing this injury report midline neck pain, particularly with flexion. Any neurologic symptoms should be further evaluated for spinal cord injury. A swimmer's view radiograph will allow for improved visualization of the lower cervical and upper thoracic spine as compared with a simple lateral cervical spine radiograph.

Management includes rest from activity as well as a soft collar to support the cervical musculature until pain decreases. Surgery is not required unless pain persists. Patients with stable, healed fractures with full, painless cervical range of motion and no neurologic deficits have no contraindications to participate in contact or collision sports.[32]

Clavicular Fracture

Clavicular fractures are very common injuries in general. Most (80%) involve the middle third of the affected clavicle, and the remaining 10% to 15% are typically in the lateral third. They can be caused by a fall on the shoulder or a direct blow from contact. A physical examination typically reveals a tender, swollen area at the fracture site. The neurovascular bundle of the subclavian and brachial plexus should be fully assessed on examination because of its proximity to the common location of this injury. Concurrent AC, rib, and scapular injuries should also be evaluated for. Radiographs with AP and AP with 30° to 45° cephalic tilt views should be obtained, as should an axillary view to assess for other possible injuries, as well as for posterior displacement of the clavicle's medial fragment. Radiographic evaluation should be repeated at 2 to 3 weeks and 6 weeks' post-injury and considered at 12 weeks if callus formation and interval healing have not been established.

Most clavicular fractures heal without surgical intervention. Figure-of-eight braces have not been shown to accelerate healing rates or decrease nonunion rates and have lower adherence than slings do, as they are typically uncomfortable. Immobilization can be discontinued in most cases after 2 to 3 weeks, and progressive range of motion exercises can be initiated. For fractures with less than 100% displacement and greater than 2 cm of shortening, surgical fixation should be considered. Any concern for an open fracture (eg, tenting of the skin, bruising over the area of fracture) should be referred for surgical consultation.

Return-to-play clearance is predicated on a combination of clinical and radiographic findings. Clinical resolution of symptoms, return of functional range of movement and strength, and radiographic evidence of healing are the most important criteria. Consideration of type of activity or sport the athlete is returning to should always be taken into account when determining the overall risk potential and types of complications that may occur. On average, most athletes with clavicular fractures can return to play between 6 and 8 weeks following injury.[33]

Wedge-Compression Fractures

The spine has 3 columns: anterior, middle, and posterior. Wedge-compression fractures occur in the anterior column alone. Involvement of the anterior and middle columns is defined as a burst fracture. L1 is the most commonly affected vertebrae by burst fractures, and C5 is the most commonly affected cervical vertebra. These usually occur because of a hyperflexion motion during tackling or collision.

Athletes will have midline pain, and neurologic assessment findings are often normal, but some athletes experience transient paresthesias or weakness, or both. Anteroposterior and lateral plain radiographs should be obtained to assess for injury, with further views of the vertebral level or higher level of imaging performed as needed on the basis of symptoms.

As with any concern for spinal injury, immobilization to prevent further or worsening of the injury is necessary until radiographs can be taken of the area. Further imaging with computed tomography (CT) scan–assisted myelography or MRI, or both, can be considered to evaluate for neural compression.

Return to play will depend on the severity of injury and the neurologic deficit. Asymptomatic athletes with normal neurologic function as well as non-displaced, stable fractures without any sagittal component on AP view and with radiographic evidence of bony healing may return to play if they achieve full strength and painless range of motion.[30]

Rib Contusions and Fractures

Collision sports definitely place athletes at risk for rib contusions and fractures. Ribs 1 to 4 are less commonly involved, as the shoulder helps protect them from impact. Injury can be from blunt trauma or from avulsion. Posterior lateral bend of the rib is a common location.

Athletes may feel a "pop" or experience a sensation such as feeling as if the wind has been knocked out of them. Assessment for more serious injury, such as pneumothorax, hemothorax, or liver, spleen, or pulmonary contusion, should be considered. A thorough cardiac and respiratory examination is necessary in addition to the musculoskeletal examination.

Plain radiographs should include a chest radiograph to assess for pneumothorax. Rib series radiographs can be helpful to identify non-displaced fractures.

Athletes should be "held out" from sport until symptoms improve, and they may use a chest binder to help with symptoms. Caution should be taken to make sure that atelectasis doesn't occur with splinting used to avoid pain. Incentive spirometry may be helpful. Surgical management is rarely indicated.

Return to play is based on the severity of pleuritic pain and pain at the site of injury. Healing generally occurs within 6 weeks, but it may take longer if there are concomitant injuries.

Chest Wall and Abdominal Injuries

Commotio Cordis

Commotio cordis is most often described in players of baseball, lacrosse, and combat sports, such as karate, although ice hockey can also be a participation risk factor. An important cause of sudden cardiac death in athletes, commotio cordis occurs in a structurally normal heart after the chest wall is struck with a blunt object. If the blow occurs during a window of cardiac repolarization, ventricular fibrillation can result. Ninety-five percent of cases involve adolescent boys, with a mean age of 14 years. Commotio cordis can occur despite the use of chest protectors. Early recognition and implementation of an automatic external defibrillator (AED) within several minutes of blunt trauma to treat the resultant cardiac arrhythmia are key components to improve survival rates, which have increased steadily to greater than 50% over the past decade, because of greater recognition of commotio cordis and improved dissemination of AEDs, as well as greater use of cardiopulmonary resuscitation and AED training in communities.[34]

Splenic and Renal Injuries

Splenic injuries are caused by a fall or direct trauma to the back or abdominal area of the left side. Common symptoms are left-sided abdominal pain, with rib tenderness and costovertebral angle tenderness, and decreased breath sounds may be found on examination. In a review of case reports of splenic rupture with infectious mononucleosis, the common clinical signs of splenic rupture were abdominal pain, left shoulder pain (Kehr sign), and syncope.[35] Severe injuries can lead to tachycardia and dyspnea. Bruising in periumbilical (Cullen sign) or flank (Turner sign) regions is a harbinger of intra-abdominal bleeding but often will be delayed for hours following injury.

Computed tomography scan is the criterion standard imaging study to assess degree of splenic injury. An ultrasound image can also show injury to the spleen and may be considered to decrease radiation exposure to the patient. Athletes may be admitted to the hospital to be monitored with serial examinations, but they may also need blood products.

Once imaging documents healing, and the athletes are asymptomatic and back to baseline fitness, they can return to play. Overall, consensus regarding full return to play is lacking, and clinical judgement is made case by case.[36]

Delayed splenic rupture from an unhealed contusion is possible, but if an athlete has been assessed with CT scan, it is unlikely an injury will be missed, as radiographic healing lags behind physiologic healing.[35]

The kidneys are in the retroperitoneal space and are thus often protected from injury because of the layers of muscle, pericapsular fat, and ribs. However, blood flow to this organ is significant, so even minor injuries can lead to great pain and unstable symptoms. Signs of renal injury could include hematuria. Symptoms include flank pain. Computed tomography scan is also the first-line imaging study to assess extent of renal injury. Return to play remains controversial, and it depends on the degree of injury. In a review of the National Football League players from 1986 to 2004 with renal contusions, most athletes were out for approximately 2 weeks, whereas those with lacerations were out for closer to 8 weeks. Players should be asymptomatic prior to return, with normalized renal function and no hematuria. Repeat imaging should be considered as well for more severe injuries, to evaluate for late complications, including hydronephrosis.[37]

Soft-Tissue Injuries

Bursitis

Bursae are potential spaces of the synovial membrane of the articular capsule, which function to reduce friction between bone and overlying soft tissue. In sports, bursitis most often results from direct trauma in areas not fully covered by protective equipment. Septic bursitis always needs to be in the differential diagnosis of soft-tissue swelling, particularly because athletes in contact sports are well-known to be methicillin-resistant *Staphylococcus aureus* carriers.[38] However, if swelling is painless and unaccompanied by warmth and erythema, infection is unlikely.

Following trauma, swelling in the setting of bursitis tends to be sudden, but range of motion is typically preserved. With olecranon injury, if elbow range of motion is limited, then causes other than bursitis should be considered, and radiographs should be obtained to assess for fracture. In a review of ice hockey injuries reported to a Finnish insurance company, the most common elbow injuries were olecranon contusion with laceration or bursitis from landing on the ice.[39]

In cases of isolated prepatellar bursitis, there is no associated joint effusion. This bursitis is a common injury seen in wrestlers not only because of bodily collisions but also because of prolonged contact with mats.

Ice and compression are first-line treatments in management. Aspiration can be considered if range of motion is affected, but performing this procedure may increase the risk of septic bursitis.

Myositis Ossificans

Myositis ossificans is a relatively common cause of thigh pain and swelling in adolescent athletes. Blunt trauma (eg, helmet to thigh, knee to thigh) as a single or repetitive trauma is recalled by the athlete, which results in hematoma development within the femoral periosteum, with subsequent rupture into adjacent muscles, releasing osteocytes from the injured bone. This release serves as a precursor for heterotopic ossification within muscle tissue. Calcification on radiograph typically appears 2 to 6 weeks' post-injury, and growth of the mass on radiograph stabilizes at 6 months. Myositis ossificans should be considered in any athlete with a firm mass at the injury site 3 to 4 weeks' post-injury. Prevention is typically effective within 10 minutes of injury and should be considered for all deep quadriceps femoris contusions. Placing the knee in 120° of flexion with an ACE wrap provides tamponade of the hemorrhage and limits muscle spasm, providing a more rapid return to reference range of motion, minimizing risk of developing myositis ossificans. Flexion should be continued for 24 to 48 hours, with partial weight bearing until pain subsides. Physical therapy (active range of motion) should be started once pain-free, and nonsteroidal anti-inflammatory drugs such as indomethacin should be considered to inhibit ossification. Return to play may be considered once the athlete demonstrates normal strength compared to the unaffected side and can achieve more than 120° of flexion. Placing a protective pad over the area is advised.[40]

Morel-Lavallée Lesions

Morel-Lavallée lesions are post-traumatic, closed soft-tissue degloving injuries most frequently involving the pelvis, thigh, and knee. In athletes, these injuries result from shear forces (eg, contact with a playing surface, direct blow from another player), which lead to the overlying skin and subcutaneous tissue separating from the underlying fascia. Perforating vessels are disrupted, resulting in a collection of fluid (eg, blood, lymph, liquefied fat) in a potential space that can lead to bacterial infection. These lesions can be associated with an underlying fracture. Clinically, these athletes present with a suprapatellar fluctuance, which often extends into the mid-thigh medially and laterally. Commonly, this lesion is misdiagnosed as prepatellar bursitis. Extension of fluctuance beyond the prepatellar bursa's anatomical boundaries is a key distinguishing feature of Morel-Lavallée lesions. Musculoskeletal ultrasound or MRI is the preferred diagnostic imaging study. Treatment including PRICEMM (protection, rest, ice, compression, and elevation) and aspiration (preferably ultrasound-guided; multiple aspirations may be indicated) followed by compressive wrapping can be effective in reducing swelling, theoretically reducing risk of superinfection, and expediting recovery, by restoring full active knee flexion. In a study of National Football League players with knee Morel-Lavallée lesions, mean time for fluid collection resolution and achievement of full active knee flexion was 16.3 days.[41] In the setting of recurrent fluid collections despite multiple aspirations, sclerodesis with doxycycline (500 mg dissolved into 5 mL of 1% lidocaine) under fluoroscopic or ultrasound guidance may be considered.[41,42] Absolute indications for surgery include association of a Morel-Lavallée lesion with an open fracture, deep infection, or severe skin necrosis.[42]

Case Files: Collision Sport Injuries

Acute Trauma

Case 1
Acute thigh injury in a 16-year-old club rugby player

Description

Office evaluation of thigh injuries on the days following injury can be challenging, as the differential diagnosis can include fracture, soft-tissue injury, or hip or knee joint injury. In this case, a 16-year-old club rugby player sustained contact with an opponent 2 days ago, while she was the ball carrier, attempting to advance the ball down the pitch. She recalls her opponent's knee striking her thigh and driving it to the ground. There was immediate pain and swelling, with bruising developing within 1 to 2 hours of injury (Figure 11-3). She presents limping into your office. She is in an all-cotton, elastic wrap, with her left knee in 120° of flexion, which was applied by her athletic trainer at time of injury.

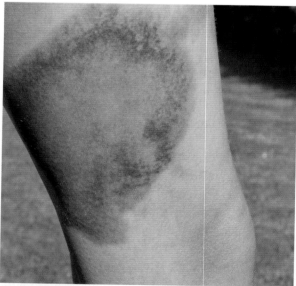

FIGURE 11-3

Thigh bruising and swelling associated with traumatic quadricep contusion. Myositis ossificans and occult fracture should be included in the differential diagnosis.

Photo by Cindy Arman, Franklin Pierce University Athletics.

Quadriceps Contusion and Myositis Ossificans

A quadriceps femoris contusion is the most likely diagnosis, but fracture must be considered, as the athlete is experiencing pain with weight bearing. Examining the hip and knee joints in addition to the affected thigh is critical. Anteroposterior and lateral views of the entire femur (if hip and knee range of motion are not painful and not limited) are indicated to assess for fracture. In this case, findings from plain radiographs were normal. The athlete is kept on crutches with partial weight bearing; an all-cotton, elastic compression wrap; and instructions to ice her thigh for the next 7 to 10 days. A physical therapy referral is given for gentle active range of motion (avoiding *aggressive* early rehabilitation) once she is pain-free. Serial evaluation continues over the next 4 to 6 weeks. Repeat radiographs at 4 weeks' post-injury reveal the following lesion (Figure 11-4). The athlete continues to demonstrate limited knee flexion (<120°). With radiographic findings supporting the clinical history and examination, myositis ossificans becomes the working diagnosis. The athlete continues in physical therapy, and indomethacin administered at 50 mg twice daily is prescribed to inhibit (further) ossification of adjacent muscle. The athlete returns at 8 weeks' post-injury with pain-free range of motion

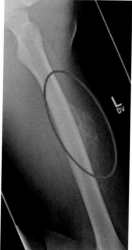

(130° knee flexion) and comparable strength to her unaffected lower extremity. She is cleared to return to play, with the stipulation that she wear a protective pad over the injured area. Indomethacin is continued, and arrangements are made for follow-up (with repeat radiographs) at 6 months' post-injury to document stabilization of the heterotopic ossification.

FIGURE 11-4

Heterotopic ossification (myositis ossificans) (circled region) identified on radiographs 2–6 wk following blunt trauma.

Thigh and Knee Contusion and Morel-Lavallée Lesion

Distal thigh and knee bruising and suprapatellar swelling in the setting of a collision sport injury can be a diagnostic challenge (Figure 11-5). A careful

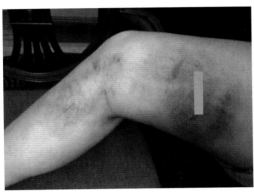

FIGURE 11-5
Diffuse bruising of the distal thigh and proximal lower leg in a collision sports athlete can pose a diagnostic dilemma.

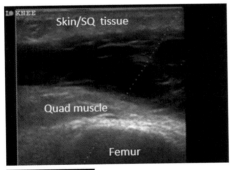

FIGURE 11-6
Musculoskeletal ultrasound imaging demonstrating a large collection of fluid (see arrow) between skin and subcutaneous tissue and underlying muscle, characteristic of a Morel-Lavallée lesion.

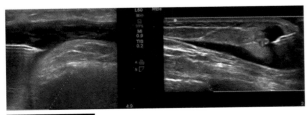

FIGURE 11-7
Ultrasound-guided aspiration of a Morel-Lavallée lesion.

and comprehensive physical examination can help narrow the differential diagnosis. Fractures, intra-articular injuries, and soft-tissue injuries can have similar presentations. Suprapatellar swelling can be caused by both intra-articular and extra-articular fluid collection. Plain radiographs should be obtained to determine whether an underlying fracture is present. Point-of-use musculoskeletal ultrasound in a clinical setting can assist with distinguishing these conditions. Magnetic resonance imaging remains the preferred imaging study to determine lesion characteristics and chronicity, but it is not necessarily indicated. In this case, a large collection of fluid (hypoechogenic signal intensity) between the skin and subcutaneous tissue and the vastus medialis (ultrasound probe location represented by blue rectangle in Figure 11-5) is identified with musculoskeletal ultrasound (Figure 11-6), indicating an extra-articular fluid accumulation in a hypovascular supra-fascial space, consistent with a Morel-Lavallée lesion.

With an underlying fracture ruled out, initial conservative treatment recommendations include activity restriction; gentle range of motion exercise; ice; all-cotton, elastic compression wrap; and monitoring for signs of infection (redness, warmth, and fever). At follow-up visit 2 weeks later, a large fluctuant mass remains over the anteromedial thigh distally. Repeat in-office limited diagnostic musculoskeletal ultrasound reveals a large fluid collection with no appreciable fibrous adhesions, despite 2 weeks of compression bandaging. Ultrasound-guided aspiration under sterile conditions is performed (Figure 11-7), yielding 60 mL of serosanguinous fluid without purulence. An additional 2 weeks of compression bandaging is recommended. At follow-up, there is no fluid reaccumulation, and the athlete has pain-free, full active range of motion of the hip and knee. The athlete is cleared for a gradual return to play, and the importance of monitoring for fluid collection recurrence is emphasized.

Case 2

Left arm numbness in a 15-year-old high school football player

Description

Upper-extremity injuries in American football players are frequent. It is common to witness an injured athlete leaving the field holding the arm, supporting the elbow or shoulder, or shaking the arm or hand because of a not-so-obvious injury. The differential diagnosis of this presentation can be broad, ranging from cervical spine injury, to AC joint injury, to brachial plexus injury, to a glenohumeral instability episode. It is imperative for team physicians to gather pertinent history and perform targeted examinations during sideline evaluation to direct further intervention and make participation decisions.

In this case, a 15-year-old football player, who swings for junior varsity and varsity, goes in for a tackle on a kick-off return in a varsity game. He runs off the field with his left arm hanging at his side. Moments later, when assessed on the bench, he reports burning and weakness in his left arm. He denies any symptoms in his right arm.

The examination is repeated after 15 minutes on the sideline, and it shows complete resolution of paresthesias and complete return of strength and range of motion. He returns for the rest of the game without recurrence of symptoms. Three games later, he again has a burning sensation in his left arm after a tackle. He admits this is the third time this season this has happened. He is restricted from further play, he is counseled on recurrent stingers, and it is suggested that he follow up in office for evaluation of his cervical spine, starting with cervical spine radiographs.

Case 3

Left-sided abdominal pain in a 14-year-old hockey player

Description

Abdominal injuries in players of collision sports can have varying degrees of severity. The initial evaluation can be challenging, and considering life-threatening injuries is important.

In this case, a 14-year-old female hockey player goes in for a loose puck against the boards and ends up getting checked from behind, resulting in her striking the left side of her trunk against the intersection of the dasher boards and the plexiglass. She has immediate left-sided pain but continues her shift. After the game, she feels more tired than usual and has worsening pain. She comes to the office the next day. On the basis of her physical examination, there is concern about a splenic injury and she is sent to the emergency department. An abdominal CT scan shows a splenic laceration (Figure 11-8A). She is admitted and undergoes serial abdominal examinations but does not undergo splenectomy. She recovers and is now 3 months out from her injury and wants to go back to hockey.

The decision is made to repeat abdominal imaging (Figure 11-8B).

The complete resolution of her splenic injury on CT scan is noted. She is cleared to return to play, her physician knowing that scan findings typically lag behind clinical healing. She completes the season without further incident.

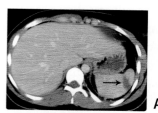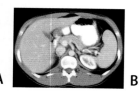

FIGURE 11-8

A, Initial abdominal CT scan demonstrating a splenic laceration in a 14-year-old female hockey player. Arrow indicates location of laceration. B, Repeat scan showed healing of laceration.

Abbreviation: CT, computed tomography.

Injury Prevention

Injury preventive strategies for collision sports include (but are not limited to)

- Protective equipment

- Rule changes and enforcement

- Limiting contact during practice

- Teaching proper bodychecking and tackling technique

- Implementing participation strategies determined by age, size, and physical maturity level

- Neck strengthening

- Changing sport culture

Protective Equipment

Protective equipment for collision sports has evolved during the modern era into sophisticated, state-of-the-art gear. Composed of lightweight durable materials, current equipment can withstand impact forces that previously would have resulted in significant morbidity to the participant.

Helmets and Headgear

American Football

Serious head injuries, including intracranial hemorrhages and skull fractures, remained prevalent in American football throughout the mid-20th century. This prompted rule changes and, ultimately, the formation of the National Operating Committee on Standards for Athletic Equipment (NOCSAE) in 1969, which implemented the first football helmet safety standards in 1973. As a result, modern-day, hard-shelled helmets have been designed primarily to respond to linear, acceleration-inducing impacts rather than rotational acceleration, the latter which is thought to cause more sport-related concussions. While helmet designs vary, similar features are incorporated: hard plastic exterior shells contain padding of variable stiffness, to absorb and dissipate collision forces, and inflating systems in the helmet's interior, to ensure proper fit. Over the past few decades, helmet manufactures have begun to design helmets with the intention of reducing concussion risk. A 2014 study involving more than 2,000 high school football players demonstrated that the incidence of sport-related concussion was similar regardless of the manufacturer or brand of helmet worn.[43] Helmet rating systems, which measure the effectiveness of football helmets to reduce forces that cause concussion, in a laboratory setting, have been developed and implemented at Virginia Tech since 2011. Prior to 2014, ratings were based only on linear acceleration and did not reflect rotational forces, leading to the rating system receiving criticism from governing bodies, including NOCSAE.[44] As of 2016, of 26 helmet models tested to date (assessing linear and rotational forces), 15 helmets have earned a 5-star rating, and 4- or 5-star helmets continue to be recommended for players, taking into account other factors such as fit and comfort.[45]

Ice Hockey

Similar to American football, ice hockey protective headgear underwent technological advances, with the introduction of plastic shells and foam liners in the 1970s, which could absorb energy and provide a comfortable fit. In 1979, the National Hockey League adopted head protection 11 years following a fatal head injury during National Hockey League play. Despite the widespread use of helmets at amateur and professional levels, brain injuries remain a serious concern. While the introduction of ice hockey helmet standards and proper helmet use have reduced fatalities and catastrophic head injuries, concussion rates have increased during this time period, likely because of better concussion awareness and reporting but possibly because of more aggressive play ("gladiator effect"). In 2014, Virginia Tech developed a helmet rating system for assessing ice hockey helmets' ability to reduce concussion risk, similar to their football helmet rating system. As of 2016, of 38 helmet models tested to date, only 2 helmets have earned a 3-star rating; none have earned a 4- or 5-star rating. Both linear and rotational accelerations were assessed in the testing parameters.[46]

Lacrosse

Helmets meeting NOCSAE standards are required for boys' and mens' lacrosse, as well as girls' and women's goalkeepers. As of 2016, Florida is the only state currently mandating headgear for high school girls' teams. However, a recommendation is currently being considered for the use of "soft" helmets during girls' lacrosse that meet ASTM standards. A 2016 independent study from Purdue University assessed 18 boys' and mens' lacrosse helmets from 6 commonly worn lacrosse helmet designs using a NOCSAE-style drop-test protocol. Nine (50%) of the helmets failed to meet the NOCSAE standard. In comparison, none of the 18 football helmets tested failed to meet the standard. The study authors concluded that lacrosse helmet modifications to better attenuate impact forces are warranted, given that prior studies have demonstrated that head impact magnitude (but not frequency) is similar between football and lacrosse.[47]

Rugby

Rugby headgear is composed of relatively sparse padding, and its use is not mandated. Commonly referred to as a "scrum cap" and originally designed for forwards, headgear is now worn by players of all positions. The primary objective of headgear is to protect the ears and prevent cauliflower ear. Alternatively, some players wear a thin strip of foam or cloth and electrical tape wrapped around the ears, similar to a headband. Secondary objectives of headgear are to protect against cuts and abrasions that occur during tackles or at rucks. Such headgear has not been shown to reduce sport-related concussion.

Mouth Guards

Currently, the National Federation of State High School Associations (NFHS) requires the use of mouth guards during football, ice hockey, and lacrosse. When properly fitted, mouth guards can greatly reduce the severity of dental and maxillofacial injuries. There are 3 main types of mouth guards: stock, boil-and-bite, and custom-made. Stock mouth guards are ready-to-wear.

Boil-and-bite mouth guards must first be heated; then they can be molded to the teeth while cooling. Custom-made mouth guards must be made by a dental professional, and they offer the best fit.

There has been great debate as to the effectiveness of mouth guards in preventing concussions. It has been postulated that mouth guards may be able to absorb some of the shock that would otherwise reach the brain. In studies comparing athletes who wear mouth guards to those who do not, no significant difference was found in concussion occurrences between those who used mouth guards and those who did not. There is also no evidence that custom-made mouth guards provide superior protection compared to stock and boil-and-bite models.[48]

Despite the lack of clear evidence as to the effectiveness of mouth guards in the prevention of concussions, the NFHS remains steadfast that mouth guards are necessary for safe participation in sports. The NFHS has determined that prior to the use of mouth guards and face masks, greater than 50% of football injuries were orofacial. That percentage has been reduced to 1% with the use of mouth guards.[49]

Tackling and Bodychecking Controversies, Rule Changes, and Fair Play

In pediatric sports medicine, there are 2 camps engaged in the contentious topic of introducing tackling (football and rugby) or bodychecking (ice hockey and lacrosse) before age 14 years, a relatively arbitrary age cutoff that has been proposed by some concussion experts. One camp contends that bodychecking and tackling should be introduced at younger than 14 so child and adolescent athletes can be taught proper tackling and bodychecking techniques before they are physically mature, before athletes get "bigger, stronger, and faster" and the laws of physics change the rules of engagement in collision sports. The other camp encourages elimination of bodychecking and tackling at younger than 14, supported by a recent landmark study conducted in Canadian child ice hockey players by Emery and colleagues in 2010, which showed that peewee (ages ≤12 years) leagues that allowed bodychecking had a threefold increased risk of concussion compared with leagues that banned bodychecking.[13] The American Academy of Pediatrics recommends the restriction of bodychecking to elite levels of boys' youth ice hockey, starting no earlier than 15 years of age.[50] Another concerning study performed by Daniel and colleagues in 2012 demonstrated that 7- and 8-year-old football players were capable of generating head impact forces (as high as 100 G of force) that have been shown to cause concussions in adult football players.[3] Because football players between 6 and 13 years of age comprise 70% of the 5 million American football participants in the United States,[3] this research undoubtedly will continue to have bearing on the future direction of collision sport participation in child and youth athletes.

Nothing is magical about ages 14 or 15 other than they are the approximate ages that most athletes enter high school. But factors such as size and physical maturity are also important considerations when parents, pediatricians, and sports medicine specialists attempt to determine, or provide counseling about, whether young athletes should enter collision sport participation.

Recently, several child and youth sports organizations have begun restricting contact during practice and instructional drills, as a consequence of Emery's child and youth ice hockey study results, Daniel's child and youth football accelerometer study results, and rule change initiatives of several collegiate football conferences, including Ivy League colleges and universities and the Pac-12. In 2011, USA Hockey eliminated bodychecking in peewee (ages ≤12 years) ice hockey. In 2012, Pop Warner Football reduced contact to one-third of practice hours, and it eliminated intentional head-to-head contact in practice. In 2012, USA Football introduced and implemented Heads Up Football, a program that teaches and reinforces proper tackling mechanics, with a focus on reducing helmet contacts. Tackling that emphasizes an ascending-blow, shoulder-strike technique, with head to the side and up, is encouraged, while launching or leaving the feet is discouraged. Similarly, USA Hockey has developed an introduction to body contact as part of its coaching education program. This initiative focuses on teaching body contact

to mite (≤8 years) and squirt (≤10) players, with a gradual phase in during peewee (≤12) play prior to permitting bodychecking at the bantam (≤14) and older levels. In 2014, the NFHS recommended reduced contact in high school–sanctioned football practices during both the regular and off-season. In 2014, US Lacrosse increased the severity of penalties for intentional collisions with defenseless players, head and neck checking, and excessive body checks. Please note that no data yet exist to support limited contact in practice as an effective intervention in reducing concussive injury from collision sports, but reducing exposure makes intuitive sense. In fall 2016, Pop Warner Football banned kickoffs in games of its 3 youngest divisions (players 5–10 years of age), because of the premise that kickoffs (and punt returns) are considered the most dangerous plays in tackle football. Finally, in 2016, USA Rugby made fends (eg, stiff-arm maneuver by ball carrier) to the head, neck, and face illegal for high school and youth rugby.

Rule changes and enforcement, rather than protective equipment advances, are likely the keys to reducing injury (and, in particular, head injury) from child and adolescent sports. In Rhode Island, a fair-play initiative, to reduce malicious hits (eg, checking from behind, hits to the head, hits on defenseless or vulnerable players), was implemented in boys' scholastic ice hockey in the 2015–2016 season, the first of its kind in any US state that sanctions boys' scholastic ice hockey. A rule change, including a 50 penalty-minute threshold for the regular season and a 70-minute threshold for both regular season and playoffs, was implemented, and a watch list of players who had exceeded 25 penalty minutes during the course of the season was posted on the league Web site. The Rhode Island Interscholastic League Hockey Committee, composed of coaches, athletic directors, referees, principals, and executive directors, approved this change prior to the 2015–2016 season. In comparison with the previous 3 seasons, game ejections during the 2015–2016 season were decreased by 65%, including virtual elimination of fighting, deliberate contact to the head, and cross- checking penalties. A formal study of the impact of rule change on injury rates associated with high school ice hockey players is currently being conducted by the senior author.[51]

References

1. Rice SG; American Academy of Pediatrics Committee on Sports Medicine and Fitness. Medical conditions affecting sports participation. *Pediatrics.* 2008;121(4):841–848

2. Langhorst P. Youth sports participation statistics and trends. Engage Sports Web site. http://www.engagesports.com/blog/post/1488/youth-sports-participation-statistics-and-trends. Published March 8, 2016. Accessed July 2, 2017

3. Daniel RW, Rowson S, Duma SM. Head impact exposure in youth football. *Ann Biomed Eng.* 2012;40(4):976–981

4. Badgeley MA, McIlvain NM, Yard EE, Fields SK, Comstock RD. Epidemiology of 10,000 high school football injuries: patterns of injury by position played. *J Phys Act Health.* 2013;10(2):160–169

5. American Academy of Pediatrics Council on Sports Medicine and Fitness. Tackling in youth football. *Pediatrics.* 2015;136(5):e1419–e1430

6. USA Hockey. *2015-2016 Season Final Registration Report.* USA Hockey Web site. http://assets.ngin.com/attachments/document/0100/7886/15-16_Final_Reports.pdf. Accessed July 2, 2017

7. King B. Are the kids alright? *Street & Smith's Sports Business Journal.* August 10, 2015. http://www.sportsbusinessdaily.com/Journal/Issues/2015/08/10/In-Depth/Lead.aspx. Accessed July 2, 2017

8. Emery CA, Meeuwisse WH. Injury rates, risk factors, and mechanisms of injury in minor hockey. *Am J Sports Med.* 2006;34(12):1960–1969

9. Roberts WO, Brust JD, Leonard B. Youth ice hockey tournament injuries: rates and patterns compared to season play. *Med Sci Sports Exerc.* 1999;31(1):46–51

10. Meehan WP III, d'Hemecourt P, Collins CL, Comstock RD. Assessment and management of sport-related concussions in United States high schools. *Am J Sports Med.* 2011;39(11):2304–2310

11. Matic GT, Sommerfeldt MF, Best TM, Collins CL, Comstock RD, Flanigan DC. Ice hockey injuries among United States high school athletes from 2008/2009-2012/2013. *Phys Sportsmed.* 2015;43(2):119–125

12. USA Hockey. *USA Hockey Official Playing Rules: Points of Emphasis; 2011-12, 2012-13 Playing Seasons.* USA Hockey Web site. http://assets.ngin.com/attachments/document/0020/3167/2011-13_USA_Hockey_Rule_Change_Summary.pdf. Accessed July 2, 2017

13. Emery CA, Kang J, Shrier I, et al. Risk of injury associated with body checking among youth ice hockey players. *JAMA.* 2010;303(22):2265–2272

14. Kerr ZY, Caswell SV, Lincoln AE, Djoko A, Dompier TP. The epidemiology of boys' youth lacrosse injuries in the 2015 season. *Inj Epidemiol.* 2016;3:3

15. Xiang J, Collins CL, Liu D, McKenzie LB, Comstock RD. Lacrosse injuries among high school boys and girls in the United States: academic years 2008-2009 through 2011-2012. *Am J Sports Med.* 2014;42(9):2082–2088

16. USA Rugby. History. USA Rugby Web site. https://www.usarugby.org/about-usa-rugby. Accessed July 2, 2017

17. Freitag A, Kirkwood G, Scharer S, Ofori-Asenso R, Pollock AM. Systematic review of rugby injuries in children and adolescents under 21 years. *Br J Sports Med.* 2015;49(8):511–519

18. Torg JS, Corcoran TA, Thibault LE, et al. Cervical cord neurapraxia: classification, pathomechanics, morbidity, and management guidelines. *J Neurosurg.* 1997;87(6):843–850

19. Safran MR. Nerve injury about the shoulder in athletes, part 2: long thoracic nerve, spinal accessory nerve, burners/stingers, thoracic outlet syndrome. *Am J Sports Med.* 2004;32(4):1063–1076

20. Kawasaki T, Ota C, Yoneda T, et al. Incidence of stingers in young rugby players. *Am J Sports Med.* 2015;43(11):2809–2815

21. Strike SA, Hassanzadeh H. Traumatic spine injuries in the athlete. In: Miller MD, ed. *Orthopaedic Knowledge Update: Sports Medicine 5.* Rosemont, IL: American Academy of Orthopaedic Surgeons; 2016:423–432

22. Vaccaro AR, Klein GR, Ciccoti M, et al. Return to play criteria for the athlete with cervical spine injuries resulting in stinger and transient quadriplegia/paresis. *Spine J.* 2002;2(5):351–356

23. Harrast MA, Weinstein SM. Cervical spine. In: Kibler WB, ed. *Orthopaedic Knowledge Update: Sports Medicine 4.* Rosemont, IL: American Academy of Orthopaedic Surgeons; 2009:295–303

24. Dickens JF, Owens BD, Cameron KL, et al. Return to play and recurrent instability after in-season anterior shoulder instability: a prospective multicenter study. *Am J Sports Med.* 2014;42(12):2842–2850

25. St. Pierre P, Gonzales R. Shoulder fractures and clavicular joint injuries. In: Seidenberg PH, Beutler AI, eds. *The Sports Medicine Resource Manual.* Philadelphia, PA: Saunders; 2008:244–252

26. Hibberd EE, Kerr ZY, Roos KG, Djoko A, Dompier TP. Epidemiology of acromioclavicular joint sprains in 25 National Collegiate Athletic Association sports: 2009-2010 to 2014-2015 academic years. *Am J Sports Med.* 2016;44(10):2667–2674

27. Pallis M, Cameron KL, Svoboda SJ, Owens BD. Epidemiology of acromioclavicular joint injury in young athletes. *Am J Sports Med.* 2012;40(9):2072–2077

28. Gardner EC, Chan WW, Sutton KM, Blaine TA. Shoulder injuries in men's collegiate lacrosse, 2004-2009. *Am J Sports Med.* 2016;44(10):2675–2681

29. Nissen CW, Chatterjee A. Type III acromioclavicular separation: results of a recent survey on its management. *Am J Orthop (Belle Mead NJ)*. 2007;36(2):89–93

30. Torg JS. Cervical spine injuries and the return to football. *Sports Health*. 2009;1(5):376–383

31. Lee P, Hunter TB, Taljanovic M. Musculoskeletal colloquialisms: how did we come up with these names? *Radiographics*. 2004;24(4):1009–1027

32. Boden BP. Cervical spine injuries. In: Seidenberg PH, Beutler AI, eds. *The Sports Medicine Resource Manual*. Philadelphia, PA: Saunders; 2008:272–284

33. Lervick GN, Klepps SK. Return to play: shoulder dislocations, clavicle fractures, and acromioclavicular separations. *Orthopaedic Knowledge Online Journal*. 2011;9(3). http://www.aaos.org/OKOJ/vol9/issue3/SHO042. Accessed July 2, 2017

34. Link MS, Estes NA III, Maron BJ; American Heart Association Electrocardiography and Arrhythmias Committee of Council on Clinical Cardiology, Council on Cardiovascular Disease in Young, Council on Cardiovascular and Stroke Nursing, Council on Functional Genomics and Translational Biology; American College of Cardiology. Eligibility and disqualification recommendations for competitive athletes with cardiovascular abnormalities: task force 13; commotio cordis: a scientific statement. *Circulation*. 2015;132(22):e339–e342

35. Bartlett A, Williams R, Hilton M. Splenic rupture in infectious mononucleosis: a systematic review of published case reports. *Injury*. 2016;47(3):531–538

36. Juyia RF, Kerr HA. Return to play after liver and spleen trauma. *Sports Health*. 2014;6(3):239–245

37. Brophy RH, Gamradt SC, Barnes RP, et al. Kidney injuries in professional American football: implications for management of an athlete with 1 functioning kidney. *Am J Sports Med*. 2008;36(1):85–90

38. Jiménez-Truque N, Saye EJ, Sooper N, et al. Association between contact sports and colonization with *Staphylococcus aureus* in a prospective cohort of collegiate athletes [published online August 31, 2016]. *Sports Med*. doi: 10.1007/s40279-016-0618-6

39. Mölsa J, Kujala U, Myllynen P, Torstila I, Airaksinen O. Injuries to the upper extremity in ice hockey: analysis of a series of 760 injuries. *Am J Sports Med*. 2003;31(5):751–757

40. Lipscomb AB, Thomas ED, Johnston RK. Treatment of myositis ossificans traumatica in athletes. *Am J Sports Med*. 1976;4(3):111–120

41. Tejwani SG, Cohen SB, Bradley JP. Management of Morel-Lavallée lesion of the knee: twenty-seven cases in the National Football League. *Am J Sports Med*. 2007;35(7):1162–1167

42. Greenhill D, Haydel C, Rehman S. Management of the Morel-Lavallée lesion. *Orthop Clin N Am*. 2016;47(1):115–125

43. McGuine TA, Hetzel S, McCrea M, Brooks MA. Protective equipment and player characteristics associated with the incidence of sport-related concussion in high school football players: a multifactorial prospective study. *Am J Sports Med*. 2014;42(10):2470–2478

44. Belson K. Researchers revise helmet rating system. *New York Times*. January 29, 2013. http://www.nytimes.com/2013/01/29/sports/football/researchers-revise-helmet-rating-system.html. Accessed July 2, 2017

45. Virginia Tech Department of Biomedical Engineering and Mechanics. Football helmet ratings. Virginia Tech Helmet Ratings Web site. http://www.beam.vt.edu/helmet/helmets_football.php. Accessed July 2, 2017

46. Virginia Tech Department of Biomedical Engineering and Mechanics. Hockey helmet ratings. Virginia Tech Helmet Ratings Web site. http://www.beam.vt.edu/helmet/helmets_hockey.php. Accessed July 2, 2017

47. Breedlove KM, Breedlove EL, Bowman TG, Nauman EA. Impact attenuation capabilities of football and lacrosse helmets. *J Biomech*. 2016;49(13):2838–2844

48. Benson BW, Hamilton GM, Meeuwisse WH, McCrory P, Dvorak J. Is protective equipment useful in preventing concussion? A systematic review of the literature. *Br J Sports Med*. 2009;43(suppl 1):i56–i67

49. National Federation of State High School Associations Sports Medicine Advisory Committee. Position statement and recommendations for mouthguard use in sports. NFHS Web site. http://www.nfhs.org/sports-resource-content/position-statement-and-recommendations-for-mouthguard-use-in-sports. Published November 21, 2014. Accessed July 2, 2017

50. American Academy of Pediatrics Council on Sports Medicine and Fitness. Reducing injury risk from body checking in boys' youth ice hockey. *Pediatrics*. 2014;133(6):1151–1157

51. Kriz PK, MacDonald J. The youth sports machine: destructive juggernaut or vehicle for success (athletic, academic, career)? Presented at American College of Sports Medicine Annual Meeting; June 2, 2016; Boston, MA

CHAPTER 12

Gymnastics and the Young Athlete

Stessie Dort Zimmerman, MD; Nicholas M. Edwards, MD, MPH, FAAP; and Teri McCambridge, MD, FAAP

Overview

Gymnastics in the United States dates to the 1820s, with gymnastic apparatuses being used in communities. As a sport, it gained popularity when YMCAs established gymnasiums in the 1860s. In the 1970s, high schools in every state had gymnastic teams for adolescent boys and adolescent girls.[1] Although the gymnastic programs for girls started later, they have persisted longer. The current women's Olympic gymnastic events are vault, floor exercise, balance beam, and uneven parallel bars.

The most elite American female gymnasts approach their prime prior to starting college, and they come from private clubs. In contrast, men tend to transition to the Olympic level after competing at the collegiate level. Currently, the National Collegiate Athletic Association (NCAA) has only 16 men's programs and 84 women's programs.

In contrast, the United States has nearly 3 million recreational gymnasts. Because of the high frequency of musculoskeletal injury, in combination with a higher than normal incidence of medial issues such as disordered eating and amenorrhea, most pediatricians will encounter gymnasts as patients in their clinical practice. This chapter provides guidance on caring for this unique population.

Physiologic Demands of Gymnastics

Gymnastics is a dynamic sport with high-intensity training programs for athletes as young as 3 or 4 years of age. Because of the rigors of gymnastics training, in conjunction with the need to specialize in the sport at a relatively young age to advance, gymnasts, their parents, and their coaches are often involved in decisions regarding sport specialization. These decisions may generate conflict, and physicians are posed to provide helpful information to the decision-makers. On the one hand, parents and coaches recognize that the benefits of child and adolescent sports include opportunities for fun, exercise, teamwork, leadership, and strengthened self-esteem. However, only 0.03% to 0.50% of high school athletes ever reach professional or Olympic level competition. Furthermore, at least 50% of athlete injuries are a result of overuse.

When physicians are counseling families and coaches, they should consider a few points. First, the primary focuses for child and youth sports are fun and developing skills. Participating in multiple sports will decrease overuse injuries and burnout, particularly before puberty. Late adolescence sport specialization may increase the probability of athletes achieving their goals. If early specialization is selected, it is important to engage in conversations about sport-related goals with the child, as well as the parents or coaches, to determine if the goals are age appropriate and attainable. As parents continue to stay actively engaged in monitoring the training environment of their child, they should ensure that the young athlete has 1 to 2 days off each week.[2]

Gymnastics requires explosive isometric muscular contractions, to generate significant mechanical power. Impressive forces are placed particularly on the upper extremities. In studies of ground reaction forces on the upper extremities, a force of 2.37 times the body weight occurs with a back-hand spring[3] and 2.38 times in a Yurchenko vault.[4] Female athletes regularly reach greater than 90% of the relative maximal heart rate while completing gymnastic routines. Although the floor and uneven bars are the most physiologically demanding, beam also generates high heart rates and lactate levels that may be associated with the isometric demands in the event.[5]

Young competitive gymnasts train year-round and practice from 10 to 25 hours per week.[6] Many gyms follow a periodization-training program with 3 phases: preparation, competition, and transition.[7] It has been well-documented that the Western world was influenced by the former success in communist countries in initiating early sport specialization, specifically in gymnastics, diving, and figure skating.[8]

The young competitive gymnast progresses gradually through levels of performance. USA Gymnastics has established 10 junior Olympic levels (level 10 being the highest prior to elite or Olympic level). The forces of impact and risks of injury increase with progression through each competitive level because the skill difficulty and training hours exponentially increase. In the United States, the incidence rate of injury, defined as "any damaged body part that would interfere with training," associated with recreational gymnastics is 4.8 injuries per 1,000 gymnasts per year for patients who seek care in emergency departments (EDs).[9] However, for collegiate women gymnasts, the rate of injury is 9.22 injuries per 1,000 athlete exposures per year. An athlete exposure is defined as one student-athlete participating in one NCAA gymnastic practice or competition.[10]

Case Files: Gymnastics Injuries

This section outlines some common injuries in female gymnasts. It is important to be cognizant of specific risk factors associated with gymnastics participation to come to the correct diagnosis, initiate the appropriate therapy, and assist the athlete in a timely return to play.

Physical Diagnoses

Case 1
Spinal injuries in a 14-year-old female level 9 gymnast

Description
A 14-year-old female level 9 gymnast presents to clinic for evaluation of 3 months of lower back pain with insidious onset. It is worsened by back walkovers and back handsprings. Her symptoms improve with rest and trunk flexion. She has no pain at rest or with normal activities of daily living. She has no systemic or neurologic symptoms.

The various skills and elements in gymnastics require a wide range of spine stressors, including traction (swinging a giant), hyperextension (back handspring), hyperflexion (roundoff), and torsion (full twist). Additionally, the elusive "hollow" position requires scapular protraction, thoracic hyper-kyphosis, and pelvic tilt. Spinal injuries accounted for 17% of injuries in elite and sub-elite female gymnasts.[11] For these athletes, it is important to include spondylolysis, spondylolisthesis, Scheuermann disease, and disk degeneration in your differential diagnosis of chronic back pain in addition to the standard differential diagnosis outlined in Box 12-1.

In athletes participating in sports that require significant repetitive hyperextension and rotational forces of the lumbar spine (eg, gymnasts, lacrosse players, ballet dancers, tennis players, football lineman), stress injuries need to be considered. These tend to be stress injuries to the vertebral arch, more specifically the pars interarticularis or pedicle (Figure 12-1).

These athletes may present with nonspecific, paraspinal lower back pain. The pain is often described as dull and achy, but it becomes sharp with certain maneuvers. Pain may radiate to the sacroiliac joint or bilateral buttocks region. Pain will be exacerbated with activities in the gym that require slow hyperextension, such as back walkovers, front walkovers, bridges, and Yurchenko-style vaults, to name a few. The physical examination might reveal a child or an adolescent with a hyperlordotic stance. These patients tend to have tenderness to palpation over paraspinal muscles, which is generally worse on one side compared with the other. Expect no

---

Box 12-1
Differential Diagnosis for Pediatric Spondylodynia

Extra-spinal and Referred Pain	Trauma or Overuse Injuries	Infections	Neoplasms	Autoimmune or Vascular
• Retrocecal appendicitis • Pyelonephritis • Psoas abscess	• Sacroiliac dysfunction • Scheuermann disease • Spondylolysis • Spondylolisthesis • Disk herniation	• Epidural abscess • Osteomyelitis • Diskitis • Pott disease	• Ewing osteosarcoma • Aneurysmal bone cyst • Leukemia • Lymphoma • Neuroblastoma • Osteoid osteoma	• Ankylosing spondylitis • Psoriatic spondylitis • Reiter syndrome • Sickle cell pain crisis

Derived from Wolfe C. Back pain. *Pediatr Rev.* 2002;23(6):221.

spinous process tenderness. Dermatologic examination findings should be normal, with no hairy patches, hyperpigmented lesions, or nevi. Results from neural tension tests, which include the straight-leg raise and slump test, should be negative. These patients also tend to

have pain with single-limb standing lumbar extension. This physical examination maneuver is called the Stork test (Figure 12-2). Findings from the neurologic assessment will be normal in the setting of isolated spondylolysis. No limitation in rotation or flexion will be appreciated.

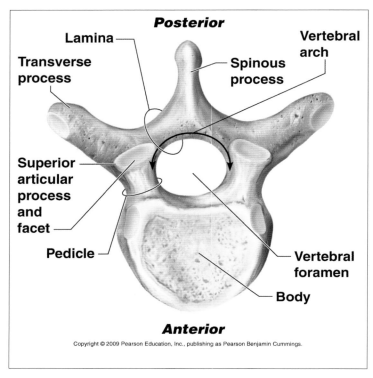

FIGURE 12-1

The vertebral arch extends from pedicle to pedicle and includes both laminae. The body of the vertebra and the vertebral arch form the vertebral foramen to allow passage of the spinal cord.

From Marieb EN, Hoehn K. *Human Anatomy & Physiology.* 7th ed. Glenview, IL: Pearson; 2007. Reproduced with permission.

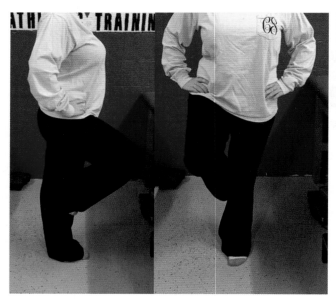

FIGURE 12-2

For the Stork test, the patient should flex one knee so the sole of the non–weight bearing leg is near the weight-bearing knee. The patient balances on the weight-bearing leg and performs a lumbar extension.

Spondylolysis

In gymnasts presenting similarly to the gymnast in case 1, unilateral spondylolysis must be included in the differential diagnosis. Spondylolysis is a fatigue fracture of the vertebral arch pars interarticularis with adjacent bone sclerosis. The pedicle is rarely involved. Spondylolysis affects around 10% of female gymnasts and is most frequently found at the L5 spinal level.[12,13]

Anteroposterior (AP) and lateral (Figure 12-3) view radiographs of the lumbar spine are often the first diagnostic images to be obtained in the workup. They are obtained to evaluate for spondylolysis or other gross bone abnormality. Oblique views were previously recommended; however, studies have shown no significant difference in sensitivity (0.59 and 0.53) and specificity (0.96 and 0.94) between 4-view and 2-view plain radiographs of the back to diagnose spondylolysis.[14] Thus, oblique views can be eliminated to substantially decrease radiation to the gonads.

If plain radiographic findings are negative, further study with magnetic resonance imaging (MRI), single-photon emission computed tomography (SPECT) scan, or computed tomography scan, or a combination of those, can be used, as effective and reliable means, to diagnose acute spondylolysis. Magnetic resonance imaging is generally preferred in the adolescent population because of the absence of radiation. The request for imaging should specifically request to rule out spondylolysis. The radiologist will then use specific thinner slice thickness MRI axial images, with the plane more parallel to the pedicles, to enhance visualization of the pars interarticularis. Some studies recommend SPECT scan, with a follow-up limited computed tomography scan of patients with positive SPECT scan findings, to best guide treatment.[15,16]

Nonoperative management for these patients includes temporary restriction from sport participation and physical therapy and may require back bracing, depending on acuity and healing potential. Untreated bilateral spondylolysis can progress to spondylolisthesis. Figure 12-4 provides examples of exercises that may be suggested by physical therapists.

Spondylolisthesis

Spondylolisthesis is defined as the translation of one vertebral segment on another. Displacement of the vertebra is called anterolisthesis (anterior displacement) or retrolisthesis (posterior displacement). Approximately 90% of cases of spondylolisthesis occur at L5-S1.[16] The Meyerding classification can be used to grade the percentage of vertebral body displacement.[17,18] This classification system ranges from grade I to V (from 0%–25% to complete displacement).

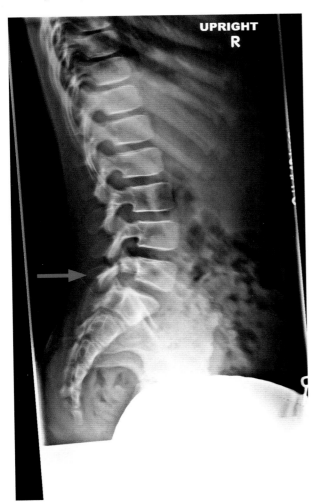

FIGURE 12-3

Lateral view plain radiographs of the spine demonstrating spondylolysis at L5 spinal level as indicated by the blue arrow.

Rehabilitation and Prevention Exercises

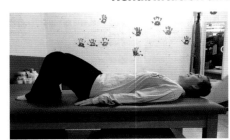

A. Isometric Abdominal Flex

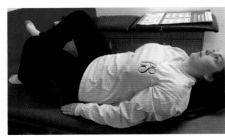

B. Bent-Leg Lift (Hook Lying)

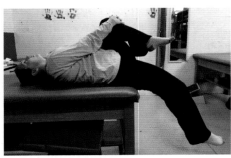

C. Pelvic Rotation: Knee to Chest (Supine)

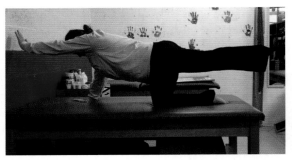

D. Upper- and Lower-Extremity Extension

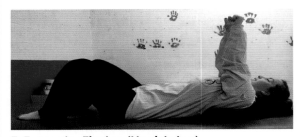

E. Extremity Flexion (Hook Lying)

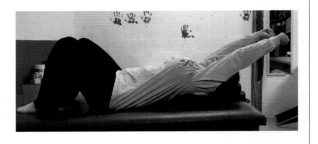

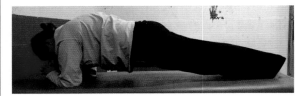

F. Plank

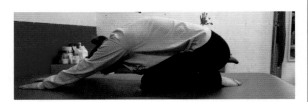

G. Middle-Back Stretch

FIGURE 12-4

These images demonstrate exercises that can be performed by the athlete without significant equipment. Repetition is used with each exercise to increase strength and stamina: A, Lie on back with knees bent; tighten stomach by pressing elbows down. Hold this position for 5 sec. B, Tighten stomach and slowly raise each leg 15 cm (6 in) from floor. Hold for 5 sec. C, With each leg hanging over side of bench and other knee to chest, relax leg as much as possible. Hold for 30 sec. D, Tighten stomach and raise each leg and opposite arm. Keep trunk rigid. Hold for 2 sec. Complete a set. E, Tighten stomach and slowly lower both arms over head until back begins to arch. Keep trunk rigid. Hold for 2 sec. Complete a set. F, Raise up on elbows, keeping back flat and stomach rigid. Hold for 30 seconds. G, Push chest toward floor, reaching forward as far as possible. Keep buttocks on heels. Hold 30 seconds.

Grade I spondylolisthesis is generally managed with rest and bracing, if the patient is symptomatic. Most patients will be pain-free within 2 to 3 weeks if adherent to these interventions. Young female gymnasts with spondylolisthesis should undergo follow-up lumbar plain radiography yearly until the age of 19 years to check for progression. Images of these patients should be obtained sooner if they have persistent symptoms or increased pain.[17]

Scheuermann Disease

Scheuermann disease, or juvenile kyphosis, is characterized by greater than 5° of anterior wedging at 3 adjacent vertebrae resulting in kyphosis. These patients have more than 45° of fixed (not positional) kyphosis. Juvenile kyphosis may be associated with Schmorl nodes, which are intervertebral disk herniations of the nucleus pulposus (Figure 12-5) into the adjacent vertebral body.[19]

The mechanism of injury is unclear, although it is thought to result from repetitive trauma in the immature spine, as might occur in young female athletes performing gymnastics. These patients generally present with cosmetic concerns. They

may also have corresponding pain. Please note that physical examination may not reveal kyphosis; however, when it is present, it will be exacerbated with forward flexion. These patients have normal neurologic assessment findings. The apex of the deformity is usually between T7 and T9 vertebrae. Patients generally present in the teenage years, between 10 and 15 years of age. There is a 2:1 male predominance in the incidence. Twenty percent to 30% of these patients also have scoliosis.[19] The initial treatment of patients with Scheuermann disease includes activity modification. For athletes with curves less than 50°, physical therapy can be effective. This would primarily include thoracic extension exercises, which might include anterior chest wall and shoulder stretches with core strengthening. For more severe disease, bracing may be indicated. However, gymnasts may be able to continue their sports as tolerated and to use their allotted out-of-brace time for practices and competition.[20]

Disk Degeneration

Disk degeneration is a less common cause of lower back pain in the pediatric and adolescent population. Gymnasts with disk degeneration may present with loss of hamstring muscle flexibility or inability to perform gymnastic maneuvers in the pike position. When the disk degeneration is severe, these gymnasts will have pain with lifting, sitting, or lying supine. Additionally, these patients may present with radiating pain or symptoms of sciatic nerve pain. Plain radiographs may show loss of disk-space height. Nevertheless, MRI is currently the criterion standard for diagnostic imaging.[15,20,21] An MRI will show a low signal intensity on T2-weighted images.

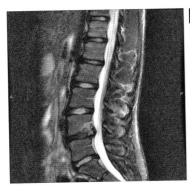

FIGURE 12-5

Herniation of the nucleus pulposis in a patient at the L4-5 intervertebral disk, although this patient does not have Scheuermann disease.

TAKE-HOME POINTS

Spondylolysis, Spondylolisthesis, and Scheuermann Disease

▶ Gymnastics puts significant traction, hyperextension, and torsion forces on the lumbar spine.

▶ Anteroposterior and lateral view plain radiographs are the initial images to obtain when attempting to rule out spondylolysis.

▶ If diagnosis is delayed, spondylolysis can progress to spondylolisthesis. Spondylolisthesis has a worse prognosis.

▶ Although scoliosis does not cause pain in the pediatric athlete, Scheuermann disease can cause pain.

Case 2

Bilateral wrist pain in a 10-year-old female level 5 gymnast

Description

A 10-year-old girl, who is a level 5 gymnast, presents with gradual onset of bilateral wrist pain, which is worse with tumbling and movements on the vault apparatus. She notes that the pain is worsened by extreme extension of the wrists and weight bearing on the hands. This is particularly concerning to her because overextension and weight bearing on the wrists are necessary in many maneuvers on the floor, on the vault, and during beam routines. In athletes with presentations like this one, physical examination often reveals tenderness to palpation over the dorsal aspect of the distal radial growth plate. There may be swelling over the dorsum of the wrist. Usually, wrist extension is limited. Given the location of the pain, the differential diagnosis includes tendinitis, distal radial epiphysitis, ganglion cyst, avascular necrosis of the capitate bone, scaphoid bone impaction syndrome, scaphoid stress fracture, or ulnar impaction syndrome.[22] Imaging is necessary for proper diagnosis.

Fundamental movements in gymnastics require athletes to bear weight on the upper extremities. These include handstands and planches, as static weight-bearing activities, and front handsprings, back handsprings, roundoffs, and cartwheels, as dynamic exercises. Upper-extremity injuries account for 50% of gymnastics-related injuries in patients presenting to the ED between the ages of 6 and 11 years.[9] The wrist is the most frequently injured region of the upper extremity in female gymnastics, followed by the elbow. The predisposing risk factors to injury in the upper extremity include improper equipment, poor technique, lack of skeletal maturity, and rapid growth spurts. Understanding these injuries is crucial to ensure proper treatment and a timely return to play.

Distal Radial Epiphysiolysis

Distal radial epiphysiolysis, or "gymnast's wrist," is an overuse injury that results in pain at the physis of the distal radius. The distal radial physes appear at 12 to 18 months and fuse at 15 to 18 years of age. The highest risk for this injury is during a growth spurt. Depending on the stage of injury, sclerosis on both sides of the physis will be seen on the AP and lateral view plain radiographs.[22] Radiographs generally show widening of the physis as well (Figure 12-6).

First-line therapy includes rest and immobilization. Fiberglass casting can be useful for initial immobilization. Mild cases may resolve in 3 to 4 weeks, while more severe cases may take 3 to 6 months to resolve. Return to play and upper-extremity weight bearing should be gradual and pain-free. Pace of improvement is directly related to adherence to the treatment plan; cutting back on some but not all upper-extremity activity often just delays recovery. Delayed diagnosis and poor management may result in radial physeal arrest, positive ulnar variance, and, in severe cases, Madelung deformity.[22,23] Figure 12-7 shows the Madelung deformity.

Avascular Necrosis of the Lunate Bone

Avascular necrosis of the lunate bone, or Kienböck disease, results in collapse of the lunate. This is secondary to vascular insufficiency resulting from singular or repetitive microtrauma to the vasculature, which compromises the blood supply to the lunate. Although this injury can occur in other athletes, it more frequently occurs in upper-extremity weight-bearing athletes, such as gymnasts. This injury most commonly occurs in the dominant hand and in athletes with negative ulnar variance (Figure 12-8).

Generally, the patient will present with dorsal wrist pain and swelling. Physical examination shows tenderness over the radiocarpal joint. Pain with passive dorsiflexion of the middle finger is characteristic. Patients will likely have decreased wrist flexion, extension, and handgrip strength. Sclerosis occurs early in the course of the disease, followed by collapse or fragmentation, or both. These findings in the lunate may be seen on AP, lateral, and oblique view plain radiographs. However, MRI may be necessary for diagnosing early disease in the absence of findings on plain radiographs. The Lichtman Classification System (Figure 12-9) can be used to stage the disease.[24]

The goal of initial treatment for stage 1 disease is to decrease the compressive forces on the lunate to permit revascularization. To achieve this, initial therapy for stage 1 disease includes temporary immobilization and nonsteroidal anti-inflammatory drugs. However, surgical procedures are indicated for more severe disease. To prevent worsening and potential debilitation, patients with more advanced disease warrant referral to a pediatric orthopedic surgeon, for surgical evaluation.

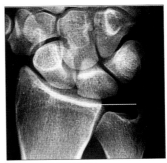

FIGURE 12-8

Ulnar variance. The degree of variance is determined by projecting a line perpendicular from the carpal joint surface of the distal end of the radius toward the ulna. Negative variance with the distal edge of the ulna proximal to the distal articular surface of the radius.

From Cerezal L, del Piñal F, Abascal F, García-Valtuille R, Pereda T, Canga A. Imaging findings in ulnar-sided wrist impaction syndromes. *Radiographics.* 2002;22(1):105–121. Reproduced with permission.

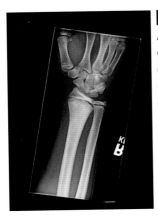

FIGURE 12-6

AP view plain radiograph of the right wrist that demonstrates widening of the radial growth plate and sclerosis.

Abbreviation:
AP, anteroposterior.

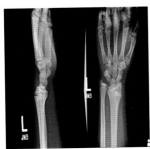

FIGURE 12-7

Left AP and lateral plain film images of the wrist demonstrating Madelung deformity. With this deformity in the coronal plane there is increasing radial inclination as well as the sagittal plane. Note how the lunate and first row of carpal bones adapt into an inverted triangle.

From Kozin S, Zlotolow DA. Madelung deformity. *J Hand Surg Am.* 2015;40(10):2090–2098. Reproduced with permission.

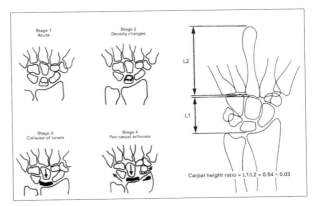

FIGURE 12-9

Lichtman Classification System.

From Keith PP, Nuttall D, Trail I. Long-term outcome of nonsurgically managed Kienböck's disease. *J Hand Surg.* 2004;29(1):63–67. Reproduced with permission.

Forearm Splints

Forearm splints, or radial periostitis, present similarly to shin splints in the leg, with dull mid-diaphysis pain of the radius. Patients may have mild pain initially that becomes more severe with increasing activity. In addition to gymnasts, weight lifters are also at increased risk because of the large loads and forces placed on the forearms during their lifts. On physical examination, there is pain with resisted wrist extension. Plain radiographic findings of the forearm are negative. A bone scan with technetium Tc 99m medronate is necessary to rule out stress fracture and may demonstrate linear periosteal uptake to confirm forearm splints.[25] Treatment for forearm splints includes temporary rest from inverted weight bearing, icing, and stretching and strengthening of the flexor and extensor muscles of the forearm. Athletes will be able to gradually return to play.

In gymnasts who may need added wrist support during practice and competition, wrist taping or braces may be helpful. Tiger Paw and Lion Paw wrist supports are specifically developed for use in gymnastics (Figure 12-10).

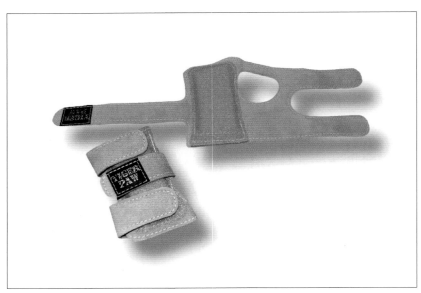

FIGURE 12-10

Tiger Paw wrist support brace.

From Tiger paw wrist supports. Tiger Paws Web site. http://www.tigerpawwristsupports.com/tiger-paw-wrist-supports. Accessed July 2, 2017. Reproduced with permission.

TAKE-HOME POINTS

Distal Radial Epiphysiolysis and Avascular Necrosis of the Lunate Bone

▶ Gymnasts place forces that are greater than 2 times their body weight on the upper extremities in fundamental maneuvers, including back handsprings.

▶ Chronic wrist pain in gymnasts requires further evaluation to avoid possible growth plate arrest, as may be the case with distal radial epiphysiolysis, or "gymnast's wrist."

▶ Avascular necrosis of the lunate bone, or Kienböck disease, occurs more frequently in gymnasts than in the general population. Delay in diagnosis and poor management can result in chronic wrist pain and debilitation.

Case 3
Lateral elbow pain in an 11-year-old competitive gymnast

Description

An 11-year-old competitive gymnast comes to clinic with concerns of lateral elbow pain when doing tumbling passes with rotations, such as a front handspring, full-vault maneuver, and locking sensations with flexion and extension of the elbow. Her pain has been present for 2 months. She was previously diagnosed as having lateral epicondylitis but has not improved with nonsteroidal anti-inflammatory drugs and stretching. Physical examination shows mild tenderness over the lateral elbow. She is unable to achieve full extension of the elbow. There is a mild elbow effusion. In similar patients, crepitus may be present. On plain radiograph is a well-defined subchondral lesion of the capitellum. It is important to consider osteochondritis dissecans (OCD) of the capitellum and Panner disease in the differential diagnosis for this presentation.

Osteochondritis Dissecans of the Capitellum

Similar to OCD lesions in the knee, OCD of the capitellum can be debilitating for young gymnasts. Although the mechanism of injury is uncertain, it is thought to be secondary to repetitive microtrauma. With recurrent weight bearing on a valgus-loaded upper extremity, high compression forces are placed on the capitellum, and this can result in injury to the subchondral bone. Chronic subchondral injury can progress to loosening of the overlying cartilage, worsening the prognosis. If untreated, athletes have chronic elbow pain, limited range of motion, and permanent elbow instability. Therefore, timely diagnosis is key. Plain radiographs can usually be used to identify an OCD lesion (Figure 12-11). The Minami classification system has been demonstrated to be the most reliable when assessing the stages of OCD lesions in the capitellum.[26] However, findings on the plain radiographs may be subtle. Magnetic resonance imaging adds additional information on the stability of a lesion and direct care and prognosis.

Unstable lesions require surgical intervention. With Minami type 1 lesions, the capitellum is flattened or there may be cystic changes. With the type 2 OCD lesions, there is subchondral detachment, or a fragment of the capitellum separates.[27]

Osteochondritis dissecans has the potential for intra-articular, loose body formation. Great care should be taken when treating these patients, as OCD lesions in the elbow can result in irreversible injury to the joint. These patients should be referred to sports medicine specialists or pediatric orthopedic surgeons, to guide management. For a stable lesion, conservative treatment with rest from upper-extremity weight bearing, until the findings on imaging resolve, may be successful. Surgical management is necessary for athletes who are skeletally mature, have loose bodies, athletes with limited range of motion, athletes whose conservative treatment of 1-year duration failed, or unstable lesions.

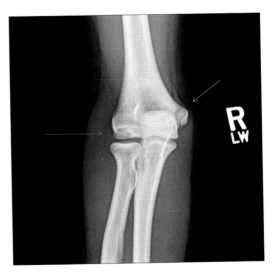

FIGURE 12-11

Radiograph demonstrates an OCD lesion of the capitellum (red arrow) of the right arm of a young athlete. Notice that some of the growth plates remain open, including the medial epicondylar apophysis (blue arrow). This is a Minami type 2 lesion.

Abbreviation: OCD, osteochondritis dissecans.

Capitellar Osteochondrosis

Capitellar osteochondrosis, or Panner disease, is an avascular necrosis of the capitellum. Osteochondrosis can be seen on plain radiographs shortly after the appearance of the ossific nucleus. Panner disease affects athletes at a younger age than OCD does and has the highest incidence at 7 to 12 years of age. Two-thirds of patients with Panner disease will present with pain; half, with a swollen elbow; and one-fourth, with limitations in extension.[28]

Plain radiographs of the elbow will show an irregularity, sclerosis, or flattening of the capitellum. Treatment for capitellar osteochondrosis is to limit all sport activity using the upper extremity until the pain has resolved and the patient has normal range of motion. This is usually a self-limiting disease and generally does not have significant sequelae.[29] However, to prevent this type of injury, gymnasts should avoid one-armed skills. They should also avoid L-grip giants on the uneven bars.

Elbow Dislocations

The elbow joint is the second most commonly dislocated major joint in the general population.[30] Dislocation makes up 10% to 25% of all elbow injuries. Boys' wrestling is the sport with the highest rate of elbow dislocations, but girls' gymnastics is second on the list. Usually, this results with a high-energy fall onto an outstretched hand. Ninety-five percent of elbow dislocations are first-time dislocations.[31] These athletes will present with a painful, swollen, and obvious deformed elbow. Physical examination usually shows a posterior deformity, with tenderness, swelling, and ecchymosis. A posterior displacement is the most common type of elbow dislocation.[32] Range of motion will be limited and result in severe pain.

It is important to evaluate for neurologic or vascular compromise. Care should be taken to evaluate the median nerve with physical examination that may include difficulty with thumb opposition; loss of sensation on the palmar surface of the index, middle, and radial half of the ring fingers; and presence of localized atrophy of the thenar eminence. Similarly, with ulnar nerve damage, patients may have difficulty with finger abduction, loss of sensation of the little finger and ulnar half of the ring finger, and localized atrophy of the hyper-thenar eminence. Plain radiographs of the elbow are diagnostic and can also be used to identify associated fractures, given 30% of elbow dislocations are associated with avulsion fractures of the medial condyle.[32] Imaging may also reveal radial head, radial neck, olecranon, coronoid bone, or other distal humerus fractures.

If the patient has neurovascular compromise, effort should be made to reduce the dislocation immediately. If this occurs out in the field, the elbow should be immobilized and splinted prior to transport to the ED. Generally, closed reductions should be done under anesthesia. Post-reduction immobilization should be limited to 5 to 7 days, with increasing range of motion for athletes with simple dislocations.[33] Handgrips and use of a pumice stone to reduce callus buildup can be helpful in preventing elbow dislocations in gymnasts.

TAKE-HOME POINTS

Osteochondritis Dissecans, Capitellar Osteochondrosis, and Elbow Dislocations

▶ In gymnasts with chronic elbow pain, it is important to consider osteochondritis dissecans of the capitellum and capitellar osteochondrosis, or Panner disease.

▶ Panner disease can be a self-limited process.

▶ Osteochondritis dissecans lesions in the elbow can result in irreversible injury to the joint if they are not managed appropriately.

▶ Elbow dislocations should be reduced promptly. It is crucial to evaluate for neurovascular compromise, with special attention given to the median and ulnar nerves.

Case 4
Heel pain in a 13-year-old female gymnast

Description

A 13-year-old female gymnast presents with heel pain that is particularly bothersome on her approach to the vault or with other sprinting during conditioning. She has a positive calcaneal squeeze test result on examination (Figure 12-12).

Calcaneal Apophysitis

Calcaneal apophysitis, or Sever disease, occurs commonly in young athletes. Gymnasts are at particular risk because they work out barefoot. These athletes will present with posterior ankle pain that is worse after activity. The physical examination findings will be unremarkable except for a positive calcaneal squeeze test result. Although the diagnosis of Sever disease in a gymnast is not unique, the approach to the management requires creativity. Heel cups used in combination with ankle neoprene supports will permit the use of heel cups in sports such as gymnastics and dance, in which the athlete does not wear shoes. Tuli's Cheetahs (Figure 12-13) are an example of an available product that provides a 2-in-1 support to produce a sure fit in the heel cup during high-velocity movements on the floor and the vault exercises.

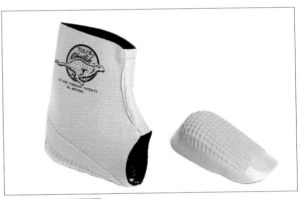

FIGURE 12-13

Tuli's Cheetahs.

From Medi-Dyne Healthcare Products. Reproduced with permission.

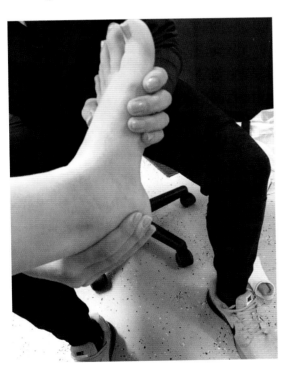

FIGURE 12-12

During the calcaneal squeeze test, pressure is applied to the medial lateral region of the calcaneal tuberosity. Pain with squeeze is a positive test result and suggestive of Sever disease or calcaneal stress fracture, depending on the patient's age.

These athletes can be permitted to continue to participate, as long as their gait is normal. Treatment should include Achilles tendon stretching (Figure 12-14), avoidance of barefoot walking at home, and ice after activity.

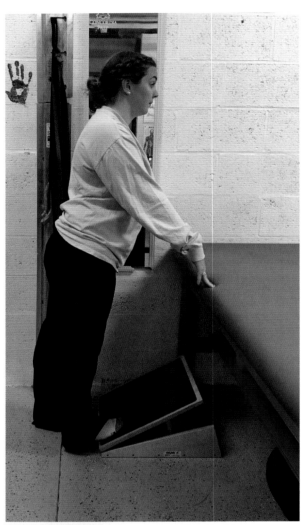

FIGURE 12-14

An example of one type of Achilles tendon stretch. Other stretches include the use of a curb or step with a similar stance.

Other Injuries

Gymnasts sustain many injuries that are common in players of other sports. For example, patellofemoral pain syndrome, Osgood-Schlatter disease, Sinding-Larsen–Johansson disease, knee ligament injuries, and ankle sprains occur frequently in gymnasts. It is important to collaborate with the athlete, to identify taping and bracing techniques that will minimize symptoms and permit participation, when considering the appropriate management of these common injuries in gymnasts.

Psychological Diagnoses

Case 5
Female gymnast with weight loss, fatigue, and weakness

A judge tells an Olympic-level athlete during competition that she is too "fluffy" for a gymnast. Desperate to advance in her athletic career, she begins avoiding fattening foods. She sees herself as overweight. She continues to lose weight and now comes to clinic with concerns of fatigue, weakness, and weight loss. This patient is demonstrating symptoms of disordered eating and potentially anorexia nervosa.

Eating Disorders

Gymnasts who aspire to be elite competitors specialize and begin intense training at an early age. Generally, they achieve peak performance during their adolescent years. This age coincides with a rise in incidence in mental disorders. Gymnastics is a sport during which tremendous demands are placed on the body and the mind. These athletes are judged on ability and aesthetics.

This sport idealizes athletes with slim physiques. The stresses of this high-performance environment can have psychological repercussions. These female athletes are at risk for low self-esteem, depression, and eating disorders.[34]

Making the diagnosis in this population may be difficult, given that characteristics such as perfectionism and obsession are frequently praised in this sport. Furthermore, many of these elite athletes are cognizant of their dietary intake and weight. Many of their coaches also supervise their diets and weight. Often, athletes will say that strict attention to their dietary intake and weight management is part of the job. These behaviors are more concerning and are likely pathological if these gymnasts lack the ability to exercise control of their response to these stimulating thoughts. It is crucial that pediatricians educate athletes, parents, and coaches about the signs and symptoms of eating disorders, as well as the female athlete triad (see case 8 in Chapter 2, Trends in Prevention of Sports Injury in the Young Athlete). The SCOFF questionnaire can be used as a screening tool to identify patients who might have an eating disorder.[35]

TAKE-HOME POINTS

Eating Disorders

▶ Even elite athletes with highly successful careers can have eating disorders.

▶ Pediatricians must be astute and thorough to avoid missing the diagnosis of eating disorders in young gymnasts, given the potential confounding signs and symptoms.

▶ Education of athletes, parents, and coaches about signs and symptoms may accelerate the diagnosis of eating disorders.

Recommendations for Keeping Young Gymnasts Healthy

What Physicians Can Do to Keep Their Gymnasts Healthy

Physicians should engage their patients and ask questions regarding frequency, duration, and intensity of training. These conversations should include discussions about goals of participation in gymnastics to ensure they are age-appropriate and attainable. Furthermore, it is important to regularly monitor growth, development, nutrition, and mental health. Regularly ask your high-level gymnasts at health supervision visits about joint pain, specifically focusing on wrist and back concerns. Learning some of the basic movements in gymnastics can help establish rapport with these patients. Frequent communication with coaches and parents may be necessary.

How Physicians Should Involve Themselves in the Gymnastics Community

Coordinating first-responder presence or physician coverage during gymnastic competitions may ensure safety of young athletes. Physicians may also approach their local gymnastics gyms about injury screening and providing lectures on nutrition, common injuries, and eating disorders. Many gyms are also looking for physicians to sign off on summer camps and first aid or cardiopulmonary resuscitation certification.

How Physicians Can Best Serve as a Resource to Their Young Gymnasts

Gymnasts will come to their health care professionals seeking input on symptom care and management. Understanding the unique features of their movements, risk for injury, unique diagnoses, and appropriate treatment plan can be improved by review of the information provided in this chapter. Further knowledge can be gained by review of the literature, beginning with the American Academy of Pediatrics and the references provided throughout this chapter.

References

1. Gross A. A history of United States artistic gymnastics. *Sci Gymnastics J.* 2010;2(2):5–28

2. Brenner JS; American Academy of Pediatrics Council on Sports Fitness. Sports specialization and intensive training in young athletes. *Pediatrics.* 2016;138(3):e20162148

3. Koh TJ, Grabiner MD, Weiker GG. Technique and ground reaction forces in the back handspring. *Am J Sports Med.* 1992;20(1):61–66

4. Seeley MK, Bressel E. A comparison of upper-extremity reaction forces between the Yurchenko vault and floor exercise. *J Sports Sci Med.* 2005;4(2):85–94

5. Marina M, Rodríguez FA. Physiological demands of young women's competitive gymnastic routines. *Biol Sport.* 2014;31(3):217–222

6. Burt LA, Naughton GA, Higham DG, Landeo R. Training load in pre-pubertal female artistic gymnastics. *Sci Gymnastics J.* 2010;2(3):5–14

7. Bompa TO, Carrera MC. *Periodization Training for Sports: Science-Based Strength and Conditioning Plans for 17 Sports.* 2nd ed. Champaign, IL: Human Kinetics; 2005

8. Malina RM. Early sport specialization: roots, effectiveness, risks. *Curr Sports Med Rep.* 2010:9(6):364–371

9. Singh S, Smith GA, Fields SK, McKenzie LB. Gymnastics-related injuries to children treated in emergency departments in the United States, 1990-2005. *Pediatrics.* 2008;121(4):e954–e960

10. Kerr ZY, Hayden R, Barr M, Klossner DA, Dompier TP. Epidemiology of National Collegiate Athletic Association women's gymnastics injuries, 2009-2010 through 2013-2014. *J Athl Train.* 2015;50(8):870–878.

11. Kolt GS, Kirkby RJ. Epidemiology of injury in elite and subelite female gymnasts: a comparison of retrospective and prospective findings. *Br J Sports Med.* 1999;33(5):312–318

12. Mohriak R, Vargas Silva PD, Trandafilov M Jr, et al. Spondylolysis and spondylolisthesis in young gymnasts. *Rev Bras Ortop.* 2010;45(1):79–83

13. Oren JH, Gallina JM. Pars injuries in athletes. *Bull Hosp Jt Dis (2013).* 2016;74(1):73–81

14. Beck NA, Miller R, Baldwin K, et al. Do oblique views add value in the diagnosis of spondylolysis in adolescents? *J Bone Joint Surg Am.* 2013;95(10):e65

15. Campbell RS, Grainger AJ, Hide IG, Papastefanou S, Greenough CG. Juvenile spondylolysis: a comparative analysis of CT, SPECT and MRI. *Skeletal Radiol.* 2005;34(2):63–73

16. Kruse D, Lemmen B. Spine injuries in the sport of gymnastics. *Curr Sports Med Rep.* 2009;8(1):20–28

17. Meyerding HW. Spondylolisthesis: surgical treatment and results. *Surg Gynecol Obstet.* 1932;54:371–377

18. Metz LN, Deviren V. Low-grade spondylolisthesis. *Neurosurg Clin N Am.* 2007;18(2):237–248

19. D'hemecourt PA, Hresko MT. Spinal deformity in young athletes. *Clin Sports Med.* 2012;31(3):441–451

20. Tribus CB. Scheuermann's kyphosis in adolescents and adults: diagnosis and management. *J Am Acad Orthop Surg.* 1998;6(1):36–43

21. Goldstein JD, Berger PE, Windler GE, Jackson DW. Spine injuries in gymnasts and swimmers. An epidemiologic investigation. *Am J Sports Med.* 1991;19(5):463–438

22. Difiori JP, Caine DJ, Malina RM. Wrist pain, distal radial physeal injury, and ulnar variance in the young gymnast. *Am J Sports Med.* 2006;34(5):840–849

23. Frush TJ, Lindenfeld TN. Peri-epiphyseal and overuse injuries in adolescent athletes. *Sports Health.* 2009;1(3):201–211

24. Keith PP, Nuttall D, Trail I. Long-term outcome of non-surgically managed Kienböck's disease. *J Hand Surg Am.* 2004;29(1):63–67

25. Wadhwa SS, Mansberg R, Fernandes VB, Qasim S. Forearm splints seen on bone scan in a weightlifter. *Clin Nucl Med.* 1997;22(10):711–712

26. Claessen FM, van den Ende KI, Doornberg JN, Guitton TG, Eygendaal D, van den Bekerom MP; Shoulder and Elbow Plat-form & Science of Variation Group. Osteochondritis dissecans of the humeral capitellum: reliability of four classification systems using radiographs and computed tomography. *J Shoulder Elbow Surg.* 2015;24(10):1613–1618

27. Smith MV, Bedi A, Chen NC. Surgical treatment for osteochondritis dissecans of the capitellum. *Sports Health.* 2012;4(5):425–432

28. Claessen FM, Louwerens JK, Doornberg JN, van Dijk CN, Eygendaal D, van den Bekerom MP. Panner's disease: literature review and treatment recommendations. *J Child Orthop.* 2015;9(1):9–17

29. Crowther M. Elbow pain in pediatrics. *Curr Rev Musculoskelet Med.* 2009;2(2):83–87

30. Dizdarevic I, Low S, Currie DW, Comstock RD, Hammoud S, Atanda A Jr. Epidemiology of elbow dislocations in high school athletes. *Am J Sports Med.* 2016;44(1):202–208

31. Kocher MS, Waters PM, Micheli LJ. Upper extremity injuries in the paediatric athlete. *Sports Med.* 2000;30(2):117–135

32. Martin BD, Johansen JA, Edwards SG. Complications related to simple dislocations of the elbow. *Hand Clin.* 2008;24(1):9–25

33. de Haan J, den Hartog D, Tuinebreijer WE, et al. Functional treatment versus plaster for simple elbow dislocations (FuncSiE): a randomized trial. *BMC Musculoskelet Disord.* 2010;11:263

34. Tan JO, Calitri R, Bloodworth A, McNamee MJ. Understanding eating disorders in elite gymnastics: ethical and conceptual challenges. *Clin Sports Med.* 2016;35(2):275–292

35. Luck AJ, Morgan JF, Reid F, et al. The SCOFF questionnaire and clinical interview for eating disorders in general practice: comparative study. *BMJ.* 2002;325(7367):755–756

CHAPTER 13

Running and the Young Athlete

Tracy Zaslow, MD, FAAP, CAQSM, and Suzy McNulty, MD, FAAP

Overview

Running is a basic developmental milestone achieved by 18 to 24 months of age for most children. Running is also a great form of exercise if performed directly through cross-country, track, and recreational running or as part of a running-based sport, such as soccer, basketball, lacrosse, and rugby. Young athletes have shown they can run the distance too. In the 1970s, multiple young runners (Wesley Paul, Scott Black, Howie Breinan, and Mary Etta Boitano) completed the New York City Marathon at 7 to 10 years of age, and young athletes continue to go the distance, running marathons, ultramarathons, and more.

Running is characterized by an aerial phase during which both feet are off the ground, compared with walking, during which one foot is always in contact with the ground. The running gait consists of 2 main phases: stance and swing. Stance is broken down into the absorption and foot strike and the propulsion phases, while the swing phase is composed of the initial swing and terminal swing.

The benefits of running are countless, and they include fitness and health, motor skills, strength, and decrease in obesity.

With a growing number of young runners, pediatricians are increasingly faced with questions about how to encourage safe running participation among their patients. These issues are particularly important in the developing skeleton with cartilaginous physes found on the ends of young bones. The goal of this chapter is to educate pediatricians about ways to keep young runners healthy and "on the road."

History and Demographics

Running is a very popular sports activity for children and adolescents. Twelve million children and adolescents (6–17 years of age) participated in running for exercise in a single year in the United States. Outside of school physical education classes, running is the most common activity for girls and second most common for boys. Running injuries are common, and, although usually not severe, injuries can sideline athletes for prolonged periods. Running accounted for 25.1% of injuries sustained during physical education classes that presented to the emergency department, and if you include all the activities that involve running (running [25.1%], basketball [20.3%], football [7.8%], volleyball [5.7%], and soccer [5.4%]), running accounts for more than 70%. Most runners (girls: 68%, boys: 59%) report previous overuse injury. Compared with boys, girls have increased rate of injury and girls are more likely to sustain an injury that resulted in greater disability during the season. Thus, recognizing injuries early, or preventing them entirely, is ideal to implement an individualized fitness plan to promote young runners' health and athletic success.

While children incorporate running into their regular activities from a very early age, organized and competitive running opportunities may begin as early as school age. At present, there are no evidence-based, age-specific sports participation guidelines for long-distance running by children. Endurance running events, specifically including half-marathons, marathons, and triathlons, have become more popular, and questions have been raised regarding safe participation for young athletes. Currently, no scientific evidence supports or refutes the safety of children participating in marathons. There are no recorded data on injuries sustained by children who run marathons. The only study done evaluating young long-distance runners (4–12 years of age) was a small observational study, with 16 subjects training 48 to 169 kilometers per week (30–105 miles per week) and competing in multiple marathon and ultramarathon events; this study showed no growth retardation, a high physical fitness, and a high incidence of psychological issues. Thus, no data support prohibiting a young athlete's participation in long-distance running as long as athletes remain symptom-free and enjoy the activity.

There are many warning signs to look out for that indicate a young athlete may be running "too much." First and foremost is pain. Pain experienced during or after running can indicate overuse injury (see Running Injuries section in this chapter). Injuries are more common during peak growth velocity, and poor underlying biomechanics can increase risk. Additionally, young athletes, like their adult counterparts, are at risk of overtraining syndrome. Defined as a "series of psychological, physiologic and hormonal changes that result in decreased sports performance," overtraining syndrome may present with chronic pain in the muscles or joints, personality changes, decreased performance, fatigue, or loss of enthusiasm for practice. Furthermore, changes in menstrual cycles of young girls can signal poor energy balance and resultant female athlete triad.

The female athlete triad is defined as the interrelationship of low energy availability (with or without disordered eating), menstrual dysfunction, and low bone mineral density). The triad may result in health consequences, including bone stress injuries. Factors such as prolonged training in endurance running can increase energy expenditures, leading to low energy availability, increasing the athlete's risk of developing female athlete triad. Additionally, in attempt to improve leanness to promote performance, athletes may reduce energy intake, further predisposing to female athlete triad. In general, children and adolescents should be gaining, not losing, lean body mass during these growing years; weight loss or lack of appropriate weight gain should be evaluated further. Moreover, signs such as cold hands and feet, dry skin, hair loss, absent or irregular menstrual periods, increased injury rates, prolonged injury recovery, and stress fractures may indicate development of female athlete triad. Sometimes, the first indication of female athlete triad may be psychological, including mood changes, difficulty concentrating, and depression. Menstrual irregularities have been associated with increased stress fractures in young runners. (See case 8 in Chapter 2, Trends in Prevention of Sports Injury in the Young Athlete, for more information on the female athlete triad.)

Male runners may be at risk for a parallel triad, the male athlete triad, with which male athletes exhibit deficits in nutrition (low energy availability with or without disordered eating), reduction in sex hormones (hypogonadotropic hypogonadism, paralleling functional hypothalamic amenorrhea in females), and impaired bone health (low bone mineral density).

In addition to bone density issues related to female (and male) athlete triad, a decrease in age-adjusted bone mineral density occurs before peak height velocity; this has been shown to be associated with increased risk of acute fracture but no specific associated increased stress fracture risk. Additionally, the growth cartilage at the articular surfaces, physes, and apophyses demonstrate a relative weakness; during rapid growth, growth cartilage is less resistant to tensile, shear, and compressive forces.

The cases that follow illustrate some of the common scenarios encountered in the young runner. Most commonly, pain is seen in the hip, knee, leg, ankle, or foot.

Running Injuries

Hip Pain

Case 1
Hip pain in a 13-year-old female runner

Description

A 13-year-old female runner comes into the office reporting hip pain. Her chart indicates she has grown 10 cm (4 in) since she was last seen, 6 months ago. She is now 170 cm (5 ft 7 in) and 54 kg (120 lb). She mentions how "lame stretching is." She reports a stabbing pain on the outside of her knee and lateral hip while running. She sometimes says she hears a pop while running as well.

Workup and Management

Swelling is noted along the distal aspect of her iliotibial band (ITB). Pain is elicited on palpation of her lateral knee approximately 2 cm above the joint line, in addition to multiple trigger points and knots all the way up to her hip. She is exquisitely tender to even gentle palpation. Her tenderness worsens when asked to stand on the affected leg and bend her knee to approximately 30°. An Ober test (Figure 13-1) is performed, with the examiner placing her in side-lying position with her affected side up, flexing her knee to 90°, and abducting and slightly extending the hip. While the examiner stabilizes her pelvis with the other hand, her leg is allowed to lower toward the table, but her leg is unable to adduct back to parallel, indicating a tight ITB at the tensor muscle of fascia lata.

A clinical diagnosis of ITB syndrome is made on the basis of the history and physical examination, and a treatment plan of acute pain control with ice and nonsteroidal anti-inflammatory drugs (NSAIDs) is prescribed, as well as a home program for stretching and foam rolling of her quadriceps femoris, hamstring muscles, gluteus muscles, and ITB. Physical therapy for active release treatment and additional stretching and strengthening exercises are also prescribed, as it is suspected that the patient will be like most 13-year-old patients and be non-adherent with the home program for ITB injury, as the treatment can be quite uncomfortable.

The differential diagnosis of hip pain can be separated into lateral, anterior, and posterior locations. Keep in mind, most injuries in runners are overuse injuries, not acute injuries.

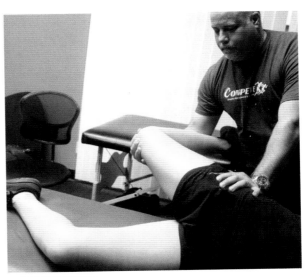

FIGURE 13-1

Ober test.

Photo by Nevia Stickney.

Lateral Pain

Iliotibial Band Syndrome (ITB Syndrome)

This runner presents with lateral hip and knee pain. The ITB is a ligament that runs down the outside of the thigh from the tensor muscle of fascia lata (which is attached to the anterior iliac crest) to its insertion on the lateral aspect of the tibia on Gerdy tubercle. When presenting as pain in the hip, the pain is caused by bursitis of the ITB over the greater trochanter. It more frequently presents as pain in the lateral knee (Figure 13-2) and is often described as a constant, stabbing pain, as if being stabbed with a knife.

The etiology of ITB syndrome is often seen with a history of dramatic increase in mileage, downhill running, and running on slanted roads (always in same direction), as well as with general overuse. It is also seen in the settings of weak or instable hips, poor flexibility, and poor biomechanical balance of leg flexors or extensors. Prevention is key; gradual increase in miles, change in direction on the track or road, and a decrease in hill terrain are all good environmental changes. Hip strengthening and flexibility are paramount to prevention as well.

Iliac Crest Apophysitis

The apophysis is the area of "growth cartilage" of the iliac spine that serves as the attachment site for the hip abductor muscles, flexors, and extensors in a child or adolescent who is skeletally immature. (Similar problems can occur over the anterior-superior iliac spine [ASIS], anterior-inferior iliac spine, and ischial tuberosity.) Apophysitis is an acute or chronic traction injury at the tendon insertion site. Patients typically present with sudden pain over the iliac crest, usually with increased demand. However, it can also have an insidious onset, with a gradual onset. Common etiologies are excessive arm swing and trunk rotation while running, or iliac crest apophysitis can be caused by a sudden change of direction. On examination, there is pain on palpation of the iliac crest as well as pain with resisted abduction of the ipsilateral side in side-lying position. Radiographs may sometimes reveal an avulsion injury of the iliac crest. Treatment consists of conservative measures of rest, NSAIDs, and ice; stretching; and a strengthening and flexibility program. Prevention can be achieved with core and hip strengthening, correction of poor biomechanics, increased flexibility, and a gradual increase in miles.

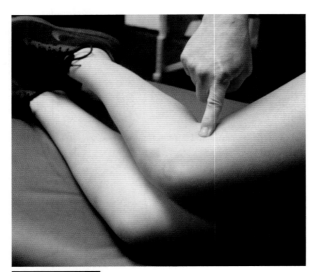

FIGURE 13-2

ITB pain location on lateral knee.

Abbreviation: ITB, iliotibial band syndrome.

Photo by Nevia Stickney.

Anterior Pain

Anterior-Superior Iliac Spine Apophysitis

Anterior-superior iliac spine apophysitis often presents with pain over the ASIS after extension of the hip and while flexing the knee. Many times, there is a gradual pain onset with no clear history of injury. This injury can be seen in any runner with an overuse injury, but, in particular, it is commonly seen in hurdlers, as hurdling requires extension of the hip and concomitant flexion of the knee. The examination often reveals localized tenderness and swelling over the ASIS, with pain with flexion and abduction of hip. Diagnosis can be made on plain hip radiographs, which may again reveal an avulsion injury. Conservative treatment is similar to that for iliac crest apophysitis.

Femoral Neck Stress Fracture

A femoral neck stress fracture is caused by weakness of the femoral neck. It is less commonly seen than apophysitis is. Failure to recognize femoral neck stress fracture may result in avascular necrosis of the femoral head. Patients often present with a vague ache or groin pain, both of which worsen when running, specifically when foot strikes the ground. Femoral neck stress fractures are often seen in female athletes with the classic triad of amenorrhea, eating disorders, and premature osteoporosis (female athlete triad), as well as in runners who have rapidly increased their miles. On examination, palpation of hip may be negative. Passive range of motion or abduction may elicit groin pain. The Trendelenburg test (Figure 13-3) result is often positive (leaning away from affected hip when standing on affected side), as is the hop test result (acute pain when hopping on the affected leg).

Oftentimes, radiographic findings of the pelvis and hip are negative until 2 to 3 weeks after injury. A magnetic resonance image is diagnostic. Treatment consists of non–weight bearing with the use of crutches, and referral to a nonoperative sports orthopedist may be helpful, to assist in management. Prevention consists of core and hip strengthening, correction of poor biomechanics, a gradual increase in miles, and avoidance of bone density problems.

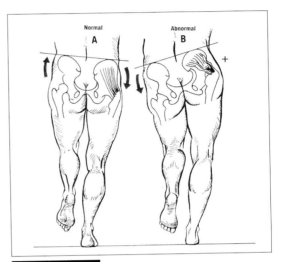

FIGURE 13-3
Trendelenburg test.
From quizlet.com. Reproduced with permission.

Labral Tear

The labrum is a crescent-shaped cartilage structure that lines the rim of the hip socket. It provides added cushion and stability to the hip joint. Patients often describe the pain of a labral tear as a deep pain in the groin, with stiffness or limited range of motion in the hip. Sometimes patients may also describe a clicking or locking sensation in their hip. Physical examination often reveals groin pain with **F**lexion, **AD**duction, and **I**nternal **R**otation (FADIR test) (Figure 13-4) as well as with **F**lexion, **AB**duction, and **E**xternal **R**otation (FABER test) (Figure 13-5).

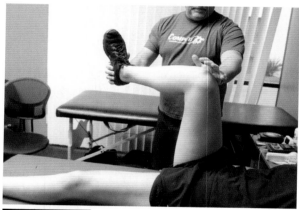

FIGURE 13-4

FADIR (**F**lexion, **AD**duction, and **I**nternal **R**otation) test with positive result.

Photo by Nevia Stickney.

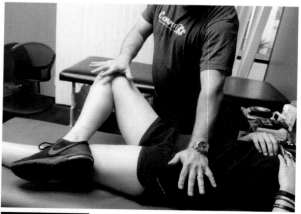

FIGURE 13-5

FABER (**F**lexion, **AB**duction, and **E**xternal **R**otation) test with positive result.

Photo by Nevia Stickney.

A plain magnetic resonance image of the hip will often reveal a labral tear, although a magnetic resonance arthrogram is more sensitive and aids in diagnosis. Repetitive motion and overuse are the main causes of labral tears. Treatment requires referral to an orthopedic surgeon, for arthroscopic repair as well as physical therapy. A gradual increase in miles and training program, once the runner returns, is important for successful return to play.

Posterior Pain

Piriformis Syndrome

Piriformis syndrome usually presents as pain that radiates or shoots down the back of the leg. (The most common cause of this kind of radiating pain is from a pinched nerve in the spine from a disk herniation, and the spine should always be evaluated at the same time if presented with these symptoms.) Patients also report pain with sitting, standing, or lying down for more than 15 to 20 minutes but that then improves with ambulation. The pain is caused by the compression of sciatic nerve as it passes through the piriformis, either from overuse of the piriformis or, more commonly, because of poor biomechanical alignment of the athlete's hips and core. On examination, the examiner will note tenderness over the piriformis on palpation, and sometimes a palpable sausage-shape mass in the ipsilateral buttocks can be felt. The FAIR test (**F**lexion, **AD**duction, and **I**nternal **R**otation of the affected hip), which is also called the piriformis test (Figure 13-6), yields pain caused by the piriformis' compression on the sciatic nerve when performed.

Treatment consists of strengthening and correcting the biomechanics of the hips and core. Specifically, the figure-of-four stretch (Figure 13-7), which can easily be done in the lying-down, seated, or standing position, works well to target this area.

Knee Pain

Case 2
Anterior knee pain in a 12-year-old girl

Description
A 12-year-old girl presents to the office reporting anterior knee pain. She recently began running the mile in physical education and has been borrowing her mom's running shoes to run in. When she forgets, she wears her Vans to run in instead. She reports pain underneath the patella, and she draws a circle around her patella with her finger ("circle sign") (Figure 13-8).

On examination, with her affected leg in full extension, the patella is displaced medially and the medial facet (undersurface) of the patella is palpitated through the retinaculum, with the examiner noting tenderness on palpation (Figure 13-9).

When comparing to the lateral side of the patella, similar pain is elicited. Similar findings are revealed on the other knee as well. The rest of the examination is unremarkable. It is recommended that she modify her running activity for the next few weeks at school, and it is suggested she get her own pair of running shoes. A physical therapy prescription is provided as well, to address imbalances of strength and flexibility.

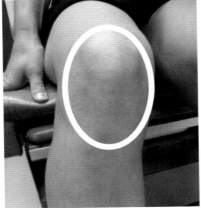

FIGURE 13-8
Circle sign.

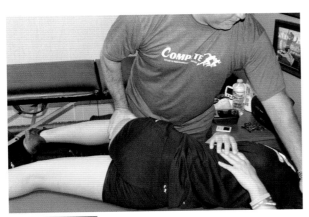

FIGURE 13-6
FAIR test (**F**lexion, **A**daduction, and **I**nternal **R**otation of the affected hip), or piriformis test.

Photo by Nevia Stickney.

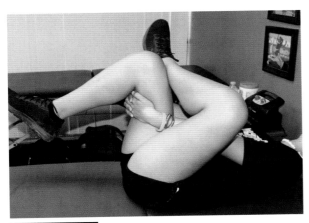

FIGURE 13-7
Figure-of-four stretch.

Photo by Nevia Stickney.

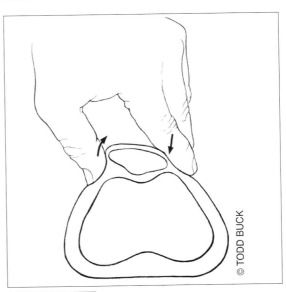

© TODD BUCK

FIGURE 13-9
Patellar tilt test.

Courtesy of Todd Buck.
Reproduced with permission.

Patellofemoral Pain Syndrome

Patellofemoral pain syndrome (PFPS) (also known as "runner's knee") causes pain associated with activities that load the patellofemoral joint, such as running, climbing or descending stairs, or prolonged sitting with knees flexed ("theater sign"). It affects primarily adolescent girls, and multifactorial etiologies are thought to contribute to the pain. Studies of the biomechanical factors that potentially contribute to PFPS demonstrate conflicting results, a lack of reproducibility, and no firm conclusions. Increased Q angle in females (anteversion of femoral neck, external rotation of tibia, and overpronation of foot) was originally thought to be a contributing factor. The Q angle theoretically increases stress in the patellofemoral joint and increases the tendency for the patella to move laterally when the quadriceps femoris is contracted, which, in turn, causes increased irritation of the underlying cartilage of the patella. Now research suggests the roll of increased Q angle in PFPS is of little importance. Pain is caused by repetitive, excessive forces, such as running on hard pavement or downhill running. These excessive forces cause chronic inflammatory changes in the cartilage or bony undersurface of the patella. Pain is often associated with a recent increase in mileage or increase in training. Patellofemoral pain syndrome can also worsen during peak height velocity, when rapid bone growth contributes to loss of quadriceps femoris, hamstring muscle, and hip muscle flexibility, putting further stress on the patellofemoral joint.

Patellofemoral pain syndrome is a clinical diagnosis primarily based on history. Possible lateral patellar tracking ("J sign") (Figure 13-10), tight lateral musculature, or poor vastus medialis tone can be appreciated as well on examination.

An effusion is usually *absent,* and it should point to another etiology if present. The patellar grind test (Figure 13-11) (direct compression of the patella into the trochlea groove inferiorly while the leg is extended and quadriceps femoris is flexed) and the patellar tilt test (Figure 13-12) (patellar facet and retinaculum tenderness with knee in full extension

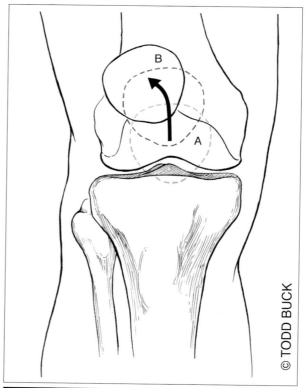

© TODD BUCK

FIGURE 13-10

"J sign."

Courtesy of Todd Buck.
Reproduced with permission.

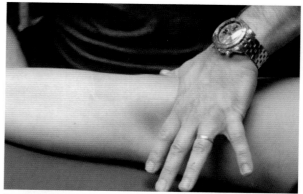

FIGURE 13-11

Patellar grind test.

Photo by Nevia Stickney.

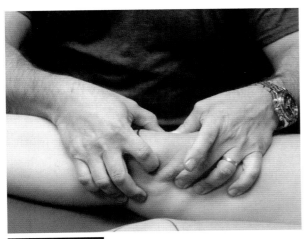

FIGURE 13-12

Patellar tilt test.

Photo by Nevia Stickney.

and quadriceps femoris relaxed; patella is displaced medially or laterally while palpating the medial or lateral facet, respectively, through the retinaculum) both have positive results.

Patellofemoral pain syndrome is a clinical diagnosis, and plain radiographs are usually unnecessary for initial management. In the absence of history of trauma, effusion, instability, or pain at rest, imaging is not performed unless there is no improvement after 1 to 2 months of appropriate, conservative treatment. If there is no improvement after 6 weeks, knee swelling is present, or pain occurs at night, 4-view knee series is indicated to rule out other etiologies of knee pain. Keep in mind, the distal femur is the most common site of bone tumors (ie, osteosarcoma) in the adolescent boy.

Treatment initially consists of pain control and activity modification, with change in running routes (to flat, uphill, or softer terrain, or a combination of those) and decrease in mileage. If the symptoms are more moderate or severe, restriction of activity while maintaining an aerobic base via stationary bike, upper-body cycle, water running, or swimming is warranted. Physical therapy is needed to strengthen the hip abductor muscles, quadriceps femoris (specifically the vastus medialis), and core muscles as well as to stretch the hip flexors, quadriceps femoris, hamstring muscles,

ITB, and gastrocnemius and soleus complex. Adjunctive therapy is often helpful. Taping and bracing of the patella to correct alignment may be indicated, if the patient is unable to tolerate the above without significant pain. Orthotic inserts may be effective as well, for patients with overpronation of the feet ("flat feet"). Prevention consists of maintaining strength and increased flexibility, focused on during the rehabilitation phases.

Osgood-Schlatter Disease (Osteochondritis of Tibial Tuberosity)

Osgood-Schlatter disease is a traction apophysitis of the proximal tibial tuberosity at the insertion of the patellar tendon. It presents as a gradual onset of pain and eventual swelling at the tibial tuberosity (point of insertion of the patellar tendon). It occurs in children and adolescents aged 9 to 14 during periods of rapid growth (11- to 12-year-old girls and 13- to 14-year-old boys). It is typically seen more in boys than in girls, although as sports participation increases in the female population, the incidence in female athletes is increasing. It is seen most in sports that require running, jumping, and cutting, as stress is placed on the apophysis during these activities because of active contraction of the quadriceps femoris. The pain subsides with closure of the growth plate at skeletal maturity.

On examination, pain is noted over the tibial tuberosity with palpation (Figure 13-13).

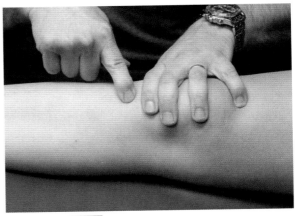

FIGURE 13-13

Pain over tibial tuberosity associated with Osgood- Schlatter disease.

Photo by Nevia Stickney.

Sometimes, the presence of a bony protuberance over the tibial tuberosity can be appreciated. Oftentimes, poor quadriceps femoris flexibility can be seen as well. Osgood-Schlatter disease is a clinical diagnosis; plain radiographs are not indicated, unless other etiologies are suspected because of the presence of symptoms such as warmth, night pain, pain with rest, mechanical symptoms (catching or locking), or systemic symptoms. Acute injury with sudden pain at the same site should be suspect for an avulsion fracture, and radiographic evaluation is warranted. Management is conservative, with recommendations for relative rest (participate to pain tolerance). Complete avoidance of sports activity is unnecessary; Osgood-Schlatter disease is one condition with which playing with pain is not contraindicated. Pain management includes relative rest, ice, and NSAIDs. Physical therapy is sometimes helpful to increase flexibility of the quadriceps femoris and hamstring muscles and strengthen the quadriceps femoris and can be preventive as well.

Sinding-Larsen–Johansson Disease (Patellar Apophysitis)

Sinding-Larsen–Johansson (SLJ) disease is another traction apophysitis of the patellar tendon. It is located at its insertion on the inferior pole of the patella. It is sometimes *incorrectly* referred to as "jumper's knee" and can be confused with patellar tendinitis (see Patellar Tendinitis section). It presents as pain over the inferior pole of the patella, especially in athletes who participate in excessive activities that involve jumping and thus repetitive traction at this location. It typically affects children and adolescents between the ages of 10 and 13 years and will spontaneously resolve after 12 to 18 months (usually once the peak height velocity has been completed).

Examination is significant for pain over the inferior pole of the patella with palpation. Patients with patellar sleeve fracture can be differentiated from those with SLJ syndrome by the inability to ambulate more than 3 to 4 steps and the presence of

significant pain with contraction of the quadriceps femoris, which can be appreciated during a straight-leg raise. Radiographs are diagnostic in this instance. However, plain radiographs are usually not otherwise indicated for pain in this location, as SLJ syndrome is a clinical diagnosis. Concerns for other etiologies would include the presence of effusion, ligamentous laxity, warmth, night pain, pain with rest, acute pain, mechanical symptoms (catching or locking), or systemic symptoms.

Treatment is conservative with relative rest (participate to pain tolerance), although a more cautious approach is needed than with Osgood-Schlatter disease, as SLJ syndrome has a more prolonged recovery. Pain management includes ice and NSAIDs. Physical therapy is helpful to increase the flexibility of the quadriceps femoris and hamstring muscles and strengthen the quadriceps femoris and also serves as prevention.

Patellar Tendinitis

Patellar tendinitis is a chronic tendinopathy and inflammation of the patellar tendon located midway between the inferior pole of the patella and the insertion on the tibial tuberosity. While it is often referred to as jumper's knee, it is more commonly seen in runners. It presents as pain over the patellar tendon and is usually seen in sports involving jumping, running, and hiking. Often, a history of overuse or rapid increase in miles over a short period of time can be elicited.

On examination, pain on palpation of the patellar tendon at midpoint between the inferior pole of the axilla and its insertion into the tibial tuberosity is noted (Figure 13-14). Patellar tendinitis is another clinical diagnosis. Plain radiographs are not indicated unless other etiologies are suspected because of presence of symptoms such are warmth, night pain, pain with rest, acute pain, mechanical symptoms (catching or locking), or systemic symptoms.

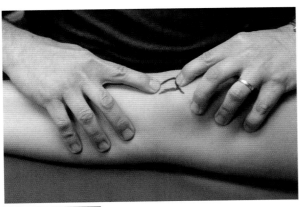

FIGURE 13-14

Location of pain over Patellar Tendon in "jumper's knee."

Photo by Nevia Stickney.

Treatment is conservative with relative rest (participate to pain tolerance) and can also include ice and NSAIDs. Physical therapy may be beneficial to increase flexibility of the quadriceps femoris and hamstring muscles and strengthen the quadriceps femoris. Sometimes, a patellar tendon strap or taping can be used to help with pain. Prevention can be achieved with a gradual increase in mileage and increased quadriceps femoris and hamstring muscle flexibility.

Lateral Knee Pain

Iliotibial Band Syndrome (ITB Syndrome)

Iliotibial band syndrome presents as pain in the lateral knee and is often described as being stabbed with a knife (please see Lateral Pain section for complete description).

Lower Leg Pain

Case 3
Lower leg pain in a 14-year-old girl

Description

A 14-year-old female freshman cross-country runner, who recently joined the team so she could participate in a school activity, presents to the office with anterior shin pain. She has never run

long distances before other than the mile run in physical education, but she thought it would be fun. She reports a dull, aching pain along the middle to distal third of her tibia during running that is relieved by rest.

Workup and Management

On examination, diffuse tenderness is noted along the medial border of distal tibia on palpation. Radiographic findings are negative for fracture and a conservative treatment plan is recommended, consisting of relative rest, ice, and NSAIDs. It is also suggested that she cross-trains with lower-impact activities such as biking, swimming, and water running. She is reminded when she returns to gradually increase her mileage and that proper shoe wear is beneficial.

Medial Tibial Stress Syndrome (Shin Splints)

Medial tibial stress syndrome is an overuse syndrome of pain in the posteromedial portion of the distal tibia. It presents as a dull, aching pain along the middle to distal third of tibia during running that is relieved by rest. Patients often report an inability to maintain speed or intensity of runs. The etiology is inflammation of the tibial periosteum caused by prolonged periods of running or sudden increases in mileage. Ankle flexors (soleus and flexor digitorum longus) that are active during running activity are adjacent to the medial tibia and possibly create repetitive motion along the periosteum. Overpronation of the foot may cause increased stress on the periosteum as well.

On examination, diffuse tenderness can be appreciated along the medial border of the distal tibia on palpation. Swelling may be seen as well. Radiographic findings are negative for fracture, but sometimes they may show periosteal reaction and scalloping of the distal tibia.

Treatment consists of relative rest; ice; NSAIDs; cross-training in lower-impact activities such as biking, swimming, and water running; a change in terrain; and orthoses if overpronation is present. Prevention can be achieved with gradual increase in mileage and proper shoe wear.

Tibial Stress Reaction (Stress Fracture)

Tibial stress reactions present as pain over the tibia during exercise, as seen with shin splints. The difference is the pain continues with rest in the setting of a stress fracture and is focal, not diffuse, pain. It is caused by the inflammation of the tibial periosteum, caused by prolonged periods of running or sudden increases in mileage. Other factors thought to contribute are female menstrual irregularities, poor calcium intake, and poor bone health.

On examination, point tenderness is appreciated over the location of the stress fracture. Plain radiography should be the first imaging study considered because of its availability and low cost. However, findings from plain radiographs are often negative initially. They may become positive over time, revealing a faint lucency (the "dreaded black line") 2 to 3 weeks after presentation. If findings from plain radiographs remain negative, magnetic resonance imaging may be considered to aid in diagnosis, as it has a high sensitivity and specificity (Figure 13-15).

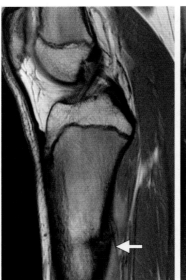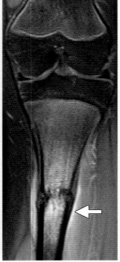

FIGURE 13-15

Tibial stress fracture: "dreaded black line."

From Jaimes C, Jimenez M, Shabshin N, Laor T, Jaramillo D. Taking the stress out of evaluating stress injuries in children. *Radiographics.* 2012;32(2):537–555. http://pubs.rsna.org/doi/full/10.1148/rg.322115022. Accessed July 31, 2017. Reproduced with permission.

Treatment consists of cessation of running and sports participation for 4 to 6 weeks. Athletes may cross-train with non–weight bearing activities such as swimming, cycling, or underwater running. Stress fractures can be prevented with proper shoe wear, proper foot and running mechanics, optimized bone density, and proper mileage increase.

Chronic Exertional Compartment Syndrome

Chronic exertional compartment syndrome is an overuse injury typically seen in a runner that causes pain in the lower leg, caused by an elevation in the pressures in 1 of the 4 compartments of the lower leg (anterior, lateral, superficial posterior, and deep posterior). It is most commonly seen in the anterior compartment. It presents with pain that is described as aching, tightening, burning, or cramping in the lower leg; worsens with exercise; and usually begins at the same time into training. Within 20 minutes of cessation of exercise, the pain will usually completely resolve. Sometimes, the athlete can also develop paresthesias, numbness, or foot drop. Compartment syndrome is caused by expansion of the muscle within the fascia of the compartment, which causes muscle ischemia.

The examination is often unremarkable, with intact pulses, full sensation in the foot, and no localized pain on palpation. Evaluation is conducted by the measurement of the intra-compartmental pressures before and after exercise performed by a sports medicine specialist. Chronic exertional compartment syndrome of the leg is present if one or more of the following intramuscular pressure criteria are met:

- Pre-exercise pressure of 15 mm Hg or greater
- One minute postexercise pressure of 30 mm Hg or greater
- Five minute postexercise pressure of 20 mm Hg or greater

Treatment consists of running on softer surfaces; use of orthoses, other shoe inserts, or better athletic shoes; and reduced training volume.

Patients may cross-train (combine cycling or swimming with reduced running) to maintain fitness, and then they may gradually increase their running, once symptoms resolve. Sometimes, complete cessation of activities may be warranted. Icing the affected area after training assists with pain management. In addition, addressing deficiencies in strength or flexibility with a physical therapist is often beneficial. If symptoms are present for more than 6 to 12 months, referral to an orthopedic surgeon, for operative management, is warranted, with a fasciotomy of the affected compartments. A gradual increase in miles works well for prevention.

Ankle and Foot Pain

Case 4
Ankle and foot pain in a 14-year-old cross-country runner

Description
A 14-year-old cross-country runner who recently finished soccer season presents to the office with heel pain. His heels have bilaterally been bothering him on and off throughout his soccer season, and now the pain is worsening and persistent since cross-country season started.

He describes posterior bilateral heel pain that worsens with activity.

Evaluation and Management
An examination is performed that involves squeezing his heels with the thumb and index finger, yielding a focal bony tenderness on the posterior-lateral aspect of the calcaneus bilaterally, at the insertion of the Achilles tendon.

Sever disease is diagnosed. Relative rest, activity modification, heel lift in shoes and cleats, and ice after exercise, with an ice cup for 5 minutes, are all prescribed. In addition, Achilles tendon stretching exercises are recommended to prevent his heel pain from recurring.

Sever Disease (Calcaneal Apophysitis)
Sever disease is an inflammation of the calcaneal apophysis, which is located on the posterior aspect of the calcaneus. It presents with posterior heel pain, is often bilateral, and worsens with activity (Figure 13-16). It is caused by repetitive micro-trauma from the pull of the Achilles tendon on its bony insertion on the calcaneus. On examination, focal bony tenderness is noted when the heel is palpated at the insertion of the Achilles tendon, on the posterior-lateral aspect of the calcaneus bilaterally. Treatment consists of ice, relative rest, activity modification, heel lift in shoes, Achilles tendon stretching exercises, and, rarely, immobilization. Prevention can be achieved with Achilles tendon stretching and improved flexibility.

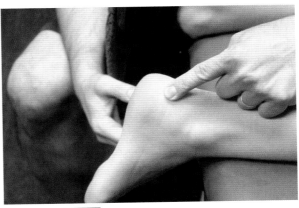

FIGURE 13-16
Pain location associated with Sever disease.
Photo by Nevia Stickney.

Metatarsal Stress Fracture
Metatarsal stress fracture is an overuse injury of one of the metatarsal bones, most commonly to the second or third metatarsal, and is seen most commonly in runners and ballet dancers because of the repetitive stress on the forefoot during these activities. Patients present with gradual, progressive pain in the forefoot, which often corresponds to an increase in intensity of training or the initiation of a new activity. Initially, the pain is intermittent, mild, diffuse, and only with activity, but, eventually, it often progresses to a more severe, localized, and constant pain, which may signal a frank fracture and should be ruled out.

On examination, point tenderness is appreciated over a particular metatarsal shaft, as well as with axial loading of the metatarsal head (hold the toe in line with its corresponding metatarsal [ie, without angulation] while pushing the toe in, toward the metatarsal [ie, in line with the long axis of the metatarsal]; this maneuver produces pain if the metatarsal is fractured, but it generally does not produce pain in patients with an isolated soft-tissue injury). A stress fracture is often a clinical diagnosis (history of recent increase in weight-bearing activity, concern of diffuse or focal fore-foot pain, and focal tenderness at a particular metatarsal shaft), as plain radiographs often do not demonstrate a stress fracture until 2 to 6 weeks after onset of symptoms. If definitive diagnosis is required, ultrasound, magnetic resonance imaging, or technetium bone scan can be performed.

Treatment consists of pain control, ice, and cessation of inciting activity for 4 to 8 weeks. A hard-soled orthopedic shoe or walking boot can be used if the pain does not subside with cessation of activity. If symptoms are severe or affect even basic ambulation, brief immobilization for several weeks may be achieved with a walking cast or non–weight-bearing cast and crutches until pain subsides. Activity modification, such as swimming, underwater running, or low resistance spinning, is helpful in this setting to maintain some cardiovascular fitness while non–weight bearing. A gradual increase in activity and mileage can aid in prevention, as can cross-training and proper footwear, with adequate cushioning.

Plantar Fasciitis

While uncommon in the young athlete, inflammation of the plantar fascia (plantar surface of foot) presents as a gradual onset of sharp, tight pain at the base of the calcaneus (Figure 13-17).

Pain is worse upon initiating walking in the morning. The pain lessens with gradually increased activity, but it worsens toward the end of the day with prolonged weight bearing, such as running.

The etiology of plantar fasciitis is poorly understood but is probably multifactorial, to include improper footwear, hard surface running, overtraining, sudden increase in mileage, and pes planus (flat feet) or pes cavus (high arch).

On examination, focal point tenderness at the base of the calcaneus is noted with pain, best elicited by dorsiflexing the patient's toes and palpating along the plantar fascia. Evaluation does not usually require radiographs initially; however, if symptoms persist, radiographs to rule out calcaneal stress fracture are warranted.

Treatment consists of ice (use frozen golf ball to roll under affected foot), NSAIDs, stretching exercises for plantar fascia and gastrocnemius and soleus, and a decrease in mileage. Arch supports can be effective during the acute inflammatory phase, but keep in mind, they are a temporary "Band-Aid" and should not be used independently of the other treatment modalities or long-term. Rarely, a steroid injection or night splint may be needed, if other therapies are not effective. Prevention involves proper shoe wear, stretching and flexibility, and a gradual increase in mileage.

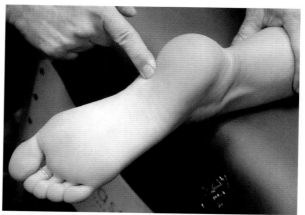

FIGURE 13-17
Location of pain associated with plantar fasciitis.
Photo by Nevia Stickney.

Achilles Tendinitis

Achilles tendinitis is an inflammation of the Achilles tendon. It can occur at the insertion of the Achilles tendon on the calcaneus or in the middle portion of the tendon. Runners will report pain (often described as burning) or stiffness along the Achilles tendon, which increases with activity and is relieved after a period of rest. Achilles tendon rupture needs to be part of the differential diagnosis when concerns of a sudden "pop" are reported by the patient. Achilles tendinitis is most commonly seen in the setting of a sudden change in activity level, such as rapid increase in training regimen or mileage, or with prolonged, rigorous training (ie, speed work or hill training). Improper footwear can also be a factor in this setting, and runners should be cognizant of "shoe mileage."

On examination, localized tenderness to palpation is usually found 2 to 6 cm proximal to the insertion site on the calcaneus. The Thompson test (squeeze test) (Figure 13-18) should always be part of the evaluation to rule out Achilles tendon rupture. The absence of plantar flexion when squeezing the gastrocnemius signals tendon rupture, and the foot and ankle should be splinted in a posterior splint and referred to an orthopedic surgeon, for repair.

Achilles tendinitis is a clinical diagnosis, and radiographs are typically not needed, except to rule out other etiologies. Treatment is mostly symptomatic treatment consisting of NSAIDs, ice, and avoidance of exacerbating activities. Taping is often beneficial as well (Figure 13-19).

Ultimately, physical therapy is usually needed to address strength and flexibility. Prevention involves a gradual increase in training, proper shoe wear, adequate warm-up, and continued strength and flexibility training.

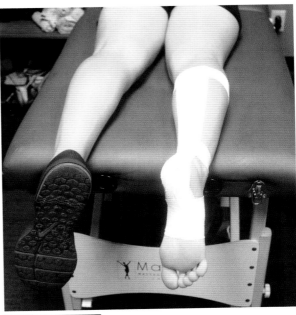

FIGURE 13-19
Taping for Achilles tendinitis.

Photo by Nevia Stickney.

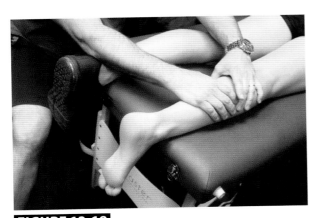

FIGURE 13-18
Thompson test.

Photo by Nevia Stickney.

Injury Prevention

Running injuries are most often overuse injuries and are thus very preventable. The pre-participation examination is the ideal time to assess risk factors and perform a focused physical examination to evaluate asymmetries, strength, and residual limitations and weaknesses from previous injury. Both intrinsic and extrinsic risk factors must be assessed and addressed to minimize injury.

Intrinsic risk factors for running refer to an athlete's biological factors, including age, sex, growth, development, muscle strength, and coordination. Developing a training program taking these intrinsic running factors into account is essential. On physical examination, focused evaluation of anatomical alignment of the spine, pelvic girdle, and lower limbs for asymmetry can aid in development of an individualized injury prevention program. Additionally, core and lower-extremity strength evaluation focused on potential deficits, including weakness of the hip abductor muscles, ankle dorsiflexors, and ankle plantar flexors, provide helpful information to further hone a prevention plan.

Home exercise programs (Table 13-1) ideally begin with muscle-specific exercises and advance to functional activities to promote healthy biomechanics. Running, as its own competitive sport and the foundation within multiple sports, necessitates proper biomechanics to prevent injury and

Table 13-1. How to Improve Localized Weakness

Area to Improve	Exercises to Improve Weakness
Spine stabilization	Bridging, side planks
Weak hip abductor muscles	Side-lying clamshells with resistance band, fire hydrants, side stepping
Weak dorsiflexors	Single-leg heel drops
Weak plantar flexors	Single-leg heel raises

maximize performance. Careful assessment and implementation of a plan to address weaknesses can make a big difference in a runner's injury-free success.

Extrinsic factors are associated with external forces related to training, footwear, sleep, and energy balance. Emphasis on skill development, rather than competition and winning, facilitates decreased risk of injury and burnout. Individualized training programs based on the athlete's age, growth rate, readiness, and injury history must be developed, as training capacity (mileage and intensity) is highly variable in young athletes.

Injury rate has been associated with hours per week of activity. Specifically, stress fracture rate increases significantly with 16 hours or more of moderate to vigorous activity. Months per year and hours per week are established as risk factors for injury. A pilot study of 10- to 14-year-old runners training for a marathon demonstrated increased reports of pain with more than 4 miles per day with a total of 12 or more miles per week. But, currently, there are no evidence-based, age-specific sports participation guidelines for long-distance running by children and adolescents, and runners are recommended to continue activity with pain as the limiting factor. Inherent in sports is the no pain, no gain mantra; however, this is not recommended for young athletes. While training can be challenging to push an individual's limits, pain must be the limiting factor for participation.

Training workload must be closely monitored, especially during the adolescent growth spurt. Training should be managed to limit mechanical stress at discrete sites of overuse injury by modulating volumes and incorporating cross-training with low-impact activities (eg, bike riding, swimming). Additionally, athletes should be encouraged to implement gradual increases into their training programs. While there are no evidence-based recommendations, generally, athletes are recommended to gradually advance training distances by about 10% per week.

Overuse injuries commonly occur when athletes have abrupt changes in their training; most studied in military recruits beginning basic training, the same issues may apply to those increasing intensity as they enter high school or transition from high school to college. A classic background story to presentation of a lower-extremity running injury is the freshman, collegiate cross-country runner; after a summer of recreational running, she or he is thrust into a 2-a-day training retreat during which runners log excessive mileage leading to shin pain and sometimes tibial stress fractures.

Overscheduling

Overscheduling, defined as participation in multiple competitive events in the same day or over multiple consecutive days, creates a high ratio of workload to recovery time for the adolescent runner, and it can put the athlete at higher risk for overuse and acute injury. Coaches and parents may need to take the lead to advocate, to ensure, adequate amount of recovery time between scheduled events, especially with respect to major competitions in which athletes attempt to push the limits of their bodies' physiologic capability. Additionally, like in other sports, early specialization is not recommended for running; no benefit in running sports performance has been demonstrated from early specialization. Discussing these issues with patients and their family help young athletes make educated choices about their training and can decrease injury rates and burnout.

Sleep

Prioritize sleep. Sleep is a safe and effective way for young athletes to decrease injury risk and potentially enhance performance. Adolescent athletes who slept less than 8 hours per night were 1.7 times more likely to sustain a sport-related injury than their peers who slept 8 or more hours per night. Sleeping 6 or fewer hours is associated with fatigue-related injury in pediatric athletes.

Shoes

While runners do not need much equipment, ensuring shoe fit is important. Athletes with poor-fitting shoes or orthoses may be more prone to poor biomechanics and injury. As young runners grow quickly, shoe fit (Box 13-1) is recommended to be reassessed regularly. Shoes should be replaced (Box 13-2) when they are showing signs of wear at the beginning of each new season or every 300 to 500 mi, or both.

Box 13-1
Getting the Right Shoe Fit

Check shoe fit frequently, especially

- During rapid growth
- Every 300–500 mi, based on training
- *Once per athletic season,* or more depending on activity
- If shoes show uneven wear when placed on a flat surface
- If shoes have creasing in the midsole
- If runner experiences new pain
  Consider inadequate shoe shock absorption.

Box 13-2
When to Replace Shoes

- Try on shoes at the end of the day, when feet are most flattened and swollen.
- Always try both shoes on.

   If feet are slightly different size, fit the larger foot.
- Make sure toes have room to splay, with a roomy toe box.
- Try on with the type of socks, braces, or other inserts to be used with the shoes.
- Shoe should bend at the ball of the foot, where the toes bend.

   If the shoe bends farther forward or behind where the toes bend, the shoe is too big or small.
- Ensure index-finger width between the longest toe and end of the shoe.
- Heel should be stable; no movement in and out of the heel counter.
- When stopping and starting, the foot should not slide back and forth.

Nutrition

Maintaining a healthy diet with appropriate caloric and nutrient intake is essential to injury prevention and athletic success for runners. Runners are considered lean sport athletes and are thus at increased risk for inadequate energy availability, a part of the female athlete triad. Ideally, a multidisciplinary approach to nutrition and eating habits includes evaluation of any inappropriate training, abnormal eating behaviors, poor nutrition, body image issues, or external stressors. Additionally, proper calcium (1,000–1,300 mg/d) and vitamin D (600 IU/d) intake through diet (4–5 servings of dairy product per day), and supplements as needed, is recommended.

Conclusion

How can you, the pediatrician, be the best "running advocate" for young runners?

1. Match individual growth and development (motor, sensory, cognitive, and social and emotional). For those new to running, review the benefits of running and importance of physical activity. For those already involved, discuss current enjoyment and short- and long-term goals.

2. Discuss current misconceptions.

3. Identify injuries early.

4. Use the pre-participation examination to discuss previous injury, identify intrinsic risk factors, review extrinsic risk factors, and promote healthy participation. Thorough examination can include evaluation for the intrinsic risk factors and a plan to improve areas of weakness.

5. Encourage appropriate expectations to avoid overscheduling, maximize sleep, and promote enjoyment.

6. Goals: Support children's interests. Emphasize skill development, rather than competition and winning.

Bibliography

Alexander CJ. Effects of growth rate on the strength of the growth plate-shaft junction. *Skeletal Radiol.* 1976;1:67–76

American Sports Data. *The Superstudy of Sports Participation.* Hartsdale, NY: American Sports Data; 2007. *Fitness Activities;* vol 1

Barrack MT, Ackerman KE, Gibbs JC. Update on the female athlete triad. *Curr Rev Musculoskelet Med.* 2013;6(2):195–204

Barrow GW, Saha S. Menstrual irregularity and stress fractures in collegiate female distance runners. *Am J Sports Med.* 1988;16(3):209–216

Batt ME. Shin splints—a review of terminology. *Clin J Sports Med.* 1995;5(1):53–57

Bennell KL, Malcolm SA, Thomas SA, et al. Risk factors for stress fractures in track and field athletes: a twelve month prospective study. *Am J Sports Med.* 1996;24(6):810–818

Brenner JS; American Academy of Pediatrics Council on Sports Medicine and Fitness. Overuse injuries, overtraining, and burnout in child and adolescent athletes. *Pediatrics.* 2007;119(6):1242–1245

Bright RW, Burstein AH, Elmore SM. Epiphyseal-plate cartilage. A biomechanical and histological analysis of failure modes. *J Bone Joint Surg.* 1974;56(4):688–703

Cobb KL, Bachrach LK, Greendale G, et al. Disordered eating, menstrual irregularity, and bone mineral density in female runners. *Med Sci Sports Exerc.* 2003;35(5):711–719

Couture CJ, Karlson KA. Tibial stress injuries: decisive diagnosis and treatment of 'shin splints.' *Phys Sportsmed.* 2002;30(6):29–36

De Souza MJ, Nattiv A, Joy E, et al; Female Athlete Triad Coalition. 2014 Female Athlete Triad Coalition consensus statement on treatment and return to play of the female athlete triad: 1st International Conference held in San Francisco, CA, May 2012, and 2nd International Conference held in Indianapolis, IN, May 2013. *Clin J Sport Med.* 2014;24(2):96–119

DiFiori JP, Benjamin HJ, Brenner JS, et al. Overuse injuries and burnout in youth sports: a position statement from the American Medical Society for Sports Medicine. *Br J Sports Med.* 2014;48(4):287–288

Dixit S, DiFiori JP, Burton M, Mines B. Management of patellofemoral pain syndrome. *Am Fam Physician.* 2007;75(2):194–202

Duri ZA, Patel DV, Aichroth PM. The immature athlete. *Clin Sports Med.* 2002;21(3):461–482, ix

Fakhouri THI, Hughes JP, Burt VL, Song M, Fulton JE, Ogden CL. *Physical Activity in U.S. Youth Aged 12–15 Years, 2012.* Hyattsville, MD: National Center for Health Statistics; 2014. NCHS data brief 141. https://www.cdc.gov/nchs/products/databriefs/db141.htm. Updated January 8, 2014. Accessed July 2, 2017

Faulkner RA, Davidson KS, Bailey DA, Mirwald RL, Baxter-Jones AD. Size-corrected BMD decreases during peak linear growth: implications for fracture incidence during adolescence. *J Bone Miner Res.* 2006;21(12):1864–1870

Flachsmann R, Broom ND, Hardy AE, Moltschaniwskyj G. Why is the adolescent joint particularly susceptible to osteochondral shear fracture? *Clin Orthop Relat Res.* 2000;(381):212–221

Hackney AC. Effects of endurance exercise on the reproductive system of men: the "exercise-hypogonadal male condition." *J Endocrinol Invest.* 2008;31(10):932–938

Jayanthi NA, LaBella CR, Fischer D, Pasulka J, Dugas LR. Sports-specialized intensive training and the risk of injury in young athletes: a clinical case-control study. *Am J Sports Med.* 2015;43(4):794–801

Loucks AB. Low energy availability in the marathon and other endurance sports. *Sports Med.* 2007;37(4-5):348–352

Loud KJ, Gordon CM, Micheli LJ, Field AE. Correlates of stress fractures among preadolescent and adolescent girls. *Pediatrics.* 2005;115(4):e399–e406

Luke A, Lazaro RM, Bergeron MF, et al. Sports-related injuries in youth athletes: is overscheduling a risk factor? *Clin J Sport Med.* 2011;21(4):307–314

Lun V, Meeuwisse WH, Stergiou P, Stefanyshyn D. Relation between running injury and static lower limb alignment in recreational runners. *Br J Sports Med.* 2004;38:576–580

Milewski MD, Skaggs DL, Bishop GA, et al. Chronic lack of sleep is associated with increased sports injuries in adolescent athletes. *J Pediatr Orthop.* 2014;34(2):129–133

Mohtadi N. Children and marathoning. *Clin J Sport Med.* 2005;15(2):110

Myburgh KH, Hutchins J, Fataar AB, Hough SF, Noakes TD. Low bone density is an etiologic factor for stress fractures in athletes. *Ann Intern Med.* 1990;113(10):754–749

Nattiv A, Loucks AB, Manore MM, Sanborn CF, Sundgot-Borgen J, Warren MP; American College of Sports Medicine. American College of Sports Medicine position stand. The female athlete triad. *Med Sci Sports Exerc.* 2007;39(10):1867–1882

Nelson NG, Alhajj M, Yard E, et al. Physical education class injuries treated in emergency departments in the US in 1997-2007. *Pediatrics.* 2009;124(3):918–925

Nudel DB, Hassett I, Gurian A, Diamant S, Weinhouse E, Gootman N. Young long distance runners. Physiological and psychological characteristics. *Clin Pediatr (Phila).* 1989;28(11):500–505

Olsen SJ II, Fleisig GS, Dun S, Loftice J, Andrews JR. Risk factors for shoulder and elbow injuries in adolescent baseball pitchers. *Am J Sports Med.* 2006;34(6):905–912

Pedowitz RA, Hargens AR, Mubarak SJ, Gershuni DH. Modified criteria for the objective diagnosis of chronic compartment syndrome of the leg. *Am J Sports Med.* 1990;18(1):35–40

Reynolds G. Phys ed: should children run marathons? *New York Times.* February 23, 2011

Rice SG, Waniewski S; American Academy of Pediatrics Committee on Sports Medicine and Fitness, International Marathon Medical Directors Association. Children and marathoning: how young is too young? *Clin J Sport Med.* 2003;13(6):369–373

Roberts WO. Children and running: at what distance is safe? *Clin J Sport Med.* 2005;15(2):109–110

Ryan MB, MacLean CL, Taunton JE. A review of anthropometric, biomechanical, neuromuscular and training related factors associated with injury in runners: review article. *Int Sportmed J.* 2006;7(2):120–137

Shaffer RA, Rauh MJ, Brodine SK, Trone DW, Macera CA. Predictors of stress fracture susceptibility in young female recruits. *Am J Sports Med.* 2006;34(1):108–115

Small E. Chronic musculoskeletal pain in young athletes. *Pediatr Clin North Am.* 2002;49(3):655–662

Tenforde AS, Barrack MT, Nattiv A, Fredericson M. Parallels with the female athlete triad in male athletes. *Sports Med.* 2016;46(2):171–182

Tenforde AS, Sayres LC, McCurdy ML, Collado H, Sainani KL, Fredericson M. Overuse injuries in high school runners: lifetime prevalence and prevention strategies. *PM R.* 2011;3(2):125–131

Wen DY. Risk factors for overuse injuries in runners. *Curr Sports Med Rep.* 2007;6(5):307–313

Zaslow TL. The effects of long-distance running on injury patterns in children 10-14 years of age. Poster presented at: 2007 American Medical Society for Sports Medicine 16th Annual Meeting; April 21–25, 2007; Albuquerque, NM

INDEX